The New Sociology of the Health Service

Health service policy and health policy have changed considerably over the past fifteen years and there is a pressing need for an up-to-date sociological analysis of these developments. Not only have policies themselves changed but new policy themes – such as evidence-based policy and practice, an increasing focus on a primary care-led health service, a growing recognition of the need to address inequalities through public health policies and a focus on the views and the voice of the user and the public – have emerged alongside some of the old.

Following up the very successful *The Sociology of the Health Service*, this all-new volume covers a broad range of key contemporary health services issues. It includes chapters on consumerism, technology, evidence-based practice, public health, managerialism and social care among others, and incorporates references to new developments, such as regulation and marketization, throughout.

The New Sociology of the Health Service provides a vital new sociological framework for analysing health policy and health care. It will be an important read for all students and researchers of medical sociology and health policy.

Jonathan Gabe is Professor of Sociology at Royal Holloway, University of London, UK.

Michael Calnan is Professor of Medical Sociology at the University of Kent, UK.

The New Sociology of the Health Service

Edited by Jonathan Gabe and
Michael Calnan

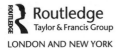
Routledge
Taylor & Francis Group

LONDON AND NEW YORK

First published 2009
by Routledge
2 Park Square, Milton Park, Abingdon, Oxon OX14 4RN

Simultaneously published in the USA and Canada
by Routledge
270 Madison Avenue, New York, NY 10016

Routledge is an imprint of the Taylor & Francis Group, an informa business

Typeset in Sabon by
Keystroke, 28 High Street, Tettenhall, Wolverhampton
Printed and bound in Great Britain by
CPI Antony Rowe, Chippenham, Wiltshire

British Library Cataloguing in Publication Data
A catalogue record for this book is available from the British Library

Library of Congress Cataloging-in-Publication Data
  The new sociology of the Health Service / edited by Jonathan Gabe and
Michael Calnan.
     p. ; cm.
  Follow up to: The sociology of the Health Service / edited by
Jonathan Gabe, Michael Calnan, and Michael Bury. 1991.
  Includes bibliographical references.
  1. National health services–Great Britain. 2. Medical policy–Great Britain.
I. Gabe, Jonathan. II. Calnan, Michael. III. Sociology of the Health Service.
[DNLM: 1. Great Britain. National Health Service. 2. National Health
Programs–Great Britain. 3. Health Policy–Great Britain. 4. Sociology, Medical–
Great Britain. WA 540 FA1 N5327 2009]
  RA395.G6N468 2009
  362.10941–dc22   2008043452

ISBN 10: 0–415–45597–9 (hbk)
ISBN 10: 0–415–45598–7 (pbk)
ISBN 10: 0–203–87974–0 (ebk)

ISBN 13: 978–0–415–45597–8 (hbk)
ISBN 13: 978–0–415–45598–5 (pbk)
ISBN 13: 978–0–203–87974–0 (ebk)

Contents

Contributors

John Abraham is Professor of Sociology and Director of the Centre for Research in Health and Medicine, University of Sussex.

Michael Calnan is Professor of Medical Sociology, School of Social Policy, Sociology and Social Research, University of Kent.

Sarah Cant is Principal Lecturer in Sociology, Department of Applied Social Sciences, Canterbury Christ Church University.

Kath Checkland is Walport Clinical Lecturer in Primary Care, National Primary Care Research and Development Centre, University of Manchester.

Sue Dopson is the Rhodes Trust Professor of Organisational Behaviour, Saïd Business School, University of Oxford.

Mary Ann Elston is Reader Emerita in Medical Sociology, Department of Health and Social Care, Royal Holloway, University of London and Visiting Reader at Surrey University.

Jonathan Gabe is Professor of Sociology, Department of Health and Social Care, Royal Holloway, University of London.

Caroline Glendinning is Professor of Social Policy and Research Director (Adults, Older People and Carers) in the Social Policy Research Unit, University of York.

Stephen Harrison is Professor of Social Policy, School of Social Sciences and National Primary Care Research and Development Centre, University of Manchester.

Carl May is Professor of Medical Sociology, Institute of Health and Society, Newcastle University.

Timothy Milewa is Lecturer in Sociology and Communications, Department of Sociology and Communications, School of Social Sciences, Brunel University.

John Mohan is Professor of Social Policy, School of Social Sciences, University of Southampton.

Jennie Popay is Professor of Sociology and Public Health, Institute of Health Research, Lancaster University.

Gareth Williams is Professor of Sociology, Cardiff School of Social Sciences, Cardiff University.

Preface

For some years now health and health care have occupied a central place in the cultures of late modern societies. At the same time, health and health care have become a key focus for politicians and policy makers in Britain and elsewhere and stand at the meeting point of a range of social conflicts. These in turn relate to profound changes in the social, economic and political map of Britain and other countries.

The health policy issues which these changes have generated were initially paid relatively little attention by medical sociologists. This realization led us to organize a seminar in London, twenty years ago, to facilitate the development of a sociological analysis of health policy. The papers from this seminar were subsequently published in a book edited by ourselves called *The Sociology of the Health Service* and published by Routledge.

While the need for a sociological analysis of health policy has now been recognized over the last decade or more, there have been considerable changes in health service policy and health policy in general. This has involved changes to existing policies and the development of new policy themes. The latter have included the emergence of evidence-based policy and practice, an increasing focus on a primary care-led health service, a growing recognition of the need to address inequalities through public health policies, a heightened awareness of the influence of the pharmaceutical industry and a focus on the views and/or the voice of the user and the public.

These developments suggested the need for a further seminar which was held at Royal Holloway, University of London, in September 2007, with financial support from the Foundation for the Sociology of Health and Illness.

The seminar included some of those who contributed to the original meeting and some new speakers to focus on emergent themes. Those invited to speak at the seminar subsequently turned their presentations into chapters for the new edition of our book, entitled *The New Sociology of the Health Service*. We should like to thank all those who attended the seminar at Royal Holloway for their helpful contributions and hope that the points they raised have been taken into account in the following pages.

We believe that the new edition offers a sociologically informed perspective on a wide range of health policy issues which are not covered collectively in any other text currently available. As such we hope the book will appeal not only to medical sociologists but also to a wider audience, including policy analysts, health service workers, medical journalists and interested members of the public.

Jonathan Gabe and Michael Calnan

Introduction

Jonathan Gabe and Michael Calnan

The essays which comprise this volume seek to highlight the contribution which sociologists and policy analysts with a sociological orientation can make to understanding a range of crucial issues currently facing the health service in the countries which collectively make up Great Britain. These issues are presently high on the political agenda and are a topic of considerable media and popular concern although they have only become the focus of sociological attention relatively recently. Consequently we want to spend some time mapping the history of this concern and relating it to developments in sociology generally and to the changing health policy context. In so doing we shall be providing a historical framework for the chapters which follow.

To facilitate this task we shall distinguish four broad phases of activity in British sociology. The first concerns the period from the end of the Second World War through to the early 1960s, during which sociology began to develop a distinctive disciplinary base in Britain. The second deals with the period of the late 1960s and 1970s which saw a number of currents running through sociological enquiry. The third covers the period from the late 1970s to the mid-1990s when sociology operated in a cold political climate. And the fourth takes us from there to the present – the context of current activity and debate.

Sociology in post-war Britain

The first period followed hard on the establishment of the welfare state in Britain, including, of course, the founding of the National Health Service. Sociologists at this time were preoccupied with two basic sets of questions. On the one hand, they were concerned with studies of poverty and community life, and with surveys of the impact of class-based inequalities which underpinned both of these. On the other hand, policy-oriented work was preoccupied with the equitable distribution and uptake of welfare and health services. In sum they were concerned with the limitations imposed by social inequalities on citizenship (Turner 2006).

Challenges to this largely empirical tradition came during this period from more theoretically informed American sociologists, most notably Edward Shils and Talcott Parsons (Halsey 1982). Not only did these theorists point to the limits of an empiricist sociology, but they also challenged the substantive pre-occupations of sociologists in Britain. Shils, for example, argued that some of the most popular institutions in British public life, such as the royal family, had never been taken seriously. Indeed, Edward Shils and Michael Young (1953) published a paper on the subject at the time of the coronation.

At this time medical sociology only existed in an embryonic form. Those sociologists concerned with health and health care worked largely in the Fabian tradition of social reform and occupied themselves with the task of consolidating the health service. They were thus concerned with how the service operated, what inhibitors there were to an equitable access to and distribution of the service and to increase understanding among participants in the service (Stacey with Homans 1978).

Many of the problems on which medical sociologists worked were defined by others, particularly public health specialists within the medical profession (Seale 2008), or were set by the agenda of the medically dominated funding agencies (Illsley 1975). Not surprisingly, therefore, medical definitions of health and health care problems were largely taken for granted. Moreover, sociologists who worked on health questions were not generally regarded as in the mainstream of the parent discipline and, isolated from departments of sociology (Johnson 1975), were seen to have a medical 'bias'. They remained 'curiously incurious' about the assumptions on which medical care was based (Jefferys 1980), as their analysis of the health care system remained separate from capitalist society.

In some ways the messages coming from American colleagues were themselves ambivalent on this point. Parsons (1951), for example, had used health and medical care as fruitful examples of the overall working of the social system. In this context health became sociologically defined as central to the value system of post-war American life, with its emphasis on productive capacity and instrumentalism (Shilling 2002), and doctoring to its pattern of social control. Other sociologists incorporated mental health and medicine as key social problem areas, but writers such as C. Wright Mills (1959) and Howard Becker (1963) specifically excluded physical ill health from their analyses of the sociological imagination and deviancy.

In this first period, then, medical sociology was struggling to find both its intellectual footing and an independent approach to both medical and policy issues. Health policy was very much under the control of those wedded to traditional (in Britain, Labour Party) loyalties, who saw little to question about the nature of medical knowledge or activity as such. The emphasis on increasing availability and access to services pulled in the opposite direction.

However, as British sociology came to take up the theoretical assaults of its American counterparts, and pay greater attention to fundamental issues such as conflict and power (e.g. Rex 1961) so medical sociology began to define its task in more consistently sociological terms.

The break with consensus

The second period we have marked out, namely that of the late 1960s and 1970s, saw the rapid development of a more 'critical' sociology and the growth of specialist areas such as medical sociology. During this period, structuralist Marxist thought from France, the Frankfurt school of 'critical sociology' and phenomenology, in the guise of ethnomethodology and symbolic interactionism from the United States, came to challenge the dominance of structural functionalism and empiricism in British sociology (Halsey 1989). This process was aided by the student unrest and increasing economic and cultural power of youth in the late 1960s (Dennis 1989) and by the cold war, which denied explanations of social order in terms of Parsons' ultimate social values.

For many conservative-minded sociologists and social policy analysts, these developments confirmed their worst fears about the discipline. For others it gave the discipline a new injection of energy and broke its cosy relationship with the (Labour) establishment, and with so-called 'positivist' survey methods (Bulmer 1989). The resurgence of feminism and the growth of interest in such areas as deviancy attracted a widespread following among younger sociologists, providing them with a new territory on which to establish their own line of enquiry.

One consequence of this theoretical pluralism, however, was that sociological 'positivism' was transformed into 'one form or another of sociological "negativism"' (Dennis 1989: 427). The assumption that society was basically benign, suffering from evils which were reformable, was replaced by an anti-authoritarianism which did not lend itself to sociologically informed, policy-orientated research. Instead, those advocating these new theoretical approaches were primarily concerned with critique and the unmasking of a previously taken-for-granted benign reality.

Medical sociology also developed rapidly in this period, with a new-found confidence that could challenge both the conservatism of Parsonian theory and the acceptance of medical definitions in the health field itself. Of the theoretical alternatives mentioned, phenomenology proved the most influential, with much work focusing on the patient's viewpoint and the nature of doctor–patient interaction (Gerhardt 1989).

At a macro level, a more critical perspective towards medical power was developed, with an emphasis on medicine as an agent of social control. In particular, Freidson's (1970) wide-ranging critique of medicine's monopoly over the definition and treatment of illness and different forms of Marxist analysis of medical power (e.g., Navarro 1976; Johnson 1977) encouraged

medical sociologists in Britain to stop seeing the medical profession's claim
to expertise and power as a legitimate and benign form of social control, as
in the earlier period. Instead, it was seen as oppressive, being characterized as either a mask for unaccountable professional power (in the case of
Freidson), or wider class interests (in the case of Marxists such as Navarro).
From either standpoint the medical profession's dominance needed to
be curtailed or made more accountable, and, if necessary, regulated by the
state.

This view of the power of the medical profession as oppressive subsequently influenced those micro sociologists employing both interactionist
(e.g. Bloor 1976) and feminist (Barrett and Roberts 1978) perspectives
and ironically led to the claim that medical sociology itself had become
imperialistic: searching for, focusing on and exaggerating the negative
aspects of medical practice for its own professional purposes (Strong 1979).
The use of symbolic interactionism in empirical work was popular for a
number of reasons not least because its portrayal of negotiations between
key actors made sense of why there was little evidence of overt conflict in
every day encounters which might have been expected giving the prevailing
theoretical approaches which emphasized a 'clash of perspectives' (Freidson
1970). However, this work tended to show how the structures, strategies and
routines found in different clinical and organizational settings reinforced
professional power and control and mitigated against patient involvement
and influence.

Equally significant, 'negativism' and naïve anti-authoritarianism encouraged medical sociologists to ignore more policy-related questions, and this
tendency was enhanced by the lack of any major public conflict over health
care. For the majority of sociologists during this period, their 'critical' preoccupation with medical power and medicalization seemed a potent enough
issue, and one which could be tackled by means of structural analysis or
ethnographic field work rather than by studying either policy development
or policy enactment.

Retrenchment in adversity

From the late 1970s until the mid-1990s, sociology in Britain operated in
a cold political climate and in the face of hostility from neoconservative
politicians who looked upon proponents of the discipline as 'folk devils'
responsible for inducing 'moral panic' (Halsey 1989). In such a climate it is
hardly surprising that government support for sociological teaching and
independent research was meagre.

Faced with such uncertainty, sociologists looked to their laurels and
recovered their interest in the classic traditions in theory and method. As
Bulmer (1989) noted, there was a proliferation of theoretical essays
concerned with what had been said previously about a phenomenon (e.g. the
nature of capitalism or anomie) or about a body of knowledge (such as the

work of classic theorists). At the same time, and with the encouragement of the ESRC (Economic and Social Research Council), there was a resurgence of interest in quantitative methods and in secondary analysis in particular (Dale *et al.* 1988). And some of those associated with the anti-positivism of the 1970s now rejected the quantitative/qualitative distinction as a false polarity (Silverman 1985, 2000) or argued that ethnographers should be more concerned with testing theories in the same way as quantitative sociologists (Hammersley 1992).

The sociology of health and illness in many ways mirrored these developments. For instance, there were a number of attempts to develop the sub-discipline's theoretical base by showing how the work of particular theorists illuminated the study of health, disease and medicine (Scambler 1987) and by establishing the different theoretical paradigms employed in explaining illness and their relationship to general sociological theory (Gerhardt 1989). These were taken a step further under the impact of Foucault's writings and this led to renewed theoretical debate about illness and its definitions (Armstrong 1983; Bury 1986). Likewise, quantitative methods made a comeback in, for example, secondary analyses of health care data contained in the Office of Population Censuses and Survey's (OPCS) General Household Survey (e.g. Arber and Gilbert 1989).

At the same time, medical sociology, unlike its parent discipline, was protected to some extent from the worst consequences of retrenchment by its historical relationship with social medicine and epidemiology. This was a mixed blessing, however. On the one hand, such an association provided employment opportunities in an otherwise shrinking job market, as funding for medical sociology research units was progressively withdrawn. On the other hand, those working as sociologists 'in medicine' (Straus 1957) had to surrender much of the responsibility for selecting topics for investigation to physicians and civil servants. Moreover, as Scambler (1987) argued, the combination of government cutbacks in research funding, together with its commitment to the more efficient allocation of health resources, resulted in an increasing number of medical sociologists doing research which was policy led and accepting of medical diagnostic categories. For example, the large-scale funding of research on HIV/AIDS in the late 1980s and early 1990s, whilst providing new opportunities for medical sociology and the use of innovative methodologies, illustrated the danger of a return to research being defined primarily by policy makers and clinicians. Such a context provided few opportunities to develop a rigorous, reflexive sociological analysis of health policy issues, at a time when health and health policy had come to occupy a more central place in debates about the future of the welfare state and the impact of consumerism, and as the social consensus over the NHS was under severe strain.

Consolidation

Since the mid 1990s, sociology has operated in a milder political climate, with some sociologists, notably Anthony Giddens, helping to shape public culture and the political agenda (Turner 2006). In turn the discipline has been able to consolidate its position and has become increasingly specialized as a result of the conditions of academic production (Payne 2007). New issues in sociological theory have developed such as the growing theoretical interest in sociological aspects of embodiment (Williams and Bendelow 1998), emotions (Williams 2001), biotechnologies, communication technologies and networks (Castells 2000; Brown and Webster 2004), risk (Lupton 1999; Denney 2005) and trust (Sztompka 1999). Consumption has also been paid more attention alongside production (Warde 1996), with increasing interest in consumption as performance and as a key aspect of lifestyle and identity, reflecting the cultural turn in British sociology (Rojek and Turner 2000). At the same time, there has been a call for a more publically engaged sociology. First articulated by Burawoy (2005) in a now famous presidential address to the American Sociological Association, the call has been favourably received in Britain, with a general endorsement of an engaged approach which has a clear connection to publicly relevant issues (Holmwood and Scott 2007).

As before, medical sociology has mirrored many of these developments and contributed to them. For instance, recognition that trust is becoming increasingly conditional and in need of being earned in particular situations (Calnan and Rowe 2008) has been taken up by sociologists interested in the current status of the medical profession and its elite's concern about the public's loss of trust in the profession and their call for a 'new professionalism'. Indeed, some sociologists have come to the defence of trust in medicine, often after having previously been critical of medicine's dominance (e.g. Freidson 2001). Consumption has been taken up by those interested in studying health promotion and the way in which the consumption of goods and services such as alcohol, fitness and leisure activities contribute to people's body image and sense of health (Bunton and Burrows 1995). Others have employed Warde's (1990) model of production/consumption cycles to see what impact changing modes of provision have for users of health care and for citizens' rights (e.g. Gabe and Calnan (2000)). Similarly, risk has become a particular interest of sociologists of health and illness who have focused on the cultural factors which have shaped risk perception of hazards to health and its management (Green 1997; Bellaby and Lawrenson 2001). Likewise consideration has been given to the ways in which material factors and social interests have shaped responses to health risks (Flynn 2006).

Medical sociologists have also taken up the call for a publicly engaged sociology and have argued that the sub-discipline needs to do more to provide a distinctive sociological perspective on health policy and the organization of health (Seale 2008). Of course it can be argued that medical sociologists have already been doing just this by analysing a variety of aspects of the current Labour government's 'modernization agenda' for the health service. One such example is Pope's (2003) study of the development of evidence-based medicine as a social movement with team spirit, a clear ideology and a strategy to pursue its goals. Another is the evaluation of innovative methods to engage citizens in participating in health care decision making, such as the use of citizens' juries and forums (Gooberman *et al.* 2008). This emphasis in policy discourse on the need for citizen participation might be a response to the optimistic call for more 'generative politics' with the emphasis on deliberative decision making, in an attempt to freshen up or democratize current political debates which, it is argued, are dominated by ideological interests and positions. However, more simply for the NHS, there is believed to be a continuing need to compensate both for the 'democratic deficit' and for the power of stakeholders such as professional medicine and the drug companies by setting up various mechanisms for users and/or citizens to be consulted or even be involved in decision making about health care. One such study (Davies *et al.* 2006) evaluated an initiative in citizen participation, the Citizens' Council, which was set up by the health service standard and priority setting body, the National Institute for Clinical Excellence (NICE). It was modelled on the idea of a citizens' jury where jurors from diverse backgrounds are 'informed' through a series of expert witnesses and then are expected to deliberate and make recommendations. Others have engaged with devolved government and have sought to inform debates about public health by undertaking relevant policy research. An example is Elliott and Williams' (2008) work on health impact assessment relating to a proposed housing renewal initiative in a former mining community. They explore the dynamics of the process and their role as public sociologists in mediating between the accounts of lay participants and published evidence.

Despite the above examples there is some merit in Seale's call for medical sociologists to engage further with health policy and the organization of health care. An aim of this book has been to encourage such engagement by inviting a variety of sociologists and social policy analysts to reflect on a variety of current policy debates, although they also address issues of long-standing concern. Some were considered in the first edition – such as community/social care and managerialism – whilst others such as the development of evidence-based practice and consumerism are included for the first time here. It could be argued that we have simply chosen topics which reflect the interests of government and the health care professions. To a considerable extent this is true, as these are the dominant interests that shape the health policy agenda. At the same time we have included a chapter on 'non-orthodox' medicine which arguably offers a challenge to a biomedicalized view of health care policy and practice, although shaped by similar structuring mechanisms and practices. And we have encouraged our contributors to take a critical view of these dominant interests, be they the state, the medical profession or the pharmaceutical industry. It is also the case that we have been forced through constraints of space to ignore other pressing policy issues such as occupational and environmental health concerns. These and other policy issues deserve serious consideration in their own right but have not been central to the current policy agenda, at least in the UK, as the dominant interest groups have not seen them as significant.

Each contributor has been asked to analyse their subject in terms of changes in the social context of health service provision since the early 1990s. In this way it is hoped that the book will provide a useful update to the first edition of *The Sociology of the Health Service* (Gabe *et al.* 1991). It will be noted that some of our contributors have framed their work by drawing on theories which first became influential in the UK during the break with consensus described earlier. Here we are thinking of neo-Weberian theories of professional dominance, Marxian-inspired political economy, interpretive and feminist perspectives and Foucauldian concerns with surveillance and governmentality. Others, however, have (also) engaged with themes which have become more prevalent during the recent period of consolidation, relating to consumption and identity, new technologies and the way they shape and are shaped by social context, the role of networks and the situated nature of trust.

In the first chapter, Mary Ann Elston considers the latter theme. She provides an overview of the emerging medical discourse on trust and the 'new professionalism', relating this discourse to general sociological analyses of trust and professionalism. Unlike much of the literature on trust in health care, which focuses on the patient's perspective, Elston concentrates instead on trust relationships between medicine and the state, and in particular those within medicine. She considers how the foundations for the professional promise of 'extraordinary trustworthiness' are being amended as a result of both exogenous and internal changes affecting the profession. And she also notes adjustments in the relationship between medical sociologists and the medical profession. Elston argues that calls for a 'new professionalism' should not be seen simply as defensive claims on the part of an occupation faced with widespread distrust in the eyes of the public and the state. While this is no doubt a major part of the story, the new professionalism can also be understood in part as an attempt from within the profession to develop new disciplinary mechanisms following a recognition that the foundations for its claims to be trustworthy require updating and making more explicit.

The next chapter, by Sue Dopson, considers the major changes in the organization and management of the NHS since the 1980s and reflects on the opportunities that exist for sociologically informed work in this area. Changes in management in the NHS are discussed in relation to what has been termed 'new public management' (NPM) – involving greater competition in service provision, hands-on professional management, a private sector style of management and explicit standards and measures of performance. The chapter begins by exploring in some detail the Griffith Report, which heralded the introduction of general management into the NHS. It then explores the subsequent changes in health services management practice which were provoked by two major, politically driven interventions: the introduction of quasi markets and the desire for a more network-driven management. Creating a quasi-market involving purchasers and providers designed to impose market forces and business discipline was intended to weaken if not destroy the regulatory machinery that had protected unaccountable professional and administrative elites in the past. In practice, according to Dopson, this form of NPM mainly involved realizing the adoption of a customer-oriented and performance-driven culture, with managers responding to the demands of a more active consumer. Since 1997, and the election of a New Labour government, the preferred management form has been underpinned by networks, coupled with management by metrics. This represents a shift from government to governance, with a wider range of agencies and stakeholders from within and beyond the public sector becoming involved in health service delivery, and an emphasis on surveillance through metrics and self-disciplining. In addition there has been a move away from disaggregated service units to partnership and integrated working. However, it is argued that the contemporary network model conveniently ignores the reality of the differences in power of the members of the networks to influence change. Contrary to the view that managerialization has resulted in the medical profession losing power to managers, the picture is seen as more complex with both losses and gains for the medical profession.

In the third chapter, Michael Calnan and Jonathan Gabe examine the changes that have taken place in primary care over the last twenty-five years. As in the chapter in the first edition, the focus is once again on general practice although it is recognized that other primary care services such as dentistry and community pharmacy have also undergone significant changes in recent years. The authors outline their neo-Weberian theoretical perspective which sees the professional development of general practice as hinging on its ability to attain and maintain autonomy, and assess its power to explain recent changes, along with that of new theories. They chart the changing profile of general practice and discuss key policy developments such the marketization of care, managerialism and patient access, choice and participation. They conclude that there is little evidence of a decline in the dominance of general practitioners or that general practice has been undermined by the key policy changes they have charted. However, they accept that there are signs of restratification, as previously suggested by Freidson in the context of developments in the United States. Much of the increasingly complex division of labour in general practice in the UK reflects a type of horizontal stratification with GPs delegating tasks to nurses and differences developing between traditional GPs and entrepreneurs. However, there is also evidence of growing vertical stratification between those GPs involved as clinical leads or in managerial roles in Primary Care Trusts or in implementing the Quality and Outcomes Framework (QOF) in their practices and those who are not involved in these activities. At the same time the encouragement of private providers to offer primary care alongside NHS contracted practitioners suggests that we may be seeing the beginning of the corporatization of general practice. On the other hand, it may be that what is developing is simply a more pluralized system in which traditional professional autonomy continues to dominate.

It has been recognized for some time that there has been a 'moving frontier' between public and private health care provision in the UK. In the next chapter, John Mohan argues that since his contribution to the first edition was published there has been a further incremental shift in the balance in favour of private provision but that this does not yet represent a decisive shift in the public–private boundary. What is much more significant, he argues, is the growing significance of private interests in the commissioning and provision of publicly funded health care. He therefore devotes his chapter to considering the changing relationship between the private sector and the NHS and the effects of the former on the NHS as a result of policies designed to pluralize the supply side and create a contestable market. He focuses on two key developments: first, the expansion of the private sector's role in the finance and delivery of health care through the private finance initiative, independent sector treatment centres and new forms of provision of primary care; and second, the current Labour government's attempt to put a gloss on its policies through new forms of social ownership such as social enterprises and foundation trusts. He offers two views of such developments. In the first, the NHS is opened up to the full play of market forces, leading to its commercialization and break up. In the second, public enterprise is replaced by new social enterprises and co-operatives. He concludes that whatever the outcome, sociology will have to come to terms with a multiplicity of new organizational forms.

The fifth chapter, by John Abraham, considers the relationship between the pharmaceutical industry, state agencies and patient organizations and how this affects NHS patients and professionals. He traces this relationship over time, since the creation of the NHS, and reveals how the key issues of pharmaceutical safety, efficacy, cost-effectiveness, pricing and promotion and advertising have been dealt with. To examine these relationships he turns to political economy in order to synthesize a 'political sociology of medicine' that conceptualizes the interactions of the state with various organized interests and shows how these interests are related to ideology and real health interests. He argues that because the pharmaceutical industry was so important to the post-war UK capitalist economy, the tension between the interests of the NHS and the industry were resolved by establishing a 'corporate bias', permitting the industry privileged access to and influence over the state that was not available to other interest groups. This bias has subsequently manifested itself in the emergence, conceptualization and implementation of drug safety, efficacy and pricing regulation. In the case of cost-effective prescribing, the state has at times been able to assert its own interests, through the creation of the National Institute of Clinical Excellence. However, Abraham argues that the industry has used its power to frustrate the state's rationalization objectives, thereby achieving 'regulatory capture'.

In Chapter 6, Harrison and Checkland consider another issue which was not covered in the first edition – namely the development of evidence-based medicine (EBM), where clinical practice is based on systematically assembled research evidence about the effectiveness of therapeutic procedures. They summarize the development of this phenomenon in the UK and explain how it has been bureaucratized and institutionalized within the NHS as 'scientific-bureaucratic' medicine. They go on to discuss its impact on medicine and suggest that, despite its initial failure to bring about change, there is some evidence that its impact is increasing. In the final section of the chapter they suggest three sociological perspectives which provide a way of understanding these changes. In particular, they view EBM as a component of state government, from both a neo-Marxist political economy and Foucauldian 'governmentality' perspective, and in terms of its impact on the autonomy and status of the medical profession and as a social movement. They do not attempt to adjudicate between these perspectives but use them to support the claim that EBM is sociologically interesting and to suggest some conceptual directions from which it might be approached.

Another new theme in this edition is how new technologies become embedded in health services and how they shape and are shaped by the social contexts in which they are enacted. In Chapter 7 Carl May considers this issue by focusing on telemedicine systems in practice. These systems use specialized video-conferencing and data transfer equipment and software to allow professionals and patients to interact remotely, in real time. As such they are seen as a key resource to secure more rapid access to health care for populations that are underserved by specialist services and to make these services more responsive to policy and patients. Telemedicine is particularly interesting however, as it failed to become embedded or normalized in everyday provision despite significant support from clinicians, managers and policy makers. May therefore considers why telemedicine has in some senses 'failed' and what would need to happen for it to become embedded. Drawing on Science and Technology Studies, he identifies four domains of the work that needs to be done to achieve this: coherence – the objectives and features of telemedicine must be specified in a way that renders them comprehensible to their users and differentiates them from others; cognitive participation – the social processes of enrolment and engagement required in order to draw groups of users into its field; collective action – the work involved in implementing telemedicine as a set of clinical practices; and reflexive monitoring – developing an understanding of the processes that make telemedicine workable and integrated into everyday health care provision. For May the development and implementation of telemedicine is best understood as messy, difficult, contingent and unpredictable and the outcome of conflicts between different groups of professionals, health care managers and policy makers.

The next chapter, by Timothy Milewa, addresses another topic which was not considered in the first edition, consumerism in health care and the politics of identity. Milewa asks three questions. First, has there been a radical change in the portrayal of health service users and their ascribed identities in policy narratives since the early days of the NHS? Second, is there evidence to suggest the growth of 'consumer' consciousness on the part of health service users in recent years? Third, if this is the case, how might such a change be explained and evaluated from a sociological perspective? In order to answer these questions, Milewa offers an overview of relevant policies and examines trends in areas such as patient choice, the 'expert patient', patient and public involvement in health service planning, patient safety, complaints and litigation. He suggests that 'consumerist' aspects of the health service user can only be understood with reference to wider social perceptions and motivations around ideas such as trust, expectation, obligation and responsibility that help to cohere understandings of identity in relation to health care. In his view, appreciating the relationship between aspects of health policy, choices and preferences made by health-service users and these wider societal expectations is central to understanding the hybrid and fluid nature of consumerism in British health care.

Arguably, one of the most significant changes in the shape and practice of medical care in Britain since the publication of the first edition of this book has been the growth of complementary and alternative therapies, forms of knowledge and practitioners. In Chapter 9 Sarah Cant reviews the burgeoning demand for and ever-increasing supply of 'non-orthodox' care and assesses its significance for the configuration of the health service in Britain. On the surface it would seem that the growth of such care attests to the emergence of the 'postmodern condition', where plural knowledge systems co-exist and are invoked because of their practical benefits in meeting the needs of clients. Furthermore, the attraction of 'non-orthodox' modalities might also point to the rise of the discerning consumer who is increasingly sceptical of biomedicine and is looking for individualized care. However, having examined the consumption practices of users, the response of 'orthodox' medicine and the state to the increased popularity of these therapies and the demands that 'non-orthodox' care should seek regulation and professionalization, Cant argues that such a reading is not fully endorsed. One problem with the argument that major social and cultural change has been the major 'driver' for the development of 'non-orthodox' care is that it downplays the role of biomedicine in determining which types of complementary and alternative therapies have gained legitimacy and in controlling their practice and modes of intervention within the NHS. Furthermore, as Cant also points out, 'non-orthodox' medicine has been shaped by similar structuring mechanisms and values as biomedicine, in that it too fulfils the function of surveying the population, is becoming commodified in line with commercial imperatives, and concentrates on the individual body/behaviour rather than social, political or economic aetiology. In addition, the delivery of 'non-orthodox' care has been further shaped by the rhetoric of the safe and responsible practitioner who embodies professionalism, a preferred therapeutic relationship which contrasts the client with the 'expert' and the continued primacy given to 'scientific' evidence to establish which practices are valid. For Cant, these influences on non-orthodox care reflect a culture of uncertainty and risk which is equally concerning for orthodox medicine.

The next chapter, by Caroline Glendinning, considers the provision of care to people who, because of illness, impairment or ageing, need help that is over and above that normally given within close family relationships. It starts with an overview of theory and debate about the nature of 'care', concentrating on feminist and philosophical theories, and considers its growing salience as a key dimension of welfare state policy and analysis. It then offers insights into the provision of social care in England, both informally by families and close relatives and formally by organized social care services. Thereafter, attention shifts to the troubled relationship between social care and the NHS and various attempts to improve it, noting the potential divergence between policies in these two domains aimed at increasing, respectively, user and patient choice. Glendinning argues that this divergence risks undermining some of the improvements in collaboration that have been achieved since the late 1990s, introducing instabilities in the governance of social care and the nature of citizenship, and marginalizing the interests of close relatives and friends who are by far the largest group of providers of social care.

In the final chapter Jennie Popay and Gareth Williams move away from the sociology of health care to explore the relationship between society and population health, and the policies and practices which have been developed to address this relationship. For reasons of space they focus in particular on class and income inequalities and leave the issues of gender and ethnicity to one side. They start their chapter by exploring the dominant paradigmatic 'ways of knowing' and explaining health inequalities, considering in particular social epidemiological approaches which focus on the life-course, psycho-social pathways to ill health, and the relationship between people and place. They then consider two less visible paradigms, namely neo-Marxist analyses of the political economy of social and health inequalities, and interpretivist analyses of how people make sense of and deal with the impact of inequalities in their daily lives. They argue that together these two sociological approaches offer a powerful critique of the dominant ways of knowing about health inequalities and provide the basis for a more integrative approach. Finally they turn to the domains of public health policy and practice and how they have responded to the challenge of reducing health inequalities. They pay particular attention to the impact of devolution and the extent to which this has triggered new, locally situated ways of framing and acting to reduce such inequalities. They conclude there is some evidence that, rhetorically at least, early public health policy in Wales post-devolution was more radical in emphasizing wider social determinants in health than equivalent policies in England or Scotland, but that none of these early policies contained a strong materialist or structuralist agenda and all continued to have a strong focus on healthy behaviour and personal responsibility. Since then public health policies across the UK have all focused predominantly on trying to improve the health of the poorest people rather than develop broader, societal responses. This leads them to conclude that the history of policy responses to health inequalities in the UK has not been a marked success and that what is needed is a far more extensive application of the sociological imagination, linking personal experience of inequality to social structure in a global context in order to generate an adequate understanding for action on health inequalities.

The future for sociologists of health care would thus seem to involve undertaking further policy-led and theoretically informed policy-relevant work. If so, it is hoped that the contributors to this volume have highlighted the advances that the discipline has made in both these respects and have provided encouragement for sociologists to contribute to Burawoy's (2005) call for a public sociology.

References

Arber, S. and Gilbert, N. (1989) 'Men: the forgotten carers', *Sociology*, 23: 111–18.
Armstrong, D. (1983) *Political Anatomy of the Body. Medical knowledge in Britain in the twentieth century*, Cambridge: Cambridge University Press.
Barrett, M. and Roberts, H. (1978) 'Doctors and their patients: the social control of women in general practice', in C. Smart and B. Smart (eds) *Women, Sexuality and Social Control*, London: Routledge & Kegan Paul.
Becker, H.S. (1963) *Outsiders: Studies in the sociology of deviance*, New York: Free Press.
Bellaby, P. and Lawrenson, D. (2001) 'Approaches to the risk of riding motorcycles', *The Sociological Review*, 49: 368–88.
Bloor, M. (1976) 'Professional autonomy and client exclusion: a study in ENT clinics', in M. Wadsworth and D. Robinson (eds) *Studies in Everyday Medical Life*, London: Martin Robinson.
Brown, N. and Webster, A. (2004) *New Medical Technologies and Society. Reordering life*, Cambridge: Polity.
Bulmer, M. (1989) 'Theory and method in recent British sociology: whither the empirical impulse?', *British Journal of Sociology*, 40: 393–417.
Bunton, R. and Burrows, R. (1995) 'Consumption and health in the "epidemiological clinic" of late modern medicine', in R. Bunton, S. Nettleton and R. Burrows (eds) *The Sociology of Health Promotion*, London: Routledge.
Burawoy, M. (2005) 'For public sociology', *American Sociological Review*, 70: 4–28.

Bury, M. (1986) 'Social constructionism and the development of medical sociology', *Sociology of Health and Illness*, 8: 137–69.

Calnan, M. and Rowe, R. (2008) *Trust Matters in Health Care*, Buckingham: Open University Press.

Castells, M. (2000) 'Materials for an explanatory theory of the networked society', *British Journal of Sociology*, 15: 5–24.

Dale, A., Arber, S. and Procter, M. (1988) *Doing Secondary Analysis*, London: Allen and Unwin.

Davies, C., Wetherell, M. and Barnett, E. (2006) *Citizens at the Centre: Deliberative participation in health care decisions*, Bristol: Policy Press.

Dennis, N. (1989) 'Sociology and the spirit of sixty-eight', *British Journal of Sociology*, 40: 418–41.

Denney, D. (2005) *Risk and Society*, London: Sage.

Elliott, E. and Williams, G. (2008) 'Developing public sociology through health impact assessment', *Sociology of Health and Illness*, 30: 1101–16.

Flynn, R. (2006) 'Health and risk', in G. Mythen and S. Walklate (eds) *Beyond the Risk Society*, Maidenhead: Open University Press.

Freidson, E. (1970) *The Profession of Medicine: a study in the sociology of applied knowledge*, New York: Dodd Mead.

Freidson, E. (2001) *Professionalism: the third logic*, Cambridge: Polity.

Gabe, J. and Calnan, M. (2000) 'Health care and consumption', in S.J. Williams, J. Gabe and M. Calnan (eds) *Health, Medicine and Society. Key theories, future agendas*, London: Routledge.

Gabe, J., Calnan, M. and Bury, M. (1991) *The Sociology of the Health Service*, London: Routledge.

Gerhardt, U. (1989) *Ideas About Illness*, Basingstoke: Macmillan.

Green, J. (1997) *Risk and Misfortune: A social construction of accidents*, London: UCL Press.

Gooberman, R., Horwood, J. and Calnan, M. (2008) 'Citizen juries in planning for research priorities: process, engagement and outcome', *Health Expectations*, 11: 272–81.

Halsey, A.H. (1982) 'Provincials and professionals: the British post-war sociologists', *Archives of European Sociology*, 23: 150–75.

Halsey, A.H. (1989) 'A turning of the tide? The prospects for sociology in Britain', *British Journal of Sociology*, 40: 353–75.

Hammersley, M. (1992) *What's Wrong with Ethnography?* London: Routledge.

Holmwood, J. and Scott, S. (2007) 'Sociology and its public face(s)', *Sociology*, 41: 779–83.

Illsley, R. (1975) 'Promotion to observer status', *Social Science and Medicine*, 9: 63–7.

Jefferys, M. (1980) 'Doctors' orders. The past, present and future of medical sociology', paper to the British Sociological Association annual conference 'Practice and progress: British sociology 1950–80', Lancaster University.

Johnson, M.L. (1975) 'Medical sociology and sociological theory', *Social Science and Medicine*, 9: 227–32.

Johnson, T.J. (1977) 'The professions in the class structure', in R. Scase (ed.) *Industrial Society: Class cleavage and control*, London: Allen & Unwin.

Lupton, D. (1999) *Risk*, London: Routledge.

Mills, C.W. (1959) *The Sociological Imagination*, Oxford: Oxford University Press.

Navarro, V. (1976) *Medicine Under Capitalism*, New York: Prodist.

Parsons, T. (1951) *The Social System*, Glencoe: Free Press.

Payne, G. (2007) 'Social divisions and social mobilities: some issues after 40 years', *Sociology*, 41: 901–15.

Pope, C. (2003) 'Resisting evidence: the study of evidence-based medicine as a contemporary social movement', *Health*, 7: 267–82.

Rex, J. (1961) *Key Problems in Sociological Theory*, London: Routledge & Kegan Paul.

Rojek, C. and Turner, B.S. (2000) 'Decorative sociology: towards a critique of the cultural turn', *The Sociological Review*, 48: 629–48.

Scambler, G. (1987) *Sociological Theory and Medical Sociology*, London: Tavistock Publications.

Seale, C. (2008) 'Mapping the field of medical sociology: a comparative analysis of journals', *Sociology of Health and Illness*, 30: 677–95.

Shilling, C. (2002) 'Culture, the "sick role" and the consumption of health', *British Journal of Sociology*, 53: 621–38.

Shils, E. and Young, M. (1953) 'The meaning of coronation', *The Sociological Review*, 1: 281–307.

Silverman, D. (1985) *Qualitative Methodology and Sociology*, Aldershot: Gower.

Silverman, D. (2000) *Doing Qualitative Research. A practical handbook*, London: Sage.

Stacey, M. with Homans, H. (1978) 'The sociology of health and illness: its present state, future prospects and potential for health research', *Sociology*, 12: 281–307.

Straus, R. (1957) 'The nature and status of medical sociology', *American Sociological Review*, 22: 200–4.

Strong, P.M. (1979) 'Sociological imperialism and the profession of medicine', *Social Science and Medicine*, 13A: 613–19.

Sztompka, P. (1999) *Trust: a sociological theory*, Cambridge: Cambridge University Press.

Turner, B.S. (2006) 'British sociology and public intellectuals: consumer society and imperial decline', *British Journal of Sociology*, 57, 169–88.

Warde, A. (1990) 'Introduction to the sociology of consumption', *Sociology*, 24: 1–4.

Warde, A. (1996) 'Afterword: the future of the sociology of consumption', in S. Edgell, K. Hetherington and A. Warde (eds) *Consumption Matters: The production and experience of consumption*, Oxford: Blackwell Publishers/The Sociological Review.

Williams, S.J. (2001) *Emotion and Social Theory*, London: Sage.

Williams, S.J. and Bendelow, G. (1998) *The Lived Body: Sociological themes, embodied issues*, London: Routledge.

1 Remaking a trustworthy medical profession in twenty-first-century Britain?

Mary Ann Elston

Introduction: 'Trust me, I'm a doctor'

This aphorism invokes a connection between membership of a specific occupation and the possession of special expertise and moral authority, which warrants doctors' taking responsibility for making judgements on behalf of those who seek their services. A particular occupational identity is claimed as sufficient to guarantee ethical conduct and expertise. Historically, such claims have, as many sociologists have pointed out, been particularly associated with those occupations regarded as professions. For example, in the late eighteenth century, Adam Smith, generally associated with a 'rigorous critique of occupational monopoly' (Dingwall and Fenn 1987: 51), 'defended the privileged position of professions on the grounds that the nature of their work requires trust' (Freidson 2001: 214). Although when Smith wrote, doctors did not have a monopoly over matters of health, a century later they were well on course to achieve market control. By the time Talcott Parsons turned his attention to the professions in the middle of the twentieth century, medicine was in a very privileged position in most affluent countries (Parsons 1939, 1951). There was general acceptance of the medical profession's claims that the nature of their work and the indeterminate knowledge required of its members warranted a high (but not unlimited) degree of public trust and autonomy to take decisions without extensive external monitoring. Trust in the medical profession was (and, arguably, is) accepted as especially important, because the vulnerability and uncertainty involved in illness, and its diagnosis and treatment, render lay people (be they patients, managers or politicians) unable to make appropriate judgements.

Accordingly, in the introduction to his now-classic analysis of the rise of the Anglo-American medical profession, published almost forty years ago, the late Eliot Freidson wrote that the term 'profession' denotes both 'a special kind of occupation' and 'an avowal or promise . . . of the extraordinary trustworthiness of its members' (Freidson 1970: xvii). Professionals could, so the promise implied, be relied on to exhibit professionalism, and be uniquely trusted to be judges of what is best for their clients and of what is good professional conduct; thus, the promise implies legitimate entitlement to (usually state-backed) occupational autonomy, including professional self-regulation of members' conduct and professionally controlled restrictions on entry (licensing). Freidson suggested that medicine in the mid-twentieth century was 'the prototype' profession which other occupations sought to emulate, with its then almost unrivalled social status, and apparently general societal acceptance of its claim to be especially trustworthy (1970: xviii).

A key aim, however, of Freidson's work in the 1970s was to raise critical questions about the medical profession's promise of extraordinary trust-worthiness, and about whether medical power and status were simply a consequence of the nature of their work, and necessarily beneficent. His analysis ushered in an era of more historically grounded Weberian- or Marxist-influenced sociological analyses of the acquisition of professional privilege as a politically and socially contingent process, rather than simply following from the nature of the work (e.g. Starr 1982; Waddington 1984). This academic shift occurred in the context, on both sides of the Atlantic, of cultural and epidemiological critiques of the effectiveness of much modern medicine, new perceptions of risk, and 'consumerist' and social move-ment challenges to medical power and paternalism, such as the women's health movement and disability activism. In much of this critical literature, the medical profession's claims to trustworthiness were seen primarily in ideological terms, as part of the occupation's strategy for gaining and maintaining status and authority (Gabe *et al.* 1994).

By the end of the 1980s, there were further challenges in the form of major reforms to the funding and organization of health care services in many affluent countries; for example, the growth of managed care in the USA, which threatened external encroachment on the doctor–patient relationship (Mechanic 1996, 1998). In the UK, the election, in 1979, of a Conservative government ideologically committed to introducing market forces, patient and consumer power and internal competition to offset producer dominance in the NHS, and to reducing professional control over NHS policy-decisions suggested that the profession's claim to trustworthiness was regarded with some scepticism by government.

This was the context for the first edition of this book (Gabe *et al.* 1991). Accordingly, the chapter on the medical profession focused on the theme then emerging in sociological doctor-watching: the putative decline of medical power and autonomy, in the face of the various challenges from active consumers, from the state or other third parties responsible for health care organization and from ideologies of managerialism as an alter-native to professionalism (Elston 1991). The 1991 chapter adopted that favourite academic position, sitting on the fence, as between decline and persistence of medical power, partly on the grounds of lack of detailed empirical evidence. It did, however, draw attention to what were described as 'uncomfortable adjustments' by the medical profession's institutions in response to the various challenges and changes (Elston 1991: 83). Challenges and changes have continued in subsequent years (Kelleher *et al.* 2006). In many respects, the election of the New Labour regime in 1997 did not change the broad direction of NHS reforms, at least in England, post-devolution. Indeed, arguably, the pace of NHS reform intensified under the New Labour rubric of 'modernization'; for example, through greater emphasis on the use of clinical protocols, the implementation of institutional targets and stronger managerial oversight of professional performance, and more competition from the commercial sector (e.g. Department of Health 2000; Harrison 1999; Harrison and Ahmad 2000; Pollock 2004).

Many measures introduced since 1997 (with more in the pipeline) have direct implications for the medical profession: for example, in relation to the terms and conditions of work for doctors, including their relationships with other health care professions (Bevan 2008; Davies 2003); the systems of regulation and governance, with increased external monitoring and a major overhaul of the profession's statutory self-regulatory body, the General Medical Council (GMC) (Allsop and Saks 2002; Salter 2007); and recruitment and training, with the expansion of medical schools and the implementation of a new system of postgraduate medical training, Modernizing Medical Careers (MMC) (see e.g. Parry 2007; Tooke 2007). Part of the context for some recent developments was a series of major medical malpractice scandals which came to light in the mid-to-late 1990s, including the conviction of general practitioner (GP) Harold Shipman for the mass murder of patients, and the apparent tolerance of excessive mortality rates for paediatric cardiac surgery at the Bristol Royal Infirmary (see Chief Medical Officer (CMO) 2006). The 'scandal' of these events lay not just in the wrongdoing of a few individual doctors, but also in what was revealed, in subsequent professional and official enquiries, about the apparent failure by the NHS and the profession, both locally and nationally, to manage 'bad apples' within the medical profession (e.g. Smith 2004). The regulatory institutions charged with ensuring the trustworthiness of members of the profession were found wanting in their dealings with some individual doctors in whom patients' trust had proved misplaced.

So, since 1991, the medical profession has continued to face sustained criticism, and many sociologists would agree that there has been some reduction in medical autonomy and status in the last two decades. The concept of professionalism, however, is far from obsolete in either professional or sociological discourse. Rather, there is active discussion of what has been termed the 'new professionalism' in medicine, and of trust in the profession and how it might be restored and sustained. For example, according to the foreword to a recent Royal College of Physicians (RCP) Report, 'Events have undermined public trust in medicine . . . [however] The trust that patients have in their doctors is critical to their successful care' (RCP 2005: v). This report goes on to call not merely for reinstatement of the *status quo ante* with respect to trust, but for updating the foundations for doctors' promise of professionalism – for a 'new professionalism' as the basis for re-establishing trust.

The aim of this chapter is to provide an overview, inevitably highly selective, of this emerging medical discourse on trust and the new professionalism, linking it with general sociological analyses of trust and professionalism. Most of the literature on trust in health care focuses on the patients' perspective (Calnan and Rowe 2008; Rowe 2004). This chapter focuses instead on trust relationships between medicine and the state and, in particular, on those within medicine. Rather than seeking to measure levels of trust, it considers how the foundations for the professional promise of 'extra-ordinary trustworthiness' are being amended as a result of both exogenous and internal changes affecting the profession. The chapter also notes adjustments in the relationship between medical sociologists and the medical profession.

The concept of trust in contemporary social theory

The concept of trust and its place in contemporary society have been prominent themes in social theory in recent years, as in moral philosophy and political discourse generally (O'Neill 2002). There are many ways in which the term 'trust' is used in everyday language. As noun or verb, the term is used variously to refer to an expectation, an attitude or disposition, a relationship, an action, and to both abstract and concrete entities (as in legally constituted financial or National Health Service trusts, or, particularly in the USA, to illegal business groupings which interfere with the operation of free markets). Given this, to search the academic literature for a single definition that covers all possible usages would be fruitless. This chapter takes, as a heuristic starting point, a simple statement by Sztompka that captures fairly well the key aspects of the concept to be discussed here (but there is no suggestion that this definition would serve equally well in all contexts):

> Trust is a[n optimistic] bet about the future contingent action of others.
> (Sztompka 1999: 25)

The first point about this definition is that trust is regarded as constituting social action in a Weberian sense (attending to the intentions of others), that is, it brings individuals or institutions into a social relationship – which may be ongoing, as trusting someone can involve a continuing relationship as well as a specific action (Giddens 1990: 32). As Luhmann emphasizes, some degree of delegation ('trusting' another to take one's interests into account or to get on with the task in hand, accepting someone's statements at face value, etc.) is generally intrinsic to acts of trust – a trustee is entrusted with some responsibility by a trustor (Luhmann 1979). Patients might delegate some degree of judgement or decision-making to doctors they trust (although how much and in what circumstances could be highly contingent), just as established doctors may 'trust' their juniors to undertake procedures on their own. Conceptually, this emphasis on social action and relationships would seem to be particularly appropriate for sociologists, rather than, for example, regarding trust as primarily a mental state – although attitudes and emotions are likely to affect trust and, in practice, empirical social research on trust often takes the form of attitude surveys (e.g. Taylor-Gooby 2008). Second, under Sztompka's definition, trust involves a predictive judgement about the unknown, contingent actions of others. The reference to a 'bet' does not imply that trusting others is necessarily the consequence of explicit rational assessment of probable outcomes, but rather that a degree of contingency or uncertainty of outcome is always involved in trust relationships. 'Trust always remains a bet with a chance of losing' (Sztompka 1999: 33). Trust can reinforce social bonds, but the impact of trust being 'betrayed' can be devastating, a moral breach. Breaches, however, are not the expected outcome: trust is an 'optimistic' bet.

An important theme in much of the recent sociological literature on trust is that to distrust someone can be seen as a mirror-image of trusting (Sztompka 1999: 26). Distrust is betting based on negative (pessimistic) expectations. It is associated with taking strong protective measures against risk and uncertainty, seeking tight control over others' actions, minimizing discretion accorded to others – tightly specified contracts rather than a handshake, elaborate regulation rather than simple delegation. Senior doctors should closely supervise juniors whose competence they distrust; patients may be more likely to seek second opinions if they distrust particular doctors. More generally, exercising distrust may be time-consuming, and can create a vicious spiral of resentment and acrimony (as Garfinkel's (1963) ethnomethodology students found when they refused to 'trust' statements made by friends and family in normal social interactions). However, to define trust in terms of the complete absence of explicit accountability measures and formal regulation may be unhelpful. It implies that any move to make standards more explicit and transparent is, by definition, an indication of a decline in trust; yet, if, as will be discussed later, we currently have a situation in which the medical profession is seeking to restore public trust through increasing the formal accountability of its members. Moreover, blind trust can bring its own dangers, as indicated in Table 1.1, which summarizes some claims that might be made for and against relying on trust in daily conduct. In real situations, there are likely to be many intermediate positions between 'total trust' and 'total distrust'.

Sociological concern with trust as a social phenomenon sustaining social order has a long history: from Durkheim through to functionalism at a macro-sociological level, and, via Simmel, to Goffman, in the study of small-scale social interactions. Central, however, in much of the recent work of social theorists, in particular Luhmann (1979), Beck (1992) and Giddens

Table 1.1 Some functions (and dangers) of trust

Trusting the 'trustworthy' is functional because:	BUT misplaced trust can bring problems
• Trust reduces complexity and lowers transaction costs	• *Caveat emptor* might be better in some circumstances
• Trust allows innovation and flexibility	• Reputation and prestige may mislead
• Trust constitutes or contributes to social capital (and may be good for health)	• Trusting the 'distrustworthy' can lead to disappointment, loss or worse
• Distrust leads to gaming, corruption, endless regress of accountability	• There is honour and trust among thieves: trusts can be illegal conspiracies (US usage)
• Increased demand for accountability can lead to increasing distrust	• Monitoring and formal accountability requirements might lead to better results

(1990), have been three themes. First, they argue that trust is becoming ever more important for managing life in a rapidly changing society. Far from being a phenomenon rooted in and, by implication, fading with the decline of traditional face-to-face societies, or even modern ones, trust is a means of coping with the simultaneous increasing bureaucratic rationalization and risk associated with the transition to what they term 'late-modern' or 'post-traditional' (Giddens 1990) or 'risk societies' (Beck 1992). Second, these theorists suggest that the very changes generating more need for trust are, simultaneously, rendering more precarious the bases on which we might decide to place our trust, and increasing the risks of doing so. In particular, it is argued that, in a post-traditional society, there is a less deferent, more critical stance towards experts and authority figures than in the past. Such figures are, so it is suggested, no longer regarded as trustworthy simply on the basis of the positions they occupy. Rather, trust is said to have become 'active', and conditional, having to be earned in particular situations (Giddens 1994). Third, in such societies, there is an increase in the requirement for impersonal trust, that is, having to take bets on the workings of human-designed abstract systems, rather than interpersonal trust (betting on the intentions of known others. According to Giddens, a crucial role in fostering trust in abstract systems is played by those who occupy 'key access points' for abstract systems; junctions where trust can be built up through effective 'facework' (or, presumably, undermined by poor facework) on the part of these system representatives (Giddens 1990: 83, citing Goffman 1963).

This suggests that the point made in the RCP (2005) report cited above, that trust in the medical profession is both being undermined and vital for good health care, is a specific case of a more general development in contemporary society. Medicine is an important abstract system, highly valued as a means to coping with the uncertainties of modern life, while simultaneously generating risk and uncertainty. This is illustrated in Table 1.2. The first column lists some social changes that are claimed to be both undermining the foundations of trust and generating greater need for it. The second column suggests some specific illustrations of these changes in relation to the medical profession and the organization of its work. Thus, if we accept Giddens's analysis, it is not surprising that the trustworthiness of the profession has become more contested in recent years, nor that trust in the context of health care has become a significant topic of social science research (Rowe 2004; Rowe and Calnan 2006). Although occupants of key access points for abstract systems are not necessarily highly skilled professionals, it seems plausible to see doctors as being in these positions, representatives of the abstract system of scientific medicine, but no longer automatically being accorded trust. What Giddens does not address in detail, however, is the bases on which trust might be earned or what might constitute effective facework by those in key access points in a post-traditional society, given the social changes that he identifies. If the organizations and institutionalized practices of medicine are changing, as suggested in Table 1.2, the foundations for the medical profession's claims to trustworthiness might also require updating. This point is developed below, following an account of the emergence of the 'new professionalism' and what might be termed the 'new sociology of professionalism'.

Table 1.2 Social changes and the relevance of trust in late-modern societies

Social changes leading to trust becoming more relevant, and more precariously based *	*Changes affecting the medical profession*
• Societies' future seen as based on human agency not external 'fate'	• Disease is to be prevented and treated, not just accepted. Public and government expectations of medicine are increasing (but cannot always be met)
• Increasing global interdependence	• Globalization of health risks and health workforce. Medical science and technology part of globalized industry (e.g. big 'pharma')
• Increasing role differentiation and segmentation (division of labour).	• Medicine becoming embedded in a more complex inter-professional

continued

Table 1.2 (continued) Social changes and the relevance of trust in late-modern
societies

Social changes leading to trust becoming more relevant, and more precariously based *	Changes affecting the medical profession
Role expectations need constant renegotiating	division of labour and more internally specialized. Professional boundaries more contested. Team work replacing individualism
• New threats to social stability and prosperity are of human making	• New science and technology brings new health risks. Iatrogenic risks increasing. Patient safety a major concern
• Increasing range of options and choices	• Lifestyle choices have health implications. 'Patients' becoming 'consumers', expecting options and choices (to be presented by trusted advisers?) in place of paternalism. Health care becoming more pluralistic (e.g. rise of complementary and alternative medicines)
• Increasing opacity of social environment to all but specific experts	• More need for medical 'facework' with patients. Increasing professional specialization limits doctors' expertise to narrow fields while patients have more access to information
• Increasing reliance on anonymous and impersonal systems and institutions	• Technological and third party mediation between doctor and patient increasing, e.g. managed care systems, clinical governance. Increased clinical guidelines and protocols. Health care delivery becoming more anonymous, e.g. medical shift-work in hospitals, NHS walk-in primary care centres and proposed polyclinics. Medical education and training becoming more anonymous and impersonal
• Growing presence of strangers	• Social composition of UK medical profession changing rapidly

*This column is based on Sztompka (1999: 11–14)

The trustworthiness of the medical profession under the challenge and emergence of the 'new professionalism'

When, in 1998, the GMC's judgement on the doctors implicated in the Bristol case was announced, amidst huge publicity, an editorial in the *British Medical Journal* (*BMJ*) took its apocalyptic headline, 'All changed, changed utterly', from *Easter 1916*, Yeats' poem about the Irish Republican 'rising' and the subsequent executions of its leaders, observing that 'the trust that patients place in their doctors . . . will never be the same again' (Smith 1998: 1917). However, the public's trust in medicine was not the only trust relationship reportedly in trouble at the time. In 2002, the then President of the RCP co-authored an article with a government health policy adviser in which they described the strains placed on reciprocal trust between the public, the profession, and the government (Ham and Alberti 2002: 838). Ham and Alberti saw recent events as hastening the demise of the implicit compact between the state, the medical profession and the public on which the NHS was founded in 1948, that is, what Klein (2001) termed 'the politics of the double bed' – in which government determined the broad NHS policy framework, while leaving the medical profession free to deliver the service as they thought best, on the assumption that patients would be largely passive acceptors of whatever was provided. Thus, by 2002, after two decades of major NHS reform, it was clear that the government of the day was not inclined to trust the profession to set and enforce standards as freely as in the past, and that the organized profession was generally mistrustful of the government of the day. Tension between doctors and NHS managers at local level was widely reported, as 'new public management' took hold, demanding greater accountability and monitoring of professional performance, generally seen as indicators of managerial distrust of doctors (Harrison 1999). Furthermore, especially following the Shipman and Bristol scandals, there were major questions to be asked about intra-professional trust, and the continued validity of the profession's default stance, that all members should be presumed equally 'especially trustworthy' and competent once qualified, until proved otherwise (Irvine 2003; Stacey 1992). It appeared that some kind of a crisis in medical professionalism had been reached.

However, crises are not necessarily followed by terminal decline. The diagnosis within at least some sections of the profession was that trust and professionalism could and should be restorable, with radical intervention. Thus, a key point of the 'All is changed' *BMJ* editorial quoted above was that 'it will be a good thing' if the damage to public trust that lay 'at the heart of the [Bristol] tragedy' leads to a move 'to an active rather than a passive trust where doctors share uncertainty' (Smith 1998: 1917). Similarly, the context for Ham and Alberti's (2002) diagnosis of the demise of the old implicit compact was a call for a new, more explicit compact, which included recognition of the continuing importance of professionalism, 'albeit a professionalism adapted to the 21ˢᵗ century' (2002: 842). In other words, what was being propounded, within the profession and in health policy commentary, was a 'new professionalism', as manifested in major reports from the King's Fund (Rosen and Dewar 2004) and the RCP (2005), and many articles in the medical press. As Askham and Chisholm put it, 'Defining the "new medical professionalism" is a growth industry' (Askham and Chisholm 2006: 6), in which the emphasis is on the doctors' duty to protect patients' interests, and on partnership with rather than paternalism towards patients. According to a recent consultation exercise, the emphasis is shifting from 'autonomy' and 'self-regulation' to 'a position where the key characteristics of professionalism are greater accountability and transparency. This reflects a shift in social values where traditional assumptions around professional competence have been eroded alongside an increased expectation of what professionals should deliver' (Levenson *et al.* 2008: 12).

Given the sceptical stance, since the 1970s, of many sociologists towards the medical profession's claims to be especially trustworthy, calls for a 'new professionalism' might be seen as primarily ideological, as defensive claims-making on the part of an occupation faced with widespread distrust on the part of the public and of the state, and attempts to strip away professional prerogatives, whether through performance management or direct intervention in professional regulation. This is, no doubt, a major part of the story, but not, this chapter suggests, the whole story. For one reason, the extent to which public trust in doctors in general has declined is open to debate. Surveys of public trust mainly measure attitudes or 'felt trust' (Calnan and Sanford 2004; Rowe 2004). If there is a decline in the public's enacted trust, it is not obviously being reflected in a fall in the use of medical services. There is an increase in voiced public dissatisfaction, but interpretation of trends is difficult because of the changes in institutionalized ways of voicing dissent – and many acts of voice do not originate with the public but from within the profession or the health service (CMO 2006). Furthermore, in surveys on public trust, doctors come out as much more highly trusted than politicians (Calnan and Rowe 2008).

Perhaps government cannot entirely ignore the public's attitudes here, or the ability of the profession to enlist public support in any fight with government. Governments need some co-operation from NHS professionals to give policy proposals legitimacy, as well as to actually deliver services. So, the need for trust in professionals has been regularly re-iterated in government rhetoric, even when proposing measures which appear to curtail professional prerogatives; for example, in new proposals for regulating health professions, entitled *Trust, Assurance and Safety* (Secretary of State for Health 2007). Recently, government's espousal of partnership with the profession has been most obviously expressed in the appointment, in 2007, of an active NHS surgeon, Professor (now Lord) Ara Darzi, as junior health minister with responsibility for a national review of the NHS. Darzi's summary of his interim report (addressed to the prime minister), began, 'As you know, I'm a doctor, not a politician. That's why you asked me to take on this task – and that's why I agreed' (DH 2007: 3). The Darzi reform proposals are described as being 'patient-centred and clinically driven' (DH 2008a: 16), and emphasize the roles of clinicians as not only practitioners but also 'partners and leaders' in the health service (DH 2008b). Thus, the positioning of health care reforms as being led by trusted professionals (albeit not just doctors) is explicit, although Darzi's recommendations challenge clinicians to develop better measures of quality and envisage their rewards becoming linked more directly to performance (DH 2008a). Moreover, at the time of writing, some of Lord Darzi's proposals are meeting with considerable opposition from some of his professional peers. (Some GPs are particularly concerned about the proposals for what are often dubbed 'polyclinics'. These would be facilities, possibly owned and run by profit-making companies, offering extended hours primary care services open to all, and more extensive diagnostic facilities than are currently available at many small doctor-owned general practices, and according to critics, potentially undermining the personal links between family doctors and their patients (Roland 2008).)

Recent statements extolling the value of professionalism and of trust in professionals are not only to be found in political manoeuvring between sections of the medical profession and the state. Within medical sociology, defences of trust in the medical profession can also be found, including by the late Eliot Freidson. He who did so much to develop a Weberian analysis of professionalization as a competitive power struggle, and of professionalism as an ideology, was, in his last full-length book, extolling the advantages of professionalism, relative to bureaucracy and markets, as a means of controlling the provision of expert services to needy consumers (Freidson 2001). He is not alone. For example, in the UK, Calnan and Sanford (2004) and Harrison and Smith (2004) have expressed concern about the dangers of distrust and excessive regulation of doctors. Green (2004) has drawn attention to the neglect of embedded trust relationships, with particular 'family doctors', implicit in recent NHS primary care reforms. The influence of the more general social theory literature on trust is apparent here: like the general theorists, some medical sociologists are clearly making normative judgements about the benefits of trust in doctors, and the problems posed by its reported decline.

Current sociological interest in professionalism is not confined to defending it within health care. Several current strands of analysis within the sociology of work and occupations are particularly relevant here. The first strand, as represented by, for example, Evetts (2003, 2006) and Fournier (1999), takes seriously the persistence of references to 'professionalism' and 'trust' in the contemporary workplace, and the application of the epithet 'professional' to an apparently ever-increasing range of occupations, such as information technology specialists. However, rather than regarding these applications primarily as claims for power and status being made by aspirant occupations jockeying for position, these writers adopt a more Foucauldian approach. Professionalism is seen as a disciplinary mechanism operating through self-regulation at the individual level, as a form of 'government at a distance' – in which legitimated competence is linked to personal conduct to produce trustworthy practitioners, that is, 'professionals' are themselves the subject of governance. Thus, Fournier (1999) sees the extension of the professionalism discourse to new occupations as an external managerial control tool. Personal commitment to continuing professional development, participation in audit and appraisal, become the hallmarks of the self-disciplined contemporary professional. Training and socialization take on new importance. However, her analysis might be equally applicable to internal management within established professions, a point developed below.

A second strand in recent sociological work on professions focuses on their gendered character. Davies has suggested that the development of the professional identity espoused by the medical profession in its golden era, that is, of self-reliant and self-regulating solo practitioners, was forged through 'a project of nineteenth century middle-class masculinity' (Davies 2002: 99–100). She, too, argues against seeing the relationship between the profession and the state, or between doctors and management entirely in zero-sum power terms. To do so is to ignore what marks doctors out as different from politicians or managers, that is, that medicine 'offers us heroes' who, we hope, will act on our behalf (i.e. whom we can trust) (Davies 2006). Her choice of the masculine noun is not, of course, accidental, but immediately prompts consideration of another emerging theme in the sociology of professions: the implications, for erstwhile masculine professional citadels, of the marked increase in the entry of women into those citadels (Crompton and Le Feuvre 2003; Kuhlmann 2006a and b; Riska 2001a and b).

One feature that these two strands in the sociology of professions have in common is that they focus not on the collective power-seeking strategies of the organized profession, but on professional identity. In the final section of this chapter, I wish to draw on some of this recent work on professions and professionalism to argue that the 'new professionalism' in medicine should be understood as, at least in part, an attempt from within the profession to develop new disciplinary mechanisms, at the meso level of institutionalized procedures, and at the individual level of professional sense of self, following recognition that the foundations of the profession's claims to be trustworthy require updating and rendering more explicit.

Renewing 'trustworthiness' in a changing profession

Although references to the 'new professionalism' and to the need to renew trust in medicine have proliferated since the publication of the official enquiries into the Bristol and Shipman scandals, internal debate and argument about the need for professional reform began long before these scandals came to light. In the mid-1990s, there were significant changes; for example, in the composition and working of the GMC, as chronicled by the past president of the GMC, Sir Donald Irvine (Irvine 2003). Arguably, the impact of these scandals was not so much on the public's trust in doctors, but on the political balance between different interests within medicine, and between the profession and the state. The result was to make reform go rather further and faster than it might otherwise have done, and to allow government to take the initiative from a profession characterized by an increasing 'degree of introspection and self-doubt' (Levenson *et al.* 2008: vii). But close inspection of the many recent reform measures in relation to, for example, the GMC structure, appraisal and revalidation, medical education and training reveals that many of these were under discussion, if not being implemented in some form, within the profession or through professional–state co-operation, before the scandals of the late 1990s. Among those whom Irvine cites as convincing him that major reform of the GMC was necessary, were medical sociologists Margot Jefferys and, especially, Margaret Stacey, lay member of and sociological commentator on the GMC (Davies 2002; Irvine 2003: 11). Indeed, Stacey devoted the final chapter of her book on the GMC, published well before the Bristol scandal broke, to sketching out a vision of 'a new professionalism' (1992: 257–70).

Stacey records that, 'When I joined the [General Medical] Council in the mid-1970s, it still had some of . . . [the] air of a gentleman's club about it' (1992: 204), perhaps reflecting its origins, in 1858, as part of the nineteenth-century professionalization project which transformed the appearance, reputation and (perceived) performance of doctors, making them into gentlemen (Parry and Parry 1976). What Stacey and, subsequently, Davies bring out is the implication of becoming gentle*men*: the creation of a self-confident, autonomous professional identity, with a strong sense of being part of a distinct, relatively closed brotherhood of equals. Professional advancement was influenced by personal contacts (patronage), and discipline often exercised through the informal 'word in your ear' rather than punitive sanctions (Davies 2002: 99; Stacey 1992: 205). So, in an important sense, historically, the medical profession's claim to be trustworthy was based on its members being gentlemen, at a time when being a gentleman was widely accepted as grounds for trustworthiness.

Stacey was a stern critic of the barriers that the persistence of elements of this culture into the late twentieth century posed to the full inclusion of women and overseas-trained doctors into the professional community, and to the effective disciplining of the profession. But, being a gentleman was no longer, in itself, regarded sufficient to guarantee trustworthiness, and, furthermore, an increasing proportion of entrants to the profession were not 'gentlemen' (although some critics might still have claimed that too many still were). So, arguably, the foundations on which the medical profession once implicitly based its claims to be trustworthy are no longer so apposite, being either no longer socially acceptable as bases for 'trustworthiness' claims, or no longer applicable to the profession's members. At this point, we can return to Table 1.2 and the changes affecting the medical profession listed in the second column, focusing, because of limited space, particularly on the last two rows, which refer to changes in medical education and training and to the changing social composition of the UK medical profession.

The medical brotherhood that Stacey identified was formed, until well into the second half of the twentieth century, in medical schools that were, for the most part, distinctively separate, largely self-regulating and relatively small institutions, usually with close relationships to a single teaching hospital, where senior students spent long periods on the wards interacting with more senior members of the profession. Recruitment to schools was largely of men and disproportionately from medical families. Personal ties between schools and alumni remained strong. Today's medical schools look rather different: they are much larger and more fully absorbed into multi-faculty universities. Recruitment is mainly based on academic achievement, highly structured interviews, and aptitude tests (Parry 2006). A profession that was criticized for being overwhelmingly male and white in the 1970s has not only admitted a majority of women since the early 1990s, but also, currently, accepts about one-third minority ethnic group students to its medical schools (and increased diversity in recruitment has been an explicit government target) (Parry 2007; UCAS 2007). Teaching is increasingly shared with students on other degree programmes. Early clinical experience is usually spread between several hospitals and general practice placements. The greater diversity of UK-trained entrants has been supplemented by the influx of very substantial numbers of international medical graduates, particularly to increase capacity under the *NHS Plan* (DH 2000).

Major changes to postgraduate training and work organization have also occurred, following European Commission Directives mandating changes to specialist certification, and limiting working hours (European Working Time Directive) (EWTD). Recruitment into and progress through specialist training has become increasingly organized around standardized procedures and competence-based assessment (DH 1993; UK Departments of Health 2004). Under EWTD, the long hours of on-call duty, as part of a small 'firm' serving a particular consultant's patients, have increasingly been replaced by junior doctors working shifts and providing care for a wider range of patients, with less close contact with specific senior doctors.

These changes might reduce the scope for unfair patronage and discrimination, and for clinical errors arising from doctor fatigue. But they also mean that medical education and training is clearly becoming increasingly reliant on impersonal, relatively anonymous systems and institutions. If the intimate and insulated character of medical socialization and the social homogeneity of entrants were important in creating the sense of professional brotherhood identified by Stacey, then these are being greatly modified.

There is much talk and some research reporting generational differences in outlook among younger doctors, and concern about the fragmentation of the professional community and whether improving work–life balance is at the expense of acquiring clinical competence and professional values – perhaps a sense that professional identity is at risk by default (Jones and Green 2006; Levenson *et al.* 2008; McKee 2002).

So, in terms of recruitment and training, the medical profession is both increasingly composed of 'strangers' (relative to the past), and becoming more reliant on anonymous, impersonal bureaucratic systems – changes identified earlier (Table 1.2) as generating greater need for trust, but as also making the basis for trust more precarious. In this particular instance, it is the foundations for judging trustworthiness within the profession that are at issue. In an increasingly complex medical division of labour, doctors have to trust their clinical colleagues more, but they are less likely to come from a shared background or to know them well. If space permitted, analysis of some of the other changes identified in Table 1.2 would reveal similar challenges to the erstwhile gentlemanly culture of medicine. But if this culture has become less sustainable or legitimate as the foundation of claims to be trustworthy, this, in turn, raises the question as to what could replace it.

One answer seems to be the 'new professionalism'. Table 1.3 sets out some of the features of 'old' and 'new' professionalism, indicating that the latter

Table 1.3 Changing foundations for the promise of trustworthiness*

Old professionalism	New professionalism
• Public acceptance of 'mastery' and self-regulation	• Partnership with patients
• Elite social standing and appearance Masculine expertise	• Recruitment on merit Good communication skills
• Intensive socialization into closed collegiate institutions	• Lay involvement in regulation Inter-professional co-operation and teamwork
• Formal credentials on entry to career	• Continuous professional development
• Indeterminacy of knowledge makes professional judgement unchallengeable	• Use of evidence-based medicine and clinical guidelines (and judgement)
• Internal (self-) regulation	• Formal appraisal and revalidation (by peers)
• All professionals have equivalent status	• Management and leadership skills important within the profession

* This table draws on Davies (2003b)

is leading the profession down a path towards embracing greater formal accountability, more external, especially lay, involvement in professional regulation, and greater monitoring of clinical standards. So, rather than assuming all such demands for explicit evidence and transparency of information are externally imposed managerial tools or indicators of declining public or political trust in doctors, medical sociologists should recognize that these are sometimes being advanced, at least within some sections of the profession, as tools for professional self-discipline and governance, and as the foundation on which a more conditional promise of trustworthiness might be based (Kuhlmann 2006b). Of course, such managerial tools themselves need to be trusted by doctors in order to become incorporated into professional identity. Information on professional performance is not likely to totally supplant direct experience of the competence and integrity of professionals as a source of trust (Calnan and Rowe 2008). What the proponents of the new professionalism hope is that demonstrating commitment to self-audit and appraisal and the like increasingly come to be seen as part of good professional 'facework' – whether this happens or not remains to be seen.

Conclusions

This chapter began by suggesting that contemporary concerns about professionalism and trust in medicine can be related to more general societal changes. It has argued that professionalism, as a means of governance, may not be being eroded so much as being remade, with new foundations for trust being tortuously formulated and negotiated within the profession, as well as between the profession and the public and the state. Some of the distinctive features of medicine that sociologists identified in the mid-twentieth century may be disappearing, and professional identity may be changing. Generational differences may be emerging within the profession. The challenge for the profession is what kind of identity can be forged in the new, more fragmented conditions of training and practice, and whether this identity can serve as the foundation of publicly accepted claims of special trustworthiness.

What this chapter has also shown is that the relationship between medical sociology and the medical profession has also changed since the mid-twentieth century, at least in the UK. In the 1970s the critical portrayal of medicine's power and privilege by sociologists was one of the challenges to the then institutionalized foundations of professionalism. Thirty years later, at least some elements of the sociological critique have been incorporated into the vision of the new professionalism – and sociological attention has returned to some of the classic questions about what it means to be a professional.

Acknowledgements

I would like to thank Celia Davies and the editors for their helpful comments on earlier drafts of this chapter.

References

Allsop, J. and Saks, M. (2002) (eds) *Regulating the Health Professions*, London: Sage.

Askham, J. and Chisholm, A. (2006) *Patient-Centred Medical Professionalism: Towards an agenda for research and action*, Oxford: Picker Institute.

Beck, U. (1992) *Risk Society: Towards a new modernity*, London and Thousand Oaks: Sage.

Bevan, G. (2008) 'Changing paradigms of governance and regulation of quality of healthcare in England', *Health, Risk and Society*, 10: 85–101.

Calnan, M. and Rowe, R. (2008) *Trust Matters in Health Care*, Buckingham: Open University Press.

Calnan, M. and Sanford, E. (2004) 'Public trust in health care: the system or the doctor?' *Quality and Safety in Health Care*, 13: 92–7.

Chief Medical Officer (2006) *Good Doctors, Safer Patients. Proposals to strengthen the system to assure and improve the performance of doctors and to protect the safety of patients*, London: Department of Health. www.dh.gov.uk

Crompton, R. and Le Feuvre, N. (2003) 'Continuity and change in the gender segregation of the medical profession in Britain and France', *International Journal of Sociology and Social Policy*, 23: 36–58.

Davies, C. (2002) 'What about the girl next door? Gender and the politics of professional self-regulation', in G. Bendelow, M. Carpenter, C. Vautier and S. Williams (eds), *Gender, Health and Healing: The public/private divide*, London: Routledge.

Davies, C. (2003) (ed.) *The Future Health Workforce*, Basingstoke: Palgrave Macmillan.

Davies, C. (2006) 'Heroes of Health Care? Re-placing the medical profession in the policy process in the UK', in J.W. Duyvendak, T. Knijn and M. Kremer (eds) *Policy, People and the New Professional: Deprofessionalisation and reprofessionalisation in care and welfare*, Amsterdam: Amsterdam University Press.

Department of Health (DH) (1993) *Hospital Doctors: Training for the future. The report of the working party on specialist medical training*, London: Department of Health.

Department of Health (2000) *The NHS Plan: A plan for investment, plan for reform*, London: Department of Health.

Department of Health (2007) *Our NHS: Our Future. NHS Next Stage Review – Interim Report*, London: Department of Health.

Department of Health (2008a) *Leading Local Change*, London: Department of Health. www.ournhs.nhs.uk

Department of Health (2008b) *A High Quality Workforce: NHS Next Stage Review*, London: Department of Health.

Dingwall, R. and Fenn, P. (1987) '"A respectable profession?" Sociological and economic perspectives on the regulation of professional services', *International Review of Law and Economics*, 7: 51–64.

Elston, M.A. (1991) 'The politics of professional power: medicine in a changing health service', in J. Gabe, M. Calnan and M. Bury (eds) *The Sociology of the Health Service*, London: Routledge.

Evetts, J. (2003) 'The construction of professionalism in new and existing occupational contexts: promoting and facilitating occupational change', *International Journal of Sociology and Social Policy*, 23: 22–35.

Evetts, J. (2006) 'Introduction to "Trust and professionalism: Challenges and occupational changes"', *Current Sociology*, 54: 515–31.

Fournier, V. (1999) 'The appeal to "professionalism" as a disciplinary mechanism', *Sociological Review*, 47: 280–307.

Freidson, E. (1970) *Profession of Medicine: a study of the sociology of applied knowledge*, New York: Dodds Mead.

Freidson, E. (2001) *Professionalism: The third logic*, Cambridge: Polity.

Gabe, J., Calnan, M. and Bury, M. (1991) (eds) *The Sociology of the Health Service*, London: Routledge.

Gabe, J., Kelleher, D. and Williams, G. (1994) (eds) *Challenging Medicine*, London: Routledge.

Garfinkel, H. (1963) 'A conception of and experiments with"trust" as a condition of stable concerted actions', in O.J. Harvey (ed.) *Motivation and Social Interaction*, New York: Ronald Press.

Giddens, A. (1990) *The Consequences of Modernity*, Cambridge: Polity.

Giddens, A. (1994) 'Living in a post-traditional society', in U. Beck, A. Giddens and S. Lash (eds) *Reflexive Modernization: Politics, tradition and aesthetics in the modern social order*, Cambridge: Polity Press.

Goffman, E. (1963) *Behavior in Public Places*, New York: Free Press.

Green, J. (2004) 'Is trust an under-researched component of healthcare organisation?' *British Medical Journal*, 329: 384.

Ham, C. and Alberti, K.G.M.M. (2002) 'The medical profession, the public and the government', *British Medical Journal*, 324: 838–42.

Harrison, S. (1999) 'Clinical autonomy and health policy: past and futures', in M. Exworthy and S. Halford (eds) *Professsionals and the New Managerialism in the Public Sector*, Buckingham: Open University Press.

Harrison, S. and Ahmad, W.I.U. (2000) 'Medical autonomy and the UK state, 1975–2025', *Sociology*, 34: 129–42.

Harrison, S. and Smith, C. (2004) 'Trust and moral motivation: redundant resources in health and social care?' *Policy and Politics*, 32: 371–86.

Irvine, D. (2003) *The Doctors' Tale: Professionalism and Public Trust*, Oxford: Radcliffe Medical Press.

Jones, L. and Green, J. (2006) 'Shifting discourses of professionalism: a case study of general practitioners in the United Kingdom', *Sociology of Health & Illness*, 28: 927–50.

Kelleher, D., Gabe, J., and Williams, G. (2006) (eds) *Challenging Medicine*, second edition, London: Routledge.

Klein, R. (2001) *The New Politics of the NHS*, Harlow: Prentice Hall.

Kuhlmann, E. (2006a) *Modernising Healthcare: reinventing professions, the state and the public*, Bristol: Policy Press.

Kuhlmann, E. (2006b) 'Traces of doubt and sources of trust', *Current Sociology*, 54: 607–20.

Levenson, R., Dewar, S. and Shepherd, S. (2008) *Understanding Doctors: Harnessing Professionalis*, London: King's Fund & Royal College of Physicians.

Luhmann, N. (1979) *Trust and Power*, New York: Wiley.

McKee, A. (2002) 'Working and learning in hospitals: junior doctors adrift in fragmented communities', *Learning in Health and Social Care*, 3: 158–69.

Mechanic, D. (1996) 'Changing medical organization and the erosion of trust', *The Milbank Quarterly*, 74: 171–89.

Mechanic, D. (1998) 'The functions and limitations of trust in the provision of medical care', *Journal of Health Politics, Policy and Law*, 23: 661–86.

O'Neill, O. (2002) *A Question of Trust*, Cambridge: Cambridge University Press.

Parry, J. (2006) 'Admissions processes for five year medical courses at English schools: review', *British Medical Journal*, 332: 1005–9.

Parry, J. (2007) *Evaluation of the National Expansion of Medical Schools (NEMS) in England. Executive Summary*, London: HEFCE and Department of Health. www.hefce.ac.uk/aboutus/health/student/medical_student_numbers.pdf. Accessed 29 October 2007.

Parry, N. and Parry, J. (1976) *The Rise of the Medical Profession*, London: Croom Helm.

Parsons, T. (1939) 'The professions and social structure', *Social Forces*, 17: 457–67.

Parsons, T. (1951) *The Social System*, New York: The Free Press.

Pollock, A. (2004) *NHS plc: The privatisation of health care*, London: Verso.

Riska, E. (2001a) *Medical Careers and Feminist Agendas: American, Scandinavian and Russian Women Physicians*, New York: Aldine.

Riska, E. (2001b) 'Towards gender balance, but will women physicians have an impact on medicine', *Social Science and Medicine*, 52: 179–87.

Roland, M. (2008) 'Assessing the options available to Lord Darzi', *British Medical Journal*, 336: 625–6.

Rosen, R. and Dewar, S. (2004) *On Being a Doctor: Redefining medical professionalism for better health care*, London: King's Fund.

Rowe, R. (2004) *Trust in Health Care: A review of the literature*, London: Nuffield Foundation.

Rowe, R. and Calnan, M. (2006) 'Trust relations in health care: developing a theoretical framework for the "new" NHS', *Journal of Health Organisation and Management*, 20: 376–96.

Royal College of Physicians (2005) *Doctors in Society: Medical professionalism in a changing world*, London: Royal College of Physicians of London.

Salter, B. (2007) 'Governing UK medical performance: A struggle for policy dominance', *Health Policy*, 82: 263–75.

Secretary of State for Health (2007) *Trust, Assurance and Safety – The Regulation of Health Professionals in the 21st Century*, London: The Stationery Office. CM 7013.

Smith, J. (2004) *The Shipman Inquiry Fifth Report; safeguarding patients: lessons from the past – proposals for the future*, London: Stationery Office. Cmnd 6394.

Smith, R. (1998) 'All changed, changed utterly', *British Medical Journal*, 316: 1917–18.

Stacey, M. (1992) *Regulating British Medicine: The General Medical Council*, London: Wiley.

Starr, P. (1982) *The Social Transformation of American Medicine*, New York: Basic Books.

Sztompka, P. (1999) *Trust: A sociological theory*, Cambridge: Cambridge University Press.

Taylor-Gooby, P. (2008) 'Trust and welfare state reform: the example of the NHS', *Social Policy and Administration*, 42: 288–306.

Tooke, J. (2007) *Aspiring to Excellence: Findings and recommendations of the independent inquiry into modernising medical careers, led by Sir John Tooke*, London: Department of Health.

UK Department of Health (2004) *Modernising Medical Careers: The next steps*, London: Department of Health.

Universities and Colleges Admissions Service (UCAS) (2007) *Online Statistics on Applications and Acceptances*. www.ucas.org.uk (accessed 7 Sept 2007).

Waddington, I. (1984) *The Medical Profession in the Industrial Revolution*, Dublin: Gill and Macmillan.

2 Changing forms of managerialism in the NHS

Hierarchies, markets and networks

Sue Dopson

Introduction

David Cox in his chapter on health service management in the 1991 edition of *The Sociology of the Health Service* (Cox 1991) argues that the organization and management of health care has been relatively neglected in the sociological literature. Today the picture is a more promising one. There have been some excellent sociologically driven studies of managerial challenges; for example, Flynn's work on governmentality (Flynn 2002, 2004), Pope's study of the management of waiting lists (Pope 1991), work by Hunter (2006) and Dent (1993) on the relationship between medicine and management to name but a few. However, whilst acknowledging this growing body of scholarship, some commentators have noted that 'organization' and 'management' remain a relatively neglected area within medical sociology. Davies, for example, in her extremely rigorous review of how the concept of 'organizations' has fared in the journal *Sociology of Health and Illness* in its first twenty-five years, concludes that organizations have remained a minor theme in the journal and notes there is still no strong sense of a growing corpus of work on the theme of organizations. Dopson and Fitzgerald (2005) have also pointed to the existence of unhelpful boundaries between the writers on health policy, organizational studies of health care and medical sociology.

This chapter does not seek to review in detail the sociological work available to those of us interested in organization and management aspects of health care, rather it seeks to reflect on the major changes in organization and management of the NHS health care since the 1980s with a view to reflecting on what opportunities exist for sociologically driven work in this area.

Changes in management in the NHS are discussed in this chapter in relation to what has been termed the new public management. New Public Management (NPM) is presented by Hood and Peters (2004) as comprising the following practices:

- Greater competition in service provision
- Disaggregation of units

- Hands-on professional management in the public sector
- Private sector styles of management
- Tighter and more efficient use of resources
- Explicit standards and measures of performance
- Emphasis on output controls.

NPM has been seen by critics as a market-based ideology invading public sector organizations (Laughlin 1991), others see it as a management hybrid with a continuing emphasis on core public service values. Ferlie *et al.* (1996), for example, argue that at least four new forms of public management are in evidence and have impacted on health care management.

1. The efficiency drives form where the emphasis is on making the public sector more businesslike.
2. Downsizing and decentralization and the introduction of market mindedness.
3. The pursuit of excellence, where organizational development and culture change are stressed.
4. Public service orientation with the emphasis on service quality and consumers.

The impact on managerial and professional roles of NPM is explored in this chapter. It begins by exploring in some detail the Griffiths Report which heralded the introduction of general management into the NHS. This report and the implementation of its findings represented a radical change in the practice of managing health services in the UK and is an example of an efficiency form of NPM. Future changes in health services management practice were provoked by two major and politically driven interventions. First, the introduction of quasi markets, and, second, the desire for more network-driven management.

This chapter also looks at what a more sociological approach could offer to the study of organization and management issues. Specifically, I consider a relatively recent policy-driven initiative requiring managers to ensure health services delivery is more 'evidence based' (EBM).

The Griffiths Report and the introduction of general management

Up until 1983, the NHS had two unusual organizational characteristics: the national uniformity of its senior management structures, and the practice of 'consensus management'. Just as the dust of the NHS's second major reorganization was beginning to settle, the conservative government led by Margaret Thatcher rounded on NHS management and health care professionals' failure to achieve significant improvements in cost containment or health care. Health Minister Norman Fowler appointed four leading businessmen to conduct an 'independent' management inquiry into the:

> effective use and management of manpower and related resources in the NHS from professional managers with experience in other large organizations.
>
> (DHSS 1983)

Members of this government held an ideologically driven belief that public services such as the NHS could and should learn from private sector management practices. The Griffiths Report, as the Inquiry became known, was published in October 1983. It takes the form of a letter to the secretary of state and consists of recommendations for action as well as observations and some ten pages of background notes. Although brief, the Report sparked off a surge of interest, anxiety and controversy which continued well after the Griffiths post-mortem. The Griffith Report is an example of the efficiency drive form of NPM where the emphasis was on making the NHS more businesslike. It points to five areas of alleged weakness, documented in the 'Observations' section of the Report.

> A lack of strategic central direction.
> A lack of individual managerial responsibility.
> A failure to use objectives as a guide to managerial action.
> A neglect of performance.
> A neglect of the consumer.
>
> (Hunter *et al.* 1988: 1)

These criticisms are elaborated but not illustrated – still less validated – by various assertions scattered in the Report. First, they imply that poor central management of the NHS had led to piecemeal strategies and ad hoc interference in local management, and, second, that consensus management had failed in that the requirement to 'get agreement' had overshadowed the need to make decisions, resulting in long delays in the management process. All the criticisms of the NHS made in the Report suggest the NHS is being measured, not against private companies in the real world, but against an ideal – a typical model of how things 'ought' to be if only people would behave sensibly!

The general criticism of the lack of individual managerial responsibility was to be met by the introduction of general management defined in the Report as 'responsibility drawn together in one person, at different levels of the organization, for planning, implementation and control of performance' and the abandonment of formal consensus decision making (DHSS 1983: 11). General managers were to be 'the linchpin of dynamic management' and, importantly, could be drawn from any occupational group.

It was carefully stated that the appointment of general managers was not intended to weaken the professional responsibilities of other chief officers 'especially in relation to decision-making on matters within their own spheres of responsibility' (DHSS 1983: 17). The general manager was to be the final decision taker for decisions normally in the province of consensus teams in the hope that delay and disagreement could be avoided. The chair of the health authority was given the task of 'clarifying the general management function and identifying a general manager for every unit of management' (DHSS 1983: 6).

There were a number of proposals to meet the criticism of lack of objectives and poor implementation: fixed contracts for general managers which were later rolling contracts; the creation of the NHS management board; the extension of the review process to unit level; and, later, individual performance review and performance-related pay.

Strengthening existing performance indicators (service performance targets devised to improve the use of resources, monitor quality and ensure accountability to the public) and developing a management budgeting approach (giving units/departments clearly defined budgets, for which they are accountable) were regarded as vehicles for promoting the measurement of output in terms of patient care and dealing with the criticism that the NHS lacked a performance orientation. The Regions (these were geographically organized, strategic and monitoring bodies) were also to be strengthened as part of improving the performance orientation, although the nature of this process was not made clear.

Clinical general managers were thought to have a better chance of curbing the power of the medical profession. It was hoped clinicians, especially doctors, would take up general management posts. Although, doctors' involvement in management is intimately part of ensuring the NHS acquired a performance orientation, this was not explicitly tackled in the Report. Indeed, the only mention of this critical aspect is on page 6 of the Report, where district and regional chairs are charged with, 'involving the clinicians more closely in the management process, consistent with clinical freedom for clinical practices'. Whilst there can be no doubt that Thatcher's brand of conservatism sought to challenge the power of professional groups, there was little explicit discussion of how this was to happen. Implicit in the Report is the hope that the development of budgets at unit level would involve clinicians and allow workload and service objectives to be related to financial and manpower allocations.

The Report stressed that patients and the community were to be the focus of the planning and delivery of services. To that end, health authorities were to ascertain, and act on, public opinion surveys and the advice of Community Health Councils (CHCs) to ensure a consumer orientation for the NHS. Here we see another aspect of NPM highlighted by Ferlie *et al.* (1996): the emphasis on service quality and consumers. The National Management Board was made responsible for acting upon information regarding the experience and perceptions of patients in the community, given to them by the CHCs, market research and general practice in formulating policy and monitoring performance against it (DHSS 1983: 9).

In many senses, the Griffiths proposals were an act of faith, based on a report whose recommendations lacked substantive evidence. The Report makes a number of important assumptions, which are discussed and challenged below.

1. **Politicians will deliver clear policies which general managers will implement.** This assumes politicians are aware of the complexities involved in providing health care and ignores the political capital politicians may make from the NHS, which means that policy shifts can (and do) occur at any time and often reflect political rather than health care priorities.

2. **General management will not challenge existing arrangements for accountability.** Yet, the relationship of regional chairs to ministers changed since they were required to follow management directives from the central management board and the primary reporting relationship of functional officers was no longer to a functional head but to the general manager.

3. **Private industry is more effectively managed than the public sector.** This is clearly open to question, given the relative efficiency of the NHS by comparison to other health care systems in the world and the relatively poor performance of the British private sector as compared to its international competitors.

4. **The general manager can be the final decision taker and manage the considerable power of professional groups in the NHS.** The Griffiths recommendations assume that general managers have the authority to curb the power of the medical profession and its strong ideas about the provision of services. The general manager's task was made more difficult by consultants' contracts remaining at regional level.

5. **Output measurement is straightforward in the NHS.** Outputs of the health service are varied. It provides employment to large numbers of people. It is the major producer of medical research and of training for nurses, doctors and many other occupations. However, the most essential of health service outputs are treatments and care provided to people. An important distinction has been drawn between outputs (the treatments provided to patients) and outcomes of care (the benefits to health).

6. **The NHS consists solely of hospital services.** The community and voluntary sectors are not explicitly discussed in the Griffiths Report. This begs the question: how can general managers be responsible for the total health care of the population when the hospital sector's links with these complex important sectors are not within the scope of their authority?

The rather detailed discussion of the assumptions inherent in the Griffiths Report is not meant to convey political carping but merely to illustrate the points of debate that might have been taken up following the publication of the Report, yet rarely were these points debated in the commentary and furore which followed its publication. Rather the focus was almost exclusively on either the appointment of the new general manager, or the defence of a particular interest group. Furthermore, it is not surprising that some of these assumptions were made. A team of highly regarded and highly competent business people could not be expected to get to grips with the complexities of the NHS in the time available, particularly when there was so little available analysis of this complexity. Businessmen, like civil servants, academics, or any human being, have particular ideologies that influence the way in which they view problems, which makes it difficult to look at issues in a detached manner. Moreover, the Griffiths team did not have the luxury (as academics do) of saying they simply do not know the answer, as Sir Roy noted, the noise level in the NHS reached unprecedented heights at the time he and his team made his observations (Griffiths 1991: 2). The Griffiths team had to come up with some analysis.

The Griffiths recommendations were supplemented with a number of management changes. In 1983, the DHSS produced the first set of national NHS Performance Indicators which enabled health authorities to compare their performance on certain measures with national and regional norms. Health authorities were instructed to put cleaning, laundry and catering services out for tender. In 1984, annual reviews of hospitals were introduced; in 1987, Individual Performance Review and Performance Related Pay were introduced for general managers (see Pollitt 1990, for a thorough review of these changes). All these changes were introduced against a backdrop of increasingly tough financial constraints as the NHS sought to accommodate financial demands from advances in medical technology and an increasing aging population.

The Griffiths Report was subjected to critical examination by a number of writers. Day and Klein (1983), for example, suggested that the report signified a change away from the mobilization of consent and towards the management of conflict. Davies (1987) saw the Griffiths Report as an important part of a government strategy to gain a greater degree of centralized control and concluded that the report indicated that centralization and the creation of a market in health care are not as opposed as they might at first seem. Petchey (1986) saw the report as transferring in an uncritical way managerial concepts from the private sector, where he suggested management is less problematic.

David Cox in the first edition of this book argued 'Griffiths had caught sociologists on the hop' (Cox 1991). However, there were a number of empirical studies carried out by organizational behaviour and health policy scholars that focused on the implementation of the Griffiths proposals (Harrison *et al.* 1992; Pettigrew *et al.* 1992; Stewart *et al.* 1987). A more sociological approach to the study of the introduction of general management is Strong and Robinson (1990) a study of the NHS under new management. Such studies pointed to a trend towards greater centralization of power, accompanied by increased bureaucracy and a proliferation of policy objectives, all of which served to curtail the freedom of the health district to meet the needs of its local population. Accountability structures appeared to be more confused. Furthermore, because general management was introduced at a time when the Conservative government, led by Margaret Thatcher, was seeking dramatically to reduce public expenditure, general management and cuts became inextricably linked. These studies also found that doctors did not flock to take up management posts as government had hoped.

Improvements in quality mainly took the form of improvements in 'hotel' services, that is to say the physical appearance of hospitals improved, customer service initiatives were launched. Patterns of health care delivery did not significantly change. Such change would have involved managers challenging the power of clinicians. These studies also signal that professional groups in health care became much more interdependent, partly as a result of a general management system replacing the old functional professional hierarchies and partly because of static resources, numerous new priorities for health care and an increase in general monitoring.

Markets and managerialism

The NHS and Community Care Act (1990) heralded the introduction of quasi markets where contracts became an important means of control. Old District Health Authorities merged to form larger purchasing consortia and the vast majority of NHS hospitals adopted Trust status. In 1991, GP fund holding and a more complete GP contract were introduced. An internal purchaser–provider relationship was established with health authorities and GP fund holders acting as the former, and hospitals, newly created as trusts acting as providers.

By imposing market forces and business disciplines right across the full range of public sector provision, the ideology of neo-liberal managerialism was intended to weaken, if not totally destroy, the regulatory ethic and machinery that had protected unaccountable professional and administrative elites in the past (Freidson 1994, 2001). However, in practical terms this form of NPM consisted of a series of policy initiatives aimed at realizing the widespread adoption of a customer-oriented and performance-driven culture supporting a much 'leaner and fitter' organizational delivery system fully responsive to the threats and opportunities provided by revitalized market competition (Pollitt 2002). In-house providers were forced to compete with external, private sector contractors, placing significant downward pressures on employee terms and conditions as attempts were made to reduce costs

(Escott and Whitfield 1995). While in many instances contracts were won by in-house teams, this was a process which contributed to the 'hollowing-out' of the state (Skelcher 2000) as it became an 'enabler', commissioning services from outside contractors rather than providing them itself, creating the possibility of privatization from within. The pressure to contract out, coupled with changes in the legal framework, facilitated a decline in the power of the unions and a shift from traditional forms of collective pay bargaining to more contract and performance based on reward and appraisal.

The argument put forward by the Conservative government at this time was that for public sector organizations to compete effectively, they needed discretion over their resources. The disaggregation of service units, with the creation of self-governing Trusts in the NHS and the break-up of central government departments to establish executive agencies was designed to provide these freedoms. Seen as better able to respond to discrete product market circumstances than the former monoliths, these units were given responsibility for key resources such as budgets and employees. NHS trusts, for example, became employers of their own staff. Disaggregation and devolution could not, however, negate the ongoing need for political control and this in large part accounted for the development of more explicit performance standards and measures. If public sector organizations were to be given discretion to compete, they still needed to be held to account, encouraging the development of a tighter audit framework (Power 1997). This framework was not, however, solely related to central control and accountability. The use of performance measures and targets was also associated with attempts to provide the kind of transparency needed for service users, as consumers, to make informed choices. In a more general sense, it was reflected in the Citizen's Charter formulated by the Major government, the Conservative's successor to the Thatcher government. This elevation of 'user rights' can, in turn, be seen as part of the government's project to wrest control of the public services from professionals.

Managers in the NHS were expected to be change agents, entrepreneurs and business oriented. Unlike the Griffiths era, managers were often recruited on short-term contracts with substantially higher salaries, but required to achieve demanding performance targets. There was a desire for more visible active and individualistic forms of leadership (Ferlie 2002: 284). The numbers employed as 'general' managers dramatically rose; between 1985 and 1995 the number of employees categorized as NHS managers, for example, increased from 300 to over 23,000 (Kirkpatrick *et al.* 2005: 91).

Empirical studies exploring the impact of this wave of NPM on occupational groups involved in the delivery of health care suggest that the dynamics and power issues apparent within the new public management may be more complex than commonly supposed. Ferlie *et al.*'s (1996) evidence did not support the idea of doctors being controlled by managers as a result of the discipline of a contracting process and the quasi market. They found public health to be a rising function within medicine because of its strategic role within purchasing organizations. The introduction of GP fundholding also shifted resources and to some extent, power away from the hospital consultants to GPs. However, empowered by the doctrine that managers must manage, public sector managers are seen by researchers of management processes in the era of markets as a gaining group (Pollitt 1990; Pettigrew *et al.* 1992; Farnham and Horton 1993). As stated earlier, there had been a proliferation of operational management posts in business management, finance, audit and information functions. However, whilst senior managers are better paid, they enjoy far less job security and are part of a demanding target-oriented appraisal process.

Debate continues as to the extent to which one can state empirically that the substantial process of 'managerialization' in this period led to significant changes in the power of the medical profession. There is no doubt that there has been a fundamental shift towards the inclusion of clinical personnel in key management roles in health care in the UK. The 1990 Act induced the need for a definable, bounded organizational service/ unit basis for contracts. Acute and community trusts were re-structured into clinical directorates, virtually overnight (Fitzgerald and Sturt 1992). A clinical directorate is a team of health care professionals within a speciality or group of specialities which is responsible for the provision of patient care within allocated resources. It is usually headed by a clinician and is accountable for its management function to the Board of Management of the Trust, unit or division. Montgomery (1990) drew attention to the fact that such a change can be seen either as a defensive move – to keep the voice of the collective medical profession at the forefront – or as an opportunistic move to create prestigious new employment opportunities. There are no precise figures to substantiate the numbers of clinicians holding posts as clinical directors of a service or as medical directors of a trust during this period.

During this period, further substantial changes occurred to the management contribution of general practitioners (GPs). With the introduction of GP fundholding, GPs now held more strategic management roles in primary care and would increasingly do so as their role in the commissioning process expanded. With the change to a Labour government in 1997, GP fundholding was abolished. It was announced that 'partnerships' and 'agreements' would replace quasi-markets. Primary Care Groups (PCGs) were established evolving into Primary Care Trusts (PCTs), local GP contracts and salaried general practice appeared. By 2004, budgets for hospital referrals were being transferred back to general practices or groups of them ('practice-based commissioning'). GPs were now obliged to offer such patients a choice of hospital ('patient choice') and hospitals were now paid on a fixed tariff per referral ('payment by results'). The more successful NHS hospital trusts were given wider managerial and financial discretion and reconstituted as 'Foundation Trusts'. Another new national GP contract was introduced and PCTs were merged and their functions expanded (Sheaff *et al.* 2004).

Sheaff *et al.* (2004), reflecting on the changing role of GPs, argue that whilst the demand for services which GPs supply continues to increase, this very trend has provoked skill mix changes and diversification in the clinical and organizational models of primary health provision, tending to erode the technological centrality of the medical profession as first point of contact with primary care. The emergence of alternative professions contesting the jurisdictional boundaries of medicine reflects the rising size of the groups (a consequence of health system expansion generally) and the rising educational and technical level of these professions. GPs' impersonal sources of power have on balance, they conclude, diminished.

Sheaff's study of four PCGs in 1998–2001 described a stratum of doctors emerging who mediated between the profession and NHS management (Sheaff *et al.* 2002), and thus acquired an interest in reforms which enhanced their status, influence over other doctors and voice in NHS management. The universal but relatively weak, predominantly educational form of medical audit introduced in 1991 was supplanted from 1998. Medical audit and local professional networks were reconstituted as clinical governance networks with GP 'leads'. GP membership was compulsory. These changes shifted the emphasis of medical self-regulation from private and individual towards transparent and collegial scrutiny of medical work based upon EBM. Nevertheless, clinical governance was often initiated by a core of 'early adopter' doctors, gradually involving other GPs through peer influence, and GPs' uptake of EBM was selective. Other clinical professions, especially nursing, either had their own more fragmentary clinical governance networks or participated ad hoc as semi-detached members of the medical networks on an issue-by-issue basis. Clinical governance activities thus remained medically dominated.

This period also saw changes in nursing. In the UK, the professionalization project for nursing led to a long campaign by the nursing profession for a degree-based training for nurses and the removal of the grade of enrolled nurses (Francis and Humphreys 1999). This was an attempt to maintain exclusivity and to move the knowledge base from tacit/skill-based knowledge towards codified knowledge (Ainley 1994). It is argued that raising the qualification level has priced nurses out of organizations, reducing their managerial influence (Francis and Humphreys 1999). Currently, similar arguments are being used to suggest that nurse practitioners are being substituted for higher priced doctors.

The data from work in the UK on the clinician role in management does display a set of interrelated (and largely unresolved) issues. First, there is widespread concern that the technical autonomy granted to the individual practitioner and professional system of self-regulation have led to problems with the quality of output (Fitzgerald and Ferlie 2000; Coulter 2002). Second, the movement of doctors into management roles has highlighted the tensions between professional responsibility to the individual patient and managerial responsibility to the population, in a resource constrained system (Dopson 1993; Fitzgerald 1994). Finally, the employment of clinical professional 'hybrids' raises questions concerning the effective management of professionals. What are the appropriate and effective methods for the management of clinical professionals and indeed other forms of experts? If professions have traditionally been characterized by self-regulation, can clinical professionals' work be improved by 'hybrid' clinical managers or would general managers have greater expertise and impact? To date, the evidence remains sparse. The management of professional performance is seen as the province of the members of the profession and external scrutiny is resisted. There is more evidence to illustrate that clinical managers can address performance problems more accurately than general managers (Montgomery 1990; Fitzgerald and Dufour 1997; Kitchener 1999).

These trends of a growing number of clinical managers and the implementation of managerial systems of providing transparency in quality monitoring have fundamental implications. First, the changing nature of organizational roles may create ambiguity about role boundaries (Cassel 1997). This will require attention to issues of communication and effort to develop shared understanding of organizational (and national) priorities and the criteria for assessing 'effective' performance. Second, such trends characterized as NPM generate important questions about accountability for both individual decisions about individual patients and about accountability for systems of improvement and monitoring. For example, if the service requires evidence-based health care in which innovations are adopted and used, who is responsible for ensuring this, doctors or managers? How can the patients and the public be assured that clinical staff are up to date?

Managerialism and networks

If the traditional organizational logic in the public sector was based on bureaucracy and that under neo-liberalism was founded on markets, the emergent managerial form preferred by New Labour since its election in 1997 is now seen as being underpinned by networks coupled with management by metrics. This emphasis represents a shift from 'government' to 'governance'. Governance signals that a wider range of agencies and stakeholders from within and beyond the public sector are becoming involved in health service delivery. A New Labour government has chosen to emphasize three closely related features of public service reform or 'modernization':

- Person-centred services.
- A 'partnership' approach.
- Service quality and performance.

The emphasis on user- rather than producer-driven services has been strengthened and increasingly pushed to the fore by the government. As the then Prime Minister Tony Blair asserted in his introduction to the White Paper on community social and health care services, 'Our Health, Our Care, Our Say' (DoH 2006:1):

> These proposals . . . will allow us to accelerate the move into a new era where the service is designed around the patient rather than the needs of the patient being forced to fit around the service already provided.

In seeking to give effect to this notion of person-centred services, the government has emphasized such principles as 'choice', 'independence' and 'voice'. There has been considerable debate about whether genuine choice is possible in the public services given finite capacity and under-developed markets or indeed whether users, preferring universal access to a high standard of localized state provision, really want it. However, the government has sought to give some substance to the notion of 'choice' through such mechanisms as direct payments and individual budgets, which provide users with the funds to purchase their own care. This person-centred approach has been founded upon various sorts of partnership arrangements with bargains between different sorts of stakeholder. An important bargain has been that of the state and the service users (Kessler and Dopson 2008).

Whereas under the New Public Management of the Thatcher years the emphasis was on individual consumer entitlement to services, there has been a shift of emphasis within service charters towards collective, civic obligations (Drewry 2005). In other words, the user as a citizen rather than a consumer has responsibilities (e.g. for their health) as well as rights.

The public suspicion of professional expertise has arguably continued with high profile examples coming to light of what often appear to be professional failure, such as at Alder Hay Hospital where a medical practitioner retained children's organs without parental permission (Lamming 2003; see also Chapter 1, this volume, by Elston).

These forms of partnership mark a retreat from key elements of the New Public Management approach with a reliance on disaggregated service units giving way to a greater emphasis on integrated working. Various examples are available of different forms of partnership. The most controversial is the Public Finance Initiative. Introduced by the Major government in 1992 but embraced on a grander scale by New Labour, this initiative provides a way of funding major capital investment through the involvement of private sector consortia without immediate recourse to the public purse.

Inter-organizational working whether within the public sector or between the public, private and voluntary sectors creates a new range of managerial issues and challenges. Inevitably different, often conflicting, organizational cultures need to be managed and there are inevitably major differences in the power of organizations to influence. If the partnership principle, manifest in this range of bargains between different stakeholders, represents the novel and distinctive feature of the network model, the emphasis on organizational performance and service quality represents 'the most significant line of continuity with New Public Management' (Newman 2000: 50). Reed (2002: 3) notes that 'domination is structured and power operationalized in strategically concentrated network governance forms emerging through a number of overlapping mechanisms and their supporting control technologies'. First, the development of a cadre of 'manager professionals' at key nodes within the network governance structure. Second, the continuous surveillance and disciplining of these professional managers, via performance metrics where organizational outcomes are judged. Finally the incremental incorporation of professional provider groups into these governance regimes in which self-surveillance and self-disciplining are the long-term objectives. This, Reed argues, has put professional provider groups in a relatively new and unfamiliar position of having to struggle hard to defend their established jurisdictional work domains. The study of emerging networks is badly needed and we await the results of recent studies on this topic commissioned by NHS Service Delivery and Organisation research arm. Key research questions include: What makes for a successful network? What mechanisms need to be in place for professionals to work together? How is order negotiated? What leadership is required to manage networks? All of which lend themselves to sociological scrutiny.

Clarke (2003) has suggested that policy fads and managerial fashions in this phase of NPM oscillate between a centralizing thrust that re-affirms the power of the audit-state and a decentralizing movement that calls for customer empowerment and localized decision making.

In summary, there have been significant changes in the practice of management since the last volume of this book was published in the era of general management. The model of public service delivery was founded on hierarchy; hospital administration recognized the state as a major provider of services, ensuring organizational performance through conformity to well-established procedural rules and therefore restricting the manager to largely administrative change tasks. In such circumstances, the control of resources lay with the professional and the manager relied upon their expertise to act as the 'custodian' of the users' interest. The market-driven model relied on the discipline of the market to guarantee performance. Here the role of the manager was one of a negotiating business manager responding to the demands of a more active consumer and at the expense of the 'self-serving' professional. The more contemporary network model recognizes the range of agencies and stakeholders required to deliver public services; however, it conveniently ignores the reality of the differences in power of the members of the networks to influence change.

Over the years we can see significant change in the nature of health care management. Who are managers in the NHS has changed radically.

Prior to the Griffiths changes, the management function was executed through the health service administrator. More recently, managers in the NHS come from a range of occupational sources; hybrid managerial forms are common. What managers do has changed significantly. There are many more priorities to address, managers today have to operate within hierarchies, markets and networks, each mode of working presents very different management challenges and requires different management styles and judgements.

Debate continues as to the extent to which one can state empirically that there has been a substantial process of 'managerialization' (Osbourne and Gaebler 1992; Ferlie *et al.* 1996; Hoggett 1996). The changes have led to both gains and losses in the position and status for the medical profession vis-à-vis managers and other professions. Because of the successive waves of organizational change in health care settings, it remains difficult to estimate the current balance of power. The evidence does not support the idea of the medical profession losing power (indeed medical power remains strong and influential in health care delivery) and managers gaining it, but suggests a more complex picture with some professionals gaining, others losing ground and others adapting and taking on managerial responsibilities.

Within health care, one critical issue in debates about inter-professional power is who should take decisions with major resource implications? Given that many such decisions are clinical decisions, should they be taken by clinical professionals turned managers, that is, 'hybrids', or by general managers? Decisions about the adoption of innovations for example, however well supported by science, are almost always influenced by cost priorities. Indeed, much of the controversy concerns cost benefit analysis.

The contribution of a more sociological approach

Empirical studies of organizational and managerial developments in the NHS exist and have shed light on the complexities involved in managing the delivery of health care. Davies, whilst stating that there is still no strong sense of a growing corpus of work on the theme of organizations, acknowledges that 'it was not that organizational developments in the NHS were being ignored in the academic world'. Most of this work is shelved under management or organizational behaviour. Mark and Dopson have also highlighted the lack of exchange between this kind of work and what counts as sociology of organizations in the health fieldwork. There is indeed a gulf between the work on organizations and management done by writers on health policy and organizations and work done by sociologists of health and illness. We can speculate on the reasons for this divide. Possibilities include differences in PhD and post-doctoral training; the pressure to publish in very different types of journals; different career incentives; differences in the identity of academics are amongst the most obvious. However, this chapter, in its partial review of developments in how health services are managed, suggests that a great deal of sociologically interesting research beckons. Davies highlights the need for attention to be paid to the realignment between the health care professions and between professions, patients and the public. She argues 'it is time for sociology to re-engage with the formal organizations that are being created' and transformed to adapt to a climate of 'modernization' of public services and to tease out the impacts of this (Davies 2003: 181). In particular she suggests research into the factors prompting new organizational arrangements, the contradictions in them and the potential impact on patient and professional identities would be most welcome. A sociological perspective would help counter the criticism Mark Learmonth hurls at health service management research to date (Learmonth 2003: 110). In a piece that reviews qualitative research published since 1990, he argues that much of the established work in this field takes for granted managerial assumptions that are consequently not subjected to sustained critical examination.

A sociological-informed perspective has much to offer in unpacking the complexity of managing health services. I want to give as an example work studying relatively recent attempts by policy makers to make health care more evidence based. NHS commissioners have increasingly been trying to secure a demonstrable shift to an evidence-based approach from health care providers through the commissioning process and target setting. The emergence of Evidence Based Health Care (EBHC) was largely professionally driven, although it has not been uncontested within the medical profession (see Chapter 6 in this volume by Harrison and Checkland). Over time, politicians, managers and commissioners in the UK have taken an interest in EBHC and so see it as a key to changing clinical practice and improving health care, as well as contributing to the value for money agenda. These groups have sought to produce treatment guidelines for specific conditions and required 'managers' to implement them. New systems and organizations have been set up, devoted to the evaluation and dissemination of clinical evidence, such as the NHS Technology Assessment Programme and The National Institute for Clinical Excellence.

The majority of statements from policy makers and in policy documents on EBHC implementation draw on classic diffusion of innovation models, the most influential of which remains Rogers (1995). Rogers argues that the adoption of new ideas, practices and artefacts is influenced by the inter-action among the innovation, the adopter and the environment. In his view there are five characteristics that influence the success rate of adoption: the perception of the relative advantage of innovation; the compatibility with existing structures; the degree of difficulty involved in making the change; the extent to which innovation can be tested by potential adopters without significant resource expenditure; and the visibility of the outcomes. Advocates of EBHC, policy makers and managers have been surprised at the degree of difficulty of implementing EBHC since it seems self-evidently good and worthwhile, and also entirely consistent with the 'scientific' biomedical paradigm (a simple puzzle is explored in Chapter 7 in this volume by May). Why do policy makers and 'managers' face such difficulties? A sociological approach would seek to:

- explore 'managerial' relationships in the wider social context in which those relationships are a part and how the problem is institutionally framed
- acknowledge local contexts as multi-dimensional, multifaceted configuration of forces
- explore the complex connections, interdependencies and interactions
- explore the impact of history
- consider the capacity of individuals to influence context.

Dopson and Fitzgerald (2005) illuminate the complexity of getting such desired changes in this area, drawing on a more sociologically driven approach. Across all their case studies of the careers of EBHC initiatives, the spread and pathways of innovation were slow, complex and contested. Robust science in the form of guidelines does not naturally flow into use as policy makers assume. One major reason accounting for this is the inherent difficulty of interpreting 'the evidence'. The data demonstrated that, in many instances, scientific evidence does not appear to the beholder as clear, accepted and bounded. There is no such thing as evidence, there are simply bodies of evidence, usually competing bodies of evidence. Deciding to use new knowledge is a social and political process, which nearly always involves debate and reference to other views and involves issues of power; it is especially important to study the power of the medical profession. In this context, the randomized control is viewed as the superior source of evidence. Of course this is old news for anyone who has studied the sociology of knowledge but this source of sociological knowledge and evidence is rarely drawn upon by policy makers or managers.

Also highlighted in the work is the critical social role played by communities of practice in interpreting and translating evidence into a local context. Local professional groups work together in communities of practice which are frequently unprofessional, and the medical profession is dominant in relation to the power to influence. There are complex interactions between and across professional boundaries both at the local level and at the level of the whole institution. These boundaries affect the motivations for seeking improvement and upgrading, and the way evidence and knowledge are perceived and interpreted. Furthermore, the role of the social context in which such processes of change take place has emerged as a key theme. Health care context cannot be seen as a set of static and independent variables, rather context is more properly conceived of as a syndrome of forces typically involving elements of hierarchy, markets and networks, which interact in complex ways and lead to unintended outcomes. Furthermore, individuals make sense of such multiple contexts by drawing on a range of cognitive and emotional judgements to create for themselves an 'integral context' that informs this action.

EBHC is now in a mature phase of its policy life cycle. The work reported in Dopson and Fitzgerald (2005) argued for the need to build up local systems' capacity and leadership to support EBHC rather than a continuation of relying on the publication of guidelines alone. If the enactment of EBHC depends on a set of underlying processes, underlying system capacity is important. This argues for a switch of attention from short-term, stand-alone policy initiatives and managerial targets to drive EBHC forward, to a greater focus on long-term systems development and the development of the capacity of the system to process the issue effectively. Here the insights already available in the existing body of sociological scholarship are very useful.

Acknowledgements

Insights on public sector management in this chapter draw on Kessler and Dopson (2008).

References

Ainley, P. (1994) *Degrees of Difference*, London: Lawrence and Wishart.

Cassel, E. (1997) *Doctoring: the nature of primary care medicine*, New York: Oxford University Press.

Clarke, J. (2003) 'Performing for the public: governing public services in a dispersed state', unpublished paper, Oxford University.

Coulter, A. (2002) 'After Bristol: putting patients first', *British Medical Journal*, 324: 648–51.

Cox, D. (1991) 'Health service management – a sociological view: Griffiths and the non-negotiated order of the hospital', in J. Gabe, M. Calnan and M. Bury (eds) *The Sociology of the Health Service*, London, Routlege.

Davies, C. (1987) 'A viewpoint: things to come: the NHS in the next decade', *Sociology of Health and Illness*, 9: 302–17.

Davies, C. (2003) 'Some of our concepts are missing: reflections on the absence of sociology of organisations in Sociology of Health and Illness', *Sociology of Health and Illness*, 25: 172–90.

Day, P. and Klein, R.D. (1983) 'The mobilisation of consent versus the management of conflict: decoding the Griffiths Report', *British Medical Journal*, 1287: 1813–15.

Dent, M. (1993) 'Professionalism, educated labour and the state: hospital medicine and the new managerialism', *Sociological Review*, 41: 244–73.

Department of Health (2006) *Our Health, Our Care, Our Say*. London: HMSO.

Department of Health and Social Security (1983) (The Griffiths Report) Letter to Health Authority Chairmen *DHSS Circular* HC (84)13, 18 November.

Dopson, S. and Fitzgerald, L. (2005) *Knowledge to Action*, Oxford: Oxford University Press.

Drewry, G. (2005) 'Citizen's charters: service quality chameleons', *Public Management Review*, 7: 321–40.

Escott, K. and Whitfield, D. (1995) *The Gender Impact of CCT in Local Government*, London: HMSO.

Farnham, D. and Horton, S. (eds) (1993) *Managing the New Public Services*, Basingstoke: Macmillan.

Ferlie, E. (2002) 'Quasi strategy: strategic management in the contemporary public sector', in A. Pettigrew, H. Thomas and R. Whittington (eds) *Handbook of Strategy and Management*, London: Sage.

Ferlie, E., Ashbourner, L., Fitzgerald, L. and Pettigrew, A. (1996) *The New Public Management in Action*, Oxford: Oxford University Press.

Fitzgerald, L. (1994) 'Moving clinicians into management: a professional challenge or threat?' *Journal of Management in Medicine*, 8: 32–44.

Fitzgerald, L. and Dufour, Y. (1997) 'Clinical management as boundary management: a comparative analysis of Canadian and UK health care institutions', *International Journal of Public Sector Management*, 10: 5–20.

Fitzgerald, L. and Ferlie, E. (2000) 'Professionals: back to the future', *Human Relations*, 53: 713–38.

Fitzgerald, L. and Sturt, J. (1992) 'Clinicians into management – on the change agenda or not?', *Health Service Management Research*, 5: 137–46

Flynn, R. (2002) 'Clinical governance and governmentality', *Health Risk and Society*, 4: 155–73.

Flynn, R. (2004) 'Soft bureaucracy, governmentality and clinical governance', in A. Gray and S. Harrison (eds) *Governing Medicine*, Buckingham: Open University Press.

Francis, B. and Humphreys, J. (1999) 'Enrolled nurses and the professionalisation of nursing: a comparison of nurse education and skill mix in Australia and the UK', *International Journal of Nursing Studies*, 36: 127–35

Freidson, E. (1994) *Professional Reborn: theory, prophecy and policy*. Cambridge: Polity Press.

Freidson, E. (2001) *Professionalism, The Third Logic*. Cambridge: Polity Press.

Griffiths, R. (1991) *Seven Years of Progress – General management in the NHS*. Management Lectures, Audit Commission, No. 3, June 12.

Harris, J. (1999) 'State social work and social citizenship in Britain', *British Journal of Social Work*, 29: 915–37.

Harrison, S. (1988) *Managing the National Health Service: shifting the frontier?* London: Chapman and Hall.

Harrison, S., Hunter, D., Marnoch, G. and Pollitt, C. (1992) *Just Managing Power and Culture in the National Health Service*, London: Macmillan.

Hoggett, P. (1996) 'New modes of control in the public service', *Public Administration*, 74: 9–32.

Hood, C. and Peters, G. (2004) 'The middle aging of new public management: into the age of paradox', *Journal of Public Administration Research and Theory*, 14: 267–82.

Hunter, D.J., Harrison, S., Marnoch, G. and Pollitt, C. (1988) 'For better or worse? Assessing the impact of general management on the NHS', paper presented at ESRC Conference, 7 July.

Hunter, D. (2006) 'From tribalism to corporatism. The continuing managerial challenge to medical dominance', in D. Kelleher, J. Gabe and G. Williams (eds) *Challenging Medicine*, second edition, London: Routledge.

Kessler, I. and Dopson, S. (2008) 'Public sector management', in S. Dopson, M. Earl and P. Snow, (eds) *Mapping the Management Context*, Oxford: Oxford University Press.

Kitchener, M. (1999) 'All fur coat and no knickers: contemporary organizational change in the U.K. hospitals', in D. Brock, M. Powell, and C.R. Hinings (eds) *Restructuring the Professional Organization*, London: Routledge.

Kirkpatrick, I., Ackroyd, S. and Walker, R. (2005) *The New Managerialism and Public Service Professions*, Basingstoke: Palgrave.

Lamming, Lord (2003) *The Victoria Climbie Inquiry*. London: HMSO.

Laughlin, R. (1991) 'Can information systems for the NHS internal market work?' *Public Money and Management*, 11: 37–41.

Learmonth, M. (2003) 'Making health services research critical. A review and a suggestion', *Sociology of Health and Illness*, 25: 93–119.

Montgomery, K. (1990) 'A prospective look at the speciality of medical management', *Work and Occupations*, 17: 178–98

Newman, J. (2000) 'Beyond the New Public Management? Modernising public services' in Clarke, J. *et al.* (eds) *New Managerialism, New Welfare?* London: Sage.

Osbourne, D. and Gaebler, T. (1992) *Reinventing Government: how the entrepreneurial spirit is transforming the public sector*, Reading MA: Addison-Wesley.

Petchey, R. (1986) 'The Griffiths reorganization of the NHS; Fowlerism by stealth?', *Critical Social Policy*, 17: 87–101.

Pettigrew, A., Mckee, L. and Ferlie, E. (1992) *Shaping Strategic Change: the case of the NHS*, London: Sage.

Pollitt, C. (1990) *Managerialism and the Public Services: The Anglo-American experience*, Oxford; Blackwell.

Pollitt, C. (2002) 'New Public Management in international perspective', in K. McLaughlin, S.P. Osborne and E. Ferlie (eds) *New Public Management: current trends and future prospects*, London: Routledge.

Pope, C. (1991) 'Trouble in store: some thoughts on the management of waiting lists', *Sociology of Health and Illness*, 13: 193–212.

Power, M. (1997) *The Audit Society*, Oxford: Oxford University Press.

Rogers, E. (1995) *The Diffusion of Innovation*, New York: Free Press.

Sheaff, R., Smith, K. and Dickson, M. (2002) 'Is GP re-stratification beginning in England?' *Social Policy and Administration*, 36: 765–79.

Sheaff, R., Marshall, M., Rogers, A., Sibbald, B. and Pickard, S. (2004) 'Governmentality by network in English primary healthcare', *Social Policy and Administration*, 38: 89–103.

Skelcher, C. (2000) 'Changes in images of the state: overloaded, hollowed out, congested', *Public Policy and Administration*, 15: 3–19.

Stewart, R., Dopson, S., Gabbay, J., Smith, P. and Williams, D. (1987–8) *The Templeton College Series on District General Management, April–January*, London: National Health Service Training Authority (NHSTA) Publications.

Strong, P. and Robinson, J. (1990) *The NHS Under New Management*, Milton Keynes: Open University Press.

3 The restratification of primary care in England?

A sociological analysis

Michael Calnan and Jonathan Gabe

Introduction

The case for focusing on general practice in our chapter in the first edition of this volume nearly twenty years ago (Calnan and Gabe 1991) was that it was seen to hold a key position in the provision of health care in the UK National Health Service (NHS), mainly through its dual role as co-ordinator of patient care and gatekeeper and controller of access to specialist services, high technological care and treatment. Since then the importance of primary care in the NHS in England has, in many respects, been enhanced, although the structure and organization of general practice, as will be shown below, has altered. The aim of this chapter is to examine changes that have taken place in primary care over the last twenty-five years and to provide a sociological account of these developments. The focus once again is general practice although it is recognized that there are other primary care services such as dentistry (Calnan *et al.* 2000), opthalmology (Green and Thorogood 1998) and community pharmacy (Edmonds and Calnan 2001) which are not discussed here but have also undergone change.

In the chapter in the first edition, it was argued that the developments in general practice since the 1960s could be understood, at least in part, in terms of changes and divisions that had occurred or had been exacerbated in the medical profession in the nineteenth century. While these changes will also have had an influence on more recent developments, the intention here is not to cover the same ground again but merely to summarize these arguments and to see if the more recent policy initiatives mirror or are distinctly different to those that went before. Similarly, the intention will not be to revisit the various sociological theories of professionalism that were discussed before but to summarize the theoretical position taken and assess its power in explaining recent changes, along with that of any new theories. In the 1991 chapter, it was argued that general practice as a branch of medicine, unlike hospital medicine, had been paid little attention in terms of the sociological analysis of professionalism. However, as we shall see, this has also changed of late.

Theoretical perspectices

The theoretical approach adopted in the earlier chapter was neo-Weberian, with the professional development of general practice being seen to hinge on its ability to attain and maintain autonomy: from its powerful colleagues and rivals in hospital medicine; from other occupational groups working in the same area by controlling the boundaries between them; from the patient population by controlling patient demand through organizational change; and from the state by minimizing the latter's intrusion into clinical freedoms while benefiting from its protection to keep control over their section of the market place. This theoretical position is similar to the structural pluralist approach proposed by Alford (1975) to explain the shape of health policy. He identified three main groups of structural interests, the first of which are the dominant professional interests, made up mainly of doctors, whose powerful structural position enables them to define the values of the health care system. The second group are the challenging corporate and managerial interests whose concerns are with improving efficiency and effectiveness as well as with quality of care and the third group are the repressed interests of the public or patient population. Alford's framework was based on research carried out in New York City in the 1970s, although it has been applied to different health care systems (Duckett 1984; Cho 2000), including the NHS in the UK (North and Peckham 2001).

This general approach has also been shown to be useful in explaining recent developments in professionalism and, as Kuhlmann (2008: 47) suggests, 'the triangle comprising health professions, the state and the public must be understood as a dynamic relationship that allows for various ways to model and remodel power relations in health care systems'. While focusing on this relationship, our earlier account was concerned with the development of one branch of medicine; hence, it focused principally on how general practice developed a distinct identity from hospital medicine. It was aided in that project by the state which supported its development because a general practitioner (GP) gate-keeping system was an effective means of controlling access to expensive high-technology medicine.

More recent challenges and influences on primary care have come from the state, particularly in its attempt to introduce new public management, and its associated principles of marketization and managerialism into health care. Another common but related theme in health policy over the last two decades has been the emphasis on public participation and patient-centred care, such as the policies to improve patient access to primary care and increase patient choice of provider. This theme, as will be shown, has been driven primarily by top–down values, interests and ideologies rather than being a product of the influence of the so-called consumer health movement or patient-centred self-help groups.

These challenges or developments have been the focus of a broader debate in the sociology of professionalism which has concentrated on the extent to which medical power and authority is in decline or whether medicine has, in the face of recent challenges, managed to retain its overall dominance. Those arguing that medical power is on the wane highlight the threats generated through the impact of processes such as proletarianization, deprofessionalization, corporatization and bureaucratization. For example, Coburn *et al.* (1997) argue that manageralism has undermined the profession as a whole through the state co-option of medical organizations and elites. They suggest that medical elites are being used by external forces, such as the state, to constrain their own members and to implement policies over which they have no control.

Alternative and contrasting sociological accounts of the professionalizing strategies of medicine have argued how, at least at the elite or macro level, it has been able to respond to or anticipate possible challenges or changes and sometimes use the opportunities to maintain or even enhance its autonomy and control. For example, Freidson (1994, 2001) puts forward a theory of professional re-stratification which suggests increasing divisions between the rank and file of doctor practitioners and the 'knowledge' (research) and administrative medical elites. He argues that while the power base may have shifted within the profession towards these elite groups, the profession itself was still dominant (Freidson 1994, 2001). For example, the elite practitioners such as the Royal Colleges and medical researchers play a central role in developing the clinical protocols and guidelines being used by the rank and file practitioners, and the increasing number of medical doctors taking on managerial roles suggests that doctors may be taking back the professions' monitoring and regulatory roles (Flynn 2002). More recently Freidson (2001) has argued that professionalism should be seen as third logic where the professional acts as a mediator, officiating over the interests of the state and serving the needs and demands of the public. The benefits of such a role, according to Freidson (2001), are to ensure trust in public services and reduce the costs of governmental action and control.

Sociological theories of occupational development and control propose that there is an increasing need for professionalism as an occupational value in its own right to be restated and made explicit. As Evetts (2006) suggests, the current appeal of professionalism to occupations is markedly different from the more traditional type of occupational control which medicine exemplified over fifty years ago. The appeal to professionalism most often involves the substitution of organizational for professional values, accountability replacing trust and autonomy being constrained and controlled. However, Kuhlmann (2008) argues that this new professionalism can be a force for change. As she puts it:

> There is increasing evidence of a 'new' professionalism which is significantly different from earlier forms. Although the traditional exclusionary tactics of the professions have not been overcome,

professionalism is not necessarily a barrier to modernisation; it also carries the potential for innovation in health care.

(Kuhlmann 2008: 7)

Yet, in the context of medicine, the appeal and restatement of professional values such as the re-emphasis on the importance of trust in the doctor–patient relationship (Calnan and Rowe 2008) might also be seen as a defence against the substitution of organizational for professional values.

This analysis raises a number of questions about whether the influence of these organizational changes has been overstated and, at least at the level of the rank and file, whether these changes are being resisted or adhered to on the surface only. Alternatively, is a new type of GP emerging such as a street-level bureaucrat (Checkland 2004), who mediates between the managerial world of guidelines, evidence-based medicine and performance indicators and the professional practice of everyday medicine (e.g. Grant *et al.* 2009) or a public service entrepreneur who adopts the values of the market to meet the needs of patients while not being driven by the profit motive (Boyce 2008)? The latter would represent a hybrid of contrasting positions in the literature on professionalism, illustrating the view of occupations as driven primarily by self-interest and the need for power, status and material wealth *and* by altruism and the need to put the interests of the patient first (Saks 1995; Calnan *et al.* 2000). However, before these questions and the policy themes are explored further it is necessary to present a brief picture of the current context of primary care and the changes that have occurred in recent years.

The changing profile of general practice

The majority of GPs currently are male but the feminization of this branch of medicine is taking place with younger GPs being predominantly female (Rayner 2002). Over the past two decades there has also been a marked shift towards part-time working among men as well as women doctors (Bowler and Jackson 2002). For example, 25 per cent of GPs in the UK, in 2003, worked part time compared with 9 per cent in 1992. Coupled with this there has been a demand for greater job flexibility and a suggestion of a shift away from the traditional system of permanent full-time employment with partners owning their practices to salaried positions. This is in line with evidence that some GPs desire 'nice work' in their early career, involving innovative practice, fewer hours and a balance between work and other interests (Jones and Green 2006). It might also suggest a rejection of the core value of vocation and a preference instead for a choice of options. However, the attraction of the new personalized salaried contracts must not be overstated. They were strongly promoted by Primary Care Trusts (PCTs) through the use of incentives and only really appeared to become more prevalent as a consequence of the new General Medical Services (GMS) contract in 2003/4 when personal lists were abandoned. It was considered that patients had become attached to practices rather than doctors so a partner could be replaced by a salaried doctor without losing patients or any income. However, since the new GMS contract, Personal Medical Services (PMS) contracts have seen limited growth particularly because of the financial incentives for staying with the GMS contract, although they are still used by PCTs where vacancies are difficult to fill. More recently, Advanced Personal Medical Services (APMS) contracts are becoming more popular with PCTs because they can invite private providers to tender for them.

The introduction of the new GMS contract in 2003/4 had a number of other major consequences. Changing systems of payment and the use of financial incentives is a popular policy instrument for changing providers' practices and there is some evidence that it can be effective (Gref *et al.* 2006). It had been evident previously in policy in primary care in the UK but the 2003/4 contract was the first time that it was directly used for improving quality. While the contract included an opportunity for GPs to give up their responsibility for out-of-hours cover, its most prominent element was the Quality and Outcomes Framework (QOF), comprising 146, largely evidence-based process indicators of quality of care, mostly for chronic diseases (McDonald *et al.* 2008). Achievement of each indicator attracted a specific number of 'points', up to a maximum total of 1,050 for any practice (Roland 2004) and around a third of a GPs' income is currently dependent on their scores from the QOF indicators. The contract not only enabled flexibility but also introduced performance-related pay and had the unintended consequence of shifting work from doctors to nurses.

The GMS contract has had a mixed reception. For example, Heath (2004: 320) suggested: 'The new contract imposes changes that will serve to accelerate the fragmentation and privatisation of primary care and leave it open to commercial pressure in a manner unprecedented since the inception of the NHS in 1948'. In contrast, other evidence suggests it has been well received by rank and file GPs with little evidence of a perceived threat to professionalism or motivation, although there has been some criticism of indicators that were felt to go beyond standard clinical practice (McDonald *et al.* 2007). Others have suggested that the contract involves new regimens of surveillance of clinical practice which have been perceived as a threat to motivation, especially by nurses (McDonald *et al.* 2008).

There is also some debate about whether the contract has led GPs to position themselves as being more concerned with biomedicine than holistic or biographical medicine. This division in orientation has always been evident among rank and file GPs, as well as in the rhetoric of their representatives (Calnan and Gabe 1991), yet the emphasis in the new contract on biomedical quality indicators may have pushed them more in that direction. Evidence is mixed, with researchers agreeing that while activities may have become more biomedically orientated, the worldviews of

GPs have remained varied. Checkland *et al.* (2008) found, like Charles-Jones *et al.* (2003), that GPs delegated routine tasks to practice nurses but, unlike these authors, discovered that GPs believed or claimed that delegation freed GPs up to deal with complex problems in a holistic way rather than reconfiguring themselves as narrow, biomedical specialists. This disconnection between the discursive claims about the nature and purpose of general practice and actual practice caused little discomfort for the GPs who expressed overall satisfaction with life after the contract.

At the same time, QOF decision making and monitoring has required practices to establish internal teams of clinical and administrative staff with responsibility for making major practice-led decisions. This represents a new form of internal regulation with some clinical staff developing enhanced managerial responsibility over their clinical colleagues. Evidence from a recent study of QOF in England and Scotland (Grant *et al.* 2009) indicates that some GPs have embraced such managerialism more enthusiastically than others, reinforcing and significantly extending professional re-stratification within general practice (Sheaff *et al.* 2002).

Two further changes have taken place, although it is difficult to judge how far they have been driven by government policy or reflect a response to it. These are an increase in the size of the GP workforce and a shift in workload from GPs to other health care workers, notably practice nurses. For example, the number of non-medical staff working in general practice in England rose by around a fifth between 1994 and 2002 (Calnan 2006). More specifically, between 1992 and 2002 there was a 32 per cent increase in practice nurses, a 35 per cent increase in administrative and clerical staff and a 108 per cent increase in practitioners providing direct patient care such as physiotherapy and counselling. This might suggest that team working and shared decision making is replacing traditional hierarchical relations in the workforce of general practice (Jones and Green, 2006). However, the size of teams has increased with different occupational groups being managed by agencies other than practices, suggesting the demise of the small, close-knit team and that teamwork may now only be 'notional'. Alternatively, recent managerial reforms might lead to work being increasingly defined in terms of complexity and 'expert knowledge', with GPs creating 'hierarchies of appropriateness' and devolving hybrid tasks that do not require specialized knowledge to nurses and health care assistants, leaving existing clinical hierarchies largely intact (Charles-Jones *et al.* 2003).

There is no consistent objective evidence that there has been a major change (increase or decrease) in the volume of work undertaken by GPs, although it is claimed that this work has become more complex and GPs clearly believe they are working harder and are under increasing stress (Calnan 2006; Mechanic *et al.* 2001). This latter finding about a stated increase in the complexity and demands of the workload may be reflected, at least until very recently, in the trends in GP job satisfaction. General practice as an occupation and branch of medicine traditionally had a relatively high level of job satisfaction which peaked during the 1980s when general practice was experiencing rapid growth in its professional development. Thereafter job satisfaction decreased, although the decrease has not been linear. Sibbald *et al.* (2001) examined levels of job satisfaction in 1989, 1990, 1998 and 2001, using the same scale, and found a marked drop between 1989 and 1990 after the introduction of the new GP contract, when GPs reported increasing administration workloads. The 1990 contract was viewed by GPs as an attack on their independent contractor status and professional autonomy. Yet, by 1998, satisfaction levels had partially recovered, although not reaching the higher levels of the 1980s; illustrating that satisfaction can involve a trade-off between the positive and negative aspects of the job. There then followed a further series of organizational reforms and developments, including the introduction of Primary Care Trusts, clinical governance, Personal Medical Service contracts, walk-in centres, NHS Direct and more recently the introduction of a new national GP contract. Sibbald *et al.* (2001) found that in 2001 job satisfaction was at its lowest recorded level. Doctors were least satisfied with their hours of work and pay and most stressed by increasing workloads. Paperwork, coupled with changes imposed by health authorities and Primary Care Groups/PCTs and the overall pace of change in general practice were also perceived to be important sources of stress.

However, it cannot be assumed that job stress and job dissatisfaction go hand-in-hand: some jobs are stimulating and rewarding but also stressful or perceived as stressful. There is also a difference between self-reports of stress, which may indicate low morale, and those experiences of stress which manifest themselves in physiological signs and symptoms (Calnan and Wainwright 2002). There is some debate about how far these reports of stress reflect claims by GPs to promote their demands for better pay and conditions or are realistic accounts of the health problems resulting from the demands of working in general practice (Wainwright and Calnan 2002). The 'doing better but feeling worse' thesis implies that even though working conditions have improved (Calnan and Williams 1995), there is a deterioration in satisfaction with work. This argument has some validity in that while hours worked have decreased or at least have not increased and there has been increasing support from practice staff, there was evidence, up until very recently, of a marked decline in job satisfaction and possibly morale. This pattern might reflect a broader social change in attitudes to satisfaction with work or the fact that expectations about medical work now far exceed experience and rewards from such work (McKinlay and Marceau 2008). The alternative explanation is that the reduction in volume of workload and the implication that GPs 'have never had it so good' has been counterbalanced by increases in the complexity of work and the psychological burden of work; for example, the need to be patient-centred and to be expected to deal with a range of psycho-social problems. The plethora of organizational changes in primary care in England may have brought with them an increased administrative burden and a reduction in professional and clinical autonomy, manifested in the introduction of clinical governance. In addition to challenges and controls from management, patient expectations and demands may have risen as well as an increase in the perception of the possibility of patient complaints.

Interestingly, the 'doing better: feeling worse' thesis is not supported by more recent evidence which shows that levels of job satisfaction have increased from the low point of 2001. Evidence from a national survey carried out in 2004, prior to the introduction of the new GMS contract (Whalley *et al.* 2006), showed an increase in levels of satisfaction but concerns about the impact of the contract on time pressures, workload and job control. This upward trend in attitudes to work was found in a follow-up survey (Whalley *et al.* 2006) carried out eighteen months after the contract was introduced. Although most GPs believed that the new contract had been detrimental to their professional autonomy and work-loads, the perceived positive impact on pay and quality of care had exceeded their expectations, and the average number of hours worked was recognized as having decreased. This survey also showed that while job satisfaction had increased, job stress had decreased because of less pressure from night visits, not having 24-hour responsibility for patients' lives and no longer having to fulfil unrealistically high expectations of the role by others. These findings from the impact of the new contract seem to suggest that general practitioners' orientation towards their work has been shaped more by working conditions, financial rewards and quality of patient care than by concerns about professional freedoms, illustrating the view of occupations driven both by self-interest, such as the need for material wealth, and by altruism, such as the need to provide high-quality patient care (Saks 1995).

Policy developments in primary care: marketization or communitarianism?

Over the last two decades, as was suggested in the previous section, gov-ernment policy has placed an increasing emphasis on the notion of a primary care-led NHS (Department of Health 2001a), with an attempt to shift power and resources from secondary to primary care so as to bring planning and provision of care 'closer to patients' (Somerset *et al.* 1999). Initiatives such as fundholding, total purchasing pilots, Primary Care Groups (PCG), now Primary Care Trusts (PCTs), and the pilot salaried schemes are all attempts to tip the balance further in the direction of the primary and community sector and away from the hospital sector (Coulter and Mays 1997). Two developments that have been particularly significant and reflect the different political stances of the governments who introduced them are fundholding and the introduction of PCGs/PCTs.

Fundholding was introduced in the NHS in the early 1990s as a result of the creation of an internal market by the Conservative government. The fundholding initiative (Glennerster *et al.* 1994) allowed general practices to become fundholders who could negotiate contracts for non-emergency care for their patients. With individual patients having no purchasing rights of their own, GP fundholders were to act as proxies, purchasing services on patients' behalf. This initiative, along with earlier developments in the 1970s and 1980s that enhanced the professional status of GPs (see Calnan and Gabe 1991), attempted to give more power to GPs (through control over resources) in their negotiations with hospital doctors. Fundholding had its benefits and costs (Coulter 1995; Audit Commission 1996) but there was little evidence that the contracting process strengthened the negotiating power of GPs (Baeza and Calnan 1997; Baeza 2005). The stimulus for hospital doctors to adhere to fundholders' demands depended on the existence of other alternative sources of supply. Generally there was little evidence that this and related initiatives led to marked shifts in resources and services to primary care.

The fundholding system in England was replaced by PCGs, which have now become PCTs, in the latter part of the 1990s under the initiative of an incoming Labour government (Dixon *et al.* 1998) which was concerned to emphasize planning and collaboration rather than competition, as part of a more general policy of social inclusion. The establishment of PCGs and PCTs reflected the policy aim of developing integrated care by bringing together primary care and social care and by linking the provision of care with a major responsibility for commissioning (Ham 2004). A national network of PCGs was established in 1999, although they were to be the first stage of a process resulting in the eventual transition to free-standing PCTs. Thus, in April 2002 around 300 Primary Care Trusts were formed, with strategic health authorities leading the strategic development of the local health community and managing the performance of PCTs and NHS trusts. This left PCTs with the lead role of improving the health of the community, developing primary and community health services and commissioning secondary care services. All GPs would work in a PCT area and have a contract with them to supply services. However, the managerial control that PCTs have over GPs is limited mainly because GP contracts are centrally negotiated with the Department of Health, although PCTs do have more influence over the way practices develop as they have control over access to funds for staff, premises and new initiatives. PCTs also appear to have more leverage to promote their agenda in contracts for PMS, which are individually negotiated. In the early days gaining effective GP involvement in PCGs/PCTs was proving problematic (Regen 2002), although there were opportunities for GPs to take up managerial roles (Sheaff *et al.* 2002) and become part of what Freidson (1994) might refer to as an administrative elite. Overall, the limited evidence available about the impact of management in primary care is mixed. Harrison and Dowswells' (2002) study indicates the perceived threat to autonomy from 'top–down' managerialism, in that GPs perceived the need to respond to PCT management through careful documentation of clinical activity, although earlier research (Calnan and Williams 1995; Weiss and Fitzpatrick 1997) suggests that threats to clinical autonomy are perceived to come mainly from lay challenges to professional expertise.

A more recent development in primary care (Department of Health 2004a) has been the introduction of practice-based commissioning. Since April 2005 practices can receive an 'indicative budget' from Primary Care Trusts which they can use to improve the delivery of their services. Such an initiative appears to mirror the fundholding policy developed in the early 1990s, although this was within the different context of the quasi-market (Wainwright 1998).

A more overt indicator of the shift back to the values of marketization in government policy is the increasing number of additional providers to traditional general practice involved in primary care in England (the situation is rather different in other parts of the UK where private provision in primary care is not being encouraged (see Chapter 11, this volume, by Popay and Williams)). This development seems to have emerged out of the policy assumption that diversification of providers is more contestable and leads to greater innovation and improvement in efficiency and quality of care (Sheaff *et al.* 2006). Since 1996 other health care professionals besides GPs have been able to bid for contracts to provide primary care. This has enabled nurses to be partners in general practice businesses contracted to the NHS and to bid independently for contracts and to employ salaried GPs. More recently, in 2004, an additional type of NHS contract in primary care has become available, enabling groups of nurses to form not-for-profit social enterprises and tender for contracts with PCTs, a development supported by the recent Darzi review of the NHS. There is little empirical research exploring these developments. One exception is Lewis's (2001) evaluation of nurse-led PMS pilots which reported considerable hostility from some local general practitioners but high levels of patient satisfaction. To date, however, it seems that few nurses have taken the opportunities provided by these legislative changes and policy shifts to behave entrepreneurially and seek contracts to provide nurse-led primary care (Drennan *et al.* 2007). Consequently the opportunity for health care professionals other than GPs to provide primary care services might be seen as 'window dressing' to disguise the real agenda of enabling private providers to find a place in the market.

Private commercial and not-for-profit providers have also been encouraged by PCTs to bid for APMS contracts. There are numerous examples around England of PCTs awarding contracts to different private companies with the obvious risk of doctors following what shareholders require of them in the pursuit of profits rather than following their professional values. These types of provider are expected to increase particularly with the introduction of the 'Darzi' health centres or clinics which are to be general practices offering a wider range of services in new, purpose-built health centres and open to the public eight hours a day, seven days a week. Doctors working in these clinics will be salaried employees who are likely to be attracted by short-term sessional work with no commitment to the practice or the area (Salisbury 2008). These polyclinics will be in addition to existing provision and provides another example of a policy aimed at improving patient access by increasing points of access in primary care (other examples being walk-in centres in railway stations and GP surgeries in supermarkets).

Policy developments in primary care: managerialism and governance

The introduction of 'clinical governance' in the late 1990s was a policy which arguably had the potential to create a significant change in the relationships between clinicians and managers in the UK, and in the process adjust the political settlement agreed between the government and the medical profession in 1948 (Calnan and Rowe 2008). When the NHS was established, doctors were granted a monopoly of expertise to secure their support for a national health service, including the right to control entry to practice and freedom over their clinical work, in exchange for guaranteeing adequate standards of performance and integrating rationing decisions into clinical management (Klein 1996). Clinical autonomy ensured that fully qualified doctors should not only have control over the diagnosis and treatment of individual patients but also over the nature and volume of medical tasks and the evaluation of care (Schulz and Harrison 1986). In this professional model of accountability clinicians operated within a network system of governance, with authority relationships based not on hierarchy and line management but on professional status, coordinative competence and resource control. Accountability was sustained through relations that relied on shared values and norms and an adherence to agreed ethical codes of conduct. Thus, self-regulation protected physicians from accounting to anyone other than their professional colleagues for their clinical activity and performance or use of resources, making them invisible to public scrutiny (Evetts 1999).

The post-war consensus in the UK NHS in which trust in professionalism underpinned the relationships between the public, health professions and the state (Newman 1998) is claimed to have been weakened by the increase in consumerism, an erosion of the public service ethos arising from the promotion of entrepreneurial values in the public sector (Brereton and Temple 1999), and by political and media depictions of professional activity as paternalistic. As traditional mechanisms to ensure professional accountability have lost public confidence, the Labour government of 1997 has used this opportunity to renegotiate its agreement with the medical profession, introducing clinical governance as a mechanism to achieve clinical accountability for the quality of care provided and using performance management to influence how services are organized and provided. This has been described as a 'hard' form of narrative about the new public management (Ferlie and Geraghty 2007), which aims to control public service practitioners through the introduction of an 'accounting logic' and an emphasis on audit, performance measurement and management and performance-related pay. More recently it has been suggested that a second narrative has become popular. This is a softer version of the new public management and is linked to the human relations school of private sector management (Ferlie and Geraghty 2007). The emphasis here is on user orientation, quality enhancement and organizational and individual development and learning. It still aims to shift control and decision making away from professionals but in this case by integrating professionals into management systems. This latter form of NPM appears to be the way in which clinical governance has been implemented in the NHS, suggesting that the radical potential of clinical governance has been sacrificed to achieve clinical engagement with the policy (Calnan and Rowe 2008), although the degree to which this occurs may vary by organizational setting (see also Chapter 2, this volume, by Dopson).

Clinical governance was introduced as a framework within which local NHS organizations could work to improve and assure the quality of clinical services for patients and to minimize the risks of the negative consequences of health care outcomes (Scally and Donaldson 1998). All NHS organizations in England are now required to develop processes for regular monitoring and enhancing the quality of health care and systems of accountability for the quality of care that they provide. While quality assurance and quality improvement are the two fundamental components of clinical governance, its objective was to increase clinical accountability, although it also gave the government increased control of risk, knowledge and performance management. Up until then the medical profession had resisted political and managerial definitions of and approaches to quality assurance, suggesting that they could not be applied to the uncertainties of clinical practice (Calnan and Rowe 2008). The professional approach to quality assurance had been through medical audit which was voluntary, local and under the control of medical specialists (Pollitt 1993). Clinical audit was seen as a learning process to facilitate professional development and improve practice. Since the inception of clinical governance, quality assurance and quality improvement processes are no longer restricted activities controlled by professionals. Instead government-led definitions of quality, in the form of guidance from the National Institute of Clinical Excellence (NICE) and National Service Frameworks issued by the Department of Health, have been linked to managerial procedures to ensure clinical accountability. The quality of clinical work is compared with nationally determined standards and subject to external examination through the publication of performance data (NHSE 1999), with quality control procedures monitored by an external agency, currently the Healthcare Commission.

Clinical governance represents a significant challenge to the authority of the medical profession as in theory it requires doctors to account for what care is provided, the standards of that care, and how that care is organized and delivered. In addition, the criteria against which clinical performance is assessed are no longer exclusively determined by clinicians and their professional bodies. The state has been able to determine what services are to be provided and to what standard (Department of Health 2002), and these standards are increasingly being integrated into commissioning agreements with hospitals and GPs so that in future their income may depend on adherence to a range of highly specific quality indicators. Inspections by the Healthcare Commission, which include a review of clinical performance and the extent of compliance with NICE guidance, have increased surveillance of doctors' practices and require them to provide evidence of continuous quality improvement work.

The actual implementation and effectiveness of clinical governance in practice is difficult to gauge, although generally PCTs have a clinical governance team, often with a GP lead, to investigate concerns raised by a practice, and each area has a panel run by the PCT to investigate complaints against GPs which were not resolved locally. A study by Sheaff *et al.* (2004) of clinical governance in 12 PCG/Ts reveals that they have relied on semi-formal, collegially run, networks, with doctors thus continuing to review other doctors' work. What is different is that this GP self-regulation has become routinized and transparent, for managers as well. Clinical leads in PCTs however mediate between these GPs and managers, thereby forestalling further managerial encroachment, paralleling the role of medical leaders in NHS hospitals (Ferlie *et al.* 1996).

Policy developments in primary care: patient access, choice and participation

The previous sections have outlined the different policies aimed at changing the organization and provision of care in primary care which not only have implications for the social position and activities of the primary care work force but also for patients. However, there has also been a range of policies specifically aimed at developing patient-centred care in primary care – although the rationale for such policies has been shaped by different political philosophies (e.g. marketization and choice) and professional values (e.g. holistic care). It is possible to identify at least three distinct themes in these policies – improving patient access, increasing patient choice and developing patients as experts – and each will be considered in turn.

Policies aimed at improving patient access have involved increasing points of entry into primary care through walk-in centres (Salisbury 2004), NHS Direct call centres (Hanlon *et al.* 2005), nurse triage clinics, GPs working in larger organizations such as out-of hours cooperatives (Calnan *et al.* 2007) or in supermarkets, providing specialist services such as dermatology clinics, and the recently established polyclinics or health centres. All these developments are (and will be) dealing with an increasing proportion of the primary care workload and each of them enables the patient to have direct access to primary health care and to a variety of health professionals. This might be suitable for those patients who put a value on speed and technical care, such as the younger, healthier and infrequent user, and are happy to give up the (albeit sometimes idealized) benefits of a personal doctor. However, for those who value a 'doctor who knows you', such as those with chronic illness, this development might be seen as an additional barrier to access (Cheragi-Sohi *et al.* 2006). These policies of increasing the number of general and specialist health professionals that the patient may directly consult may be fragmenting rather than strengthening primary care as it challenges the principles of continuity of care and undermines the coordinating and gate-keeping role of the GP (Calnan *et al.* 2006). It may also be seen by general practitioners or their representatives as a threat to their 'business' and to their appeal to the professionalism of general practice where continuity of care is still a core value.

The second theme is the attempt to increase patient choice in primary care. Choice has long been a problematic concept and the focus of debates about whether an effective market for health care as a commodity can be established given the existence of externalities, uncertainty and information deficits regarding the cost, quantity and quality of care, and difficulties in entering and exiting the market (Calnan *et al.* 1993). Patient choice policy (Department of Health 2004b, 2004c, 2005), according to some commentators (Dixon *et al.* 2008), has broadened from an initiative to get patients seen more quickly to a tool for improving the efficiency of health services and their responsiveness to patients' needs and is closely tied to the government's market reforms programme in England. The concepts of equity and choice in health care seem to be incompatible, and some commentators fear that a policy of greater choice, with its emphasis on tailoring care to individual demands and preferences, will increase health inequalities (Appleby *et al.* 2003). However, according to Dixon *et al.* (2008), government patient choice policy is designed to correct inequalities in the system by giving all patients shorter waiting times and a choice of provider, and not just those who can afford to buy faster treatment from the private sector or are better able to play the system to get access to the providers of their choice (Department of Health and HMG 2004).

One example of patient choice policy is the attempt to give patients more choice over where they get referred for treatment. GPs have usually made this decision on behalf of their patients and since the 1990s have been limited to making referrals to hospitals with which their Health Authority or Primary Care Trust has a contract. However, since January 2006 patients should have been offered a choice of four or five local providers for their hospital treatment, which might include Foundation trusts, NHS trusts, General Practitioners with Special Interest (GPSIs – GPs who provide services traditionally provided by hospital or hospital-associated clinics or in so-called 'tier two' centres which are usually owned by PCTs), although take up of Choose and Book, as the computer system has been called, has been slow (Dixon *et al.* 2008). In addition, patients can now, at least in theory, choose providers from an Extended Choice Network of Foundation trusts, Independent Sector Treatment Centres (ISTCs) and approved independent hospitals across the country. From April 2008 patients should be able to choose any provider who meets Healthcare Commission standards and will provide care at the national price (Department of Health 2007). GPSIs are used here as an example of an alternative provider increasing patient choice, although in reality they may be used as a way of restricting choice as PCTs may see them as a cheaper option than hospital care and thus encourage patient referral to GPSIs.

In the recent Darzi Review (2008), choice has again featured strongly with plans announced to give patients greater choice of general practice and more information to help them choose. An NHS Choices website will be developed to provide comparative information on the range of services practices offered, their opening times, the views of local patients about the service and performance against quality indicators. These developments of course assume that patients want to exercise choice about where they are treated, even though the evidence suggests the opposite (Calnan and Gabe 2001; Forster and Gabe 2008). Furthermore, extending choice about where to obtain treatment may be disadvantageous to older people and those who lack the resources to travel to what are perceived to be the highest quality providers (Allsop and Baggott 2004; Farrington-Douglas and Allen 2005). There is also the impact of 'increased choice' and whether there will be a shift in the balance of the relationship between the patient and the general practitioner, with the latter losing their mediating role as the former gains power or control. However, the evidence from studies of patient choice and the use of private health care (Calnan *et al.* 1993) suggests little change in the relationship, with patients continuing to defer to GPs' advice about when and where to use the private sector. Evidence from a recent exploratory study (Calnan and Rowe 2008) suggests choice and trust are related: when patients exercise choice it seems to be based on trust in the doctor's competence and the cleanliness of the hospital, derived mainly from indirect or direct experience. Performance information appears to act post the referral decision to influence the extent to which patients feel comfortable with the referral rather than actively determining where patients choose to be referred.

The third theme is the development of an 'expert' patient programme to improve self-care support in the NHS. Whilst Labour's policy of involving patients in referral decisions regarding secondary care is relatively new, initiatives to involve patients in decision making about managing their own condition, particular those with chronic health problems are well established. Successful management of many chronic diseases appears to depend at least as much on changes that the patient can make as it does on specific medical interventions, and as a result requires a 'partnership' between patient and health professional. Current NHS policy in England encourages patient self-management as part of its programme to reduce the burden of chronic disease (Department of Health 2001b) and the costs to the health service (Taylor and Bury 2007). Evidence from evaluations of this programme (NPCRDC 2007) showed benefits in terms of quality of life and cost effectiveness, although taking more responsibility for health care appealed most to white, middle-class female patients but was less attractive to those living in deprived areas, who place a higher value on relationships with GPs. In order to stimulate activity in this area, chronic disease management has been identified as key to improving the quality and performance of general practice. This is reflected in the new GMS contract, which includes specific payments for practices to manage patients with chronic disease proactively through its new 'Quality and Outcomes Framework '(QOF) (Rowland 2004). The success of this policy is of course dependent on a patient's willingness and ability to participate in decision making, which in turn reflects wider changes in public attitudes and expectations of health professionals. Evidence about changes in patient perceptions is scarce, so it is difficult to judge whether patients increasingly prefer to be more involved in decision making and if the structure of the doctor–patient relationship in primary care has changed to enable this to occur (see Chapter 8, this volume, by Milewa). Likewise these professionals will need to accept the reform of the traditional paternalistic relationship with health service users and agree to work in closer partnership with them. There is some evidence of general practitioners welcoming this opportunity, especially the younger ones (Jones and Green 2006), although this favourable response needs to be interpreted with caution, as it may represent nothing more than a rhetorical expression of sectional interests (Armstrong 2002).

Finally, what general impact have these and related policies had on patient and public attitudes to primary care? Data on trends in such attitudes are in short supply although evidence from regular, national public attitude surveys since 1983 shows levels of public satisfaction with GPs remain high despite an overall decline in public satisfaction with the NHS over this period (Calnan 2006). These levels of satisfaction probably represent an under-estimate, as those with more recent experience of general practitioner care tend to report significantly higher levels of satisfaction. This favourable picture of general practice was also found in a national survey of general practice patients carried out in 1998 and repeated again in 2002 (Boreham *et al.* 2003). However, patient views about some aspects such as waiting times and responding to out-of-hours care were more critical. It has been argued that trust might be a more sensitive indicator of patient and public perception of quality and performance of health care than satisfaction. However, data about changes in trust levels over time are also in short supply, although evidence from a recent cross-sectional survey suggests that levels of public trust in general practitioners are still relatively high (Calnan and Rowe 2008). Small-scale local studies over shorter periods (1998–2001) suggest no marked changes in perceptions of quality despite organizational improvements such as improvement in access to services (see Calnan 2006). However, there is some doubt about whether access, choice and participation are aspects of care which are particularly salient to patients' perceptions of quality of primary care, as the latter tend to emphasize the quality of examination and treatment and the relationship with the clinician, such as whether the doctor knows the patient well and is interested in the patients' ideas about what is wrong (Cheraghi-Sohi *et al.* 2006).

Conclusion: a case of restratification?

This analysis has shown that there have been major policy developments which have led to significant changes in the organization and provision of primary care in England. But how useful are the theoretical positions presented earlier for explaining these changes? There is the obvious difficulty of identifying general influences on the position of the medical profession as a whole, such as the shift away from self-regulation, as a result of changes in the General Medical Council, and the specific impact of these policies on the primary care workforce. Many of these developments may have presented challenges or even threats to the professional position of general practitioners, but there is little evidence of a decline in dominance or that general practice is being undermined by managerialism or marketization, or by the so-called rise of the informed, active and demanding patient shopping around for care. While most GPs believe that the new contract has been detrimental to their professional autonomy, this has been compensated for by the positive impact on pay and quality of care and the decrease in the average number of hours worked. However, are new types of general practitioner emerging such as street-level bureaucrats (Checkland 2000) or public sector entrepreneurs (Boyce 2008) in response to these policy challenges and wider social changes? This is a difficult question to answer given the lack of detailed evidence available, although there is some evidence to suggest that a form of restratification is taking place in primary care as GPs' work and their orientation towards it becomes more diverse. Freidson (1994, 2001) proposed a form of vertical stratification between the elite at the macro-level and rank and file doctors at the micro-level but such a distinction might not be so evident in English general practice as many GPs perform a range of roles at a number of different levels and the majority are still only contracted to and not employed by the NHS. However, the increasingly complex division of labour in general practice with GPs delegating routine tasks to nurses, the limited managerial control at the PCT level, an increasing division between the traditionalists and entrepreneurs and between the paternalists, egalitarians and salaried GPs, who are more interested in a work–life balance, suggest that restratification is taking place. Much of this appears to reflect a type of horizontal stratification at the micro-level, but there is also evidence of vertical stratification between those GPs involved as clinical leads or in managerial roles in the PCTs or who are responsible for the QOF in their practices and thus have more influence and those who are not involved with these activities. Thus, while traditional professional dominance continues, there is evidence to suggest that a form of restratification is taking place in primary care. It is difficult to predict the impact of recent policies such as the encouragement of private providers to offer primary care, which has until recently been almost exclusively provided by NHS contracted practitioners, and whether it will spawn a new breed of GP working as a 'hired hand' for a private provider. Salaried positions, as our analysis has shown, are attractive to some GPs, although in the current situation where there is a surplus of general practitioners in England and difficulties in finding GP partnerships, they may have little alternative but to take up this type of employment. The future will show whether we are witnessing the beginning of the corporatization of general practice or a simply a more pluralized system in which traditional professional autonomy continues to dominate.

Acknowledgements

Thanks go to Patrick Brown, Kath Checkland and Chris Salisbury for their valuable comments on an earlier version of this chapter. We should also like to thank the participants who attended the symposium on the 'New Sociology of the Health Service' at Royal Holloway in 2007 for their suggestions.

References

Alford, R. (1975) *Health Care Politics*, Chicago: Chicago University Press.
Allsop, J. and Baggott, R. (2004) 'The NHS in England: from modernisation to marketisation?' *Social Policy Review*, 16: 29–44.
Appleby, J., Harrison, A. and Dewar, S. (2003) 'Patients choosing their hospital may not be fair and equitable', *British Medical Journal*, 326: 406–7.
Armstrong, D. (2002) 'Clinical autonomy, individual and collective: the problem of changing doctors' behaviour', *Social Science and Medicine*, 55: 1771–7.
Audit Commission (1996) *What the Doctor Ordered: A study of GP fundholders in England and Wales*, London: HMSO.
Baeza, J.I. (2005) *Restructuring the Medical Profession: The intraprofessional relations of GPs and hospital consultants*, Maidenhead: Open University Press.
Baeza, J. and Calnan, M. (1997) 'Implementing quality', *Journal of Health Services and Policy*, 2: 205–11.
Boreham, R., Airey, C., Erens, B. and Tobin, R. (2003) 'The national surveys of NHS patients', *General Practice 2002*, London: NHS Executive.
Bowler, I. and Jackson, N. (2002) 'Experiences and career intentions of general

practice registrars in Thames deaneries: postal survey', *British Medical Journal*, 324: 464–5.

Boyce, R.A. (2008) 'Professionalism meets entrepreneurialism and managerialism', in E. Kuhlmann and M. Saks (eds) *Rethinking Professional Governance*, Bristol: Policy Press.

Brereton, M. and Temple, M. (1999) 'The new public service ethos: an ethical environment for governance', *Public Administration*, 77: 455–74.

Calnan, M. (2006) 'Doing better but feeling worse', in G.P. Westert, I. Jabaaij and F.G. Schellevis (eds) *Morbidity, Performance and Quality in Health Care*, Oxford: Radcliffe.

Calnan, M. and Gabe, J. (1991) 'Recent developments in general practice: a sociological analysis', in J. Gabe, M. Calnan and M. Bury (eds) *The Sociology of the Health Service*, London: Routledge.

Calnan, M. and Gabe, J. (2001) 'From consumerism to partnership? Britain's National Health Service at the turn of the century', *International Journal of Health Services*, 31: 119–31.

Calnan, M. and Rowe, R. (2008) *Trust Matters in Health Care*, Buckingham: Open University Press.

Calnan, M. and Wainwright, D. (2002) 'Is general practice stressful?', *European Journal of General Practice*, 8: 5–17.

Calnan, M. and Williams, S. (1995) 'Challenges to professional autonomy in general practice', *International Journal of Health Services*, 25: 219–41.

Calnan, M., Cant, S. and Gabe, J. (1993) *Going Private? The use of private health insurance*. Milton Keynes: Open University Press.

Calnan, M., Hutten, J. and Tiljak, H. (2006) 'The challenge of coordination: the role of primary care professionals in promoting integration across the interface', in R.B. Saltman, A. Rico and W. Boerma (eds) *Primary Care in the Driver's Seat?* Buckingham: Open University Press.

Calnan, M., Silvester, S., Manley, G. and Taylor-Gooby, P. (2000) 'Doing business in the NHS: exploring dentists' decisions to practise in the public and private sectors', *Sociology of Health and Illness*, 22: 742–64.

Calnan, M., Payne, S., Rossdale, M., Kemple, T. and Ingram, J. (2007) 'A qualitative study exploring variations in general practitioners' out-of-hours referrals to hospital', *British Journal of General Practice*, 57: 706–13.

Charles-Jones, H., Latimer, J. and May, C. (2003) 'Transforming general practice: the redistribution of medical work in primary care', *Sociology of Health and Illness*, 25: 71–92.

Checkland, K. (2004) 'National Service Frameworks and UK general practitioners: street-level bureaucrats at work?', *Sociology of Health and Illness*, 26: 951–75.

Checkland, K., Harrison, S., McDonald, R., Grant, S., Campbell, S. and Guthrie, B. (2008) 'Biomedicine, holism and general medical practice: responses to the 2004 General Practitioner contract', *Sociology of Health and Illness*, 30: 788–803.

Cheragi–Sohi, S., Bower, P. and Mead, N. (2006) 'What are the key attributes of primary care for patients? Building a conceptual map of patient preferences', *Health Expectations*, 9: 275–84.

Cho, H.-J. (2000) 'Traditional medicine, professional monopoly and structural interests: a Korean case', *Social Science and Medicine*, 50: 123–7.

Coburn, D., Rappolt, S. and Bourgeault, I. (1997) 'Decline vs retention of medical power through restratification: the Ontario case', *Sociology of Health and Illness*, 19: 1–22.

Coulter, A. (1995) 'Evaluating general practice fundholding in the UK', *European Journal of Public Health*, 5: 233–9.

Coulter, A. and Mays, N. (1997) 'Deregulating primary care', *British Medical Journal*, 314: 510–13.

Darzi Review (2008) *High Quality Care for All*, London: Department of Health. Online. Available online: www.dh.gov.uk/en/Publicationsand statistics/Publications/PublicationsPolicyAndGuidance/DH_085825 (accessed 1 July 2008).

Department of Health (2001a) *Shifting the Balance of Power within the NHS Securing Delivery*, London: The Stationery Office.

Department of Health (2001b). *The Expert Patient: a new approach to chronic disease management in the 21st century*, London: The Stationery Office.

Department of Health (2002) *National Service Frameworks: a practical aid to implementation in primary care*, London: The Stationery Office.

Department of Health (2004a) *Practice Based Commissioning: engaging practices in commissioning*, London: The Stationery Office.

Department of Health (2004b) *Choosing Health: making healthier choices easier*. London: The Stationery Office.

Department of Health (2004c) *Building on the Best: choice, responsiveness, and equity in the NHS*. London: The Stationery Office

Department of Health (2005) *Independence, Well-being and Choice: our vision for the future of social care for adults in England*, London: The Stationery Office.

Department of Health (2007) *Choice of Referral: guidance framework for 2007/8*, London: The Stationery Office.

Department of Health and HM Government (2004) *The NHS Improvement Plan: putting people at the heart of public services*, London: The Stationery Office.

Dixon, J., Holland, P. and Mays, N. (1998) 'Developing primary care gatekeeping, commissioning and managed care', *British Medical Journal*, 317: 125–8.

Dixon, A., Robertson, R. and Bal, R. (2008) 'The experience of implementing choice at the point of referral: a comparison of the Netherlands and England', Proceedings of European Policy meeting, Dublin, unpublished.

Drennan, V., Davis, K., Goodman, C., Humphrey, C., Locke, R., Mark, A., Murray, S.F. and Traynor, M. (2007) 'Entrepreneurial nurses and midwives in the United Kingdom: an integrative study', *Journal of Advanced Nursing*, 60: 459–69.

Duckett, S.J. (1984) 'Structural interests and Australian health policy', *Social Science and Medicine*, 18: 959–65

Edmunds, J. and Calnan, M. (2001) 'The reprofessionalisation of community pharmacy', *Social Science and Medicine*, 53: 943–55.

Evetts, J. (1999) 'Professionalisation and professionalism: issues for inter-professional care', *Journal of Interprofessional Care*, 13: 119–28.

Evetts, J. (2006) 'Introduction, trust and professionalism: challenges and occupational changes', *Current Sociology*, 54: 607–20.

Farrington-Douglas, J. and Allen, J. (2005) *Equitable Choices for Health*, London: Institute for Public Policy Research.

Ferlie, E. and Geraghty, K.J. (2007) Professionals in public service organizations, in E. Ferlie, L.E. Lynn and C. Pollitt (eds) *The Oxford Handbook of Public Management*, Oxford: Oxford University Press.

Ferlie, E., Ashburner, L., Fitzgerald, L. and Pettigrew, A. (1996) *The New Public Management in Action*, Oxford: Oxford University Press.

Flynn, R. (2002) 'Clinical governance and governmentality', *Health, Risk and Society*, 4: 155–73.

Forster, R. and Gabe, J. (2008) 'Voice or choice? Patient and public involvement in the National Health Service in England under New Labour', *International Journal of Health Services*, 38: 333–56.

Freidson, E (1994) *Professionalism Reborn: theory, prophecy and policy*, Cambridge: Polity Press.

Freidson, E. (2001) *Professionalism. The third logic*, Cambridge: Polity Press.

Glennerster, H., Matsaganis, W. and Owen, P. (1994) *Implementing GP Fund Holding: wild card or winning hand?* Buckingham: Open University Press.

Grant, S. *et al.* (2009) 'The impact of pay-for-performance on professional boundaries in UK general practice: an ethnographic study', *Sociology of Health and Illness*, 31.

Green, J. and Thorogood, N. (1998) *Analysing Health Policy*, London: Longman.

Gref. S., Delnoif, D. and Groenewegen, P. (2006) 'Managing primary care behaviour through payment systems and financial incentives', in R.B. Saltman, A. Rico and W. Boerma (eds) *Primary Care in the Driver's Seat?* Buckingham: Open University Press.

Ham, C. (2004) *Health Policy in Britain*, Basingstoke: Palgrave Macmillan.

Hanlon, G., Strangelman, T., Goode, J., Luff, D., O'Cathain, A. and Greatbatch, D. (2005) 'Knowledge, technology and nursing: the case of NHS Direct', *Human Relations* 58: 147–71.

Harrison, S. and Dowswell, G. (2002) 'Autonomy and bureaucratic accountability in primary care: what English practitioners say', *Sociology of Health and Illness*, 24: 208–26.

Heath, I. (2004) 'The cawing of the crow. Cassandra-like, prognosticating woe', *British Journal of General Practice*, 54: 320–1.

Jones, L. and Green, J. (2006) 'Shifting discourses of professionalism: a case study of general practitioners in the United Kingdom', *Sociology of Health and Illness*, 28: 927–50.

Klein, R. (1996) *The New Politics of the NHS*, London: Longman.

Kuhlmann, E. (2008) 'Governing beyond markets and managerialism: professions as mediators,' in E. Kuhlmann and M. Saks (eds) *Rethinking Professional Governance*, Bristol: Policy Press.

Lewis, K. (2001) *Nurse-led Primary Care. Learning from the PMS pilots*, London: Kings Fund Publishing.

McDonald, R., Harrison S., Checkland, K., Campbell, S. and Roland, M. (2007) 'Impact of financial incentives on clinical autonomy and internal motivation in primary care: ethnographic study', *British Medical Journal*, 334: 1357–9.

McDonald, R., Harrison, S. and Checkland, K. (2008).'Incentives and control in primary health care: findings from English Pay for Performance case studies', *Journal of Health Organization and Management*, 22: 48–63.

McKinlay, J. and Marceau, L. (2008) 'When there is no doctor: Reasons for the disappearance of primary care physicians in the US during the early 21st century', *Social Science and Medicine*, 67: 1481–91.

Mechanic, D., McAlpine, D. and Rosenthal, M. (2001) 'How should hamsters run?

some observations about sufficient time in primary care', *British Medical Journal*, 323: 266–8.

National Primary Care Research and Development Centre (2007) *Spotlight on Support for Self Care in the NHS*, Manchester: NPCRDC.

Newman, J. (1998) 'The dynamics of trust', in A. Conlon (ed.) *Trust and Continuity: relationships in local government, health and public services*, Bristol: Policy Press.

NHS Executive (1999) *Clinical Governance*, HSC 1999/065, Leeds: NHS Executive.

North, N. and Peckham, S. (2001) 'Analysing structural interests in Primary Care Groups', *Social Policy and Administration*, 35: 426–40.

Pollitt, C.J. (1993) 'Audit and accountability: the missing dimension?' *Journal of the Royal Society of Medicine*, 36: 209–11.

Rayner, F. (2002) 'Are male doctors the endangered species?' *Hospital Doctor*, 30: 18–19.

Regen, E. (2002) *Driving Seat or Back Seat? GPs views on and involvement in primary care groups and trusts*, Birmingham: Health Services Management Centre.

Rowland, M. (2004) 'Linking physicians' pay to the quality of care – a major experiment in the UK', *New England Journal of Medicine*, 351: 1448–53.

Saks, M. (1995) *Professions and the Public Interest: medical power, altruism and alternative medicine*, London: Routledge.

Salisbury, C. (2004) 'Does advanced access work for patients and practices?' *British Journal of General Practice*, 54: 330–1.

Salisbury, C. (2008) 'The involvement of private companies in NHS general practice', *British Medical Journal*, 336: 400–1.

Scally, G. and Donaldson, L. (1998) 'Clinical governance and the drive for quality improvement in the new NHS in England', *British Medical Journal*, 317: 61–5.

Schulz, R.I. and Harrison, S. (1986) 'Physician autonomy in the Federal Republic of Germany, Great Britain and the United States', *International Journal of Health Planning and Management*, 1: 1213–28.

Sheaff, R., Smith, K. and Dickson, M. (2002) 'Is GP restratification beginning in England?' *Social Policy and Administration*, 36: 765–79.

Sheaff, R., Marshall, M., Rogers, A., Sibbald, B. and Pickard, S. (2004) 'Governmentality by network in English primary healthcare', *Social Policy and Administration*, 38: 89–103.

Sheaff, R., Gene-Badia, J., Marshall, M. and Svab, I. (2006) 'The evolving public-private mix', in R.B. Saltman, A. Rico and W. Boerma (eds) *Primary Care in the Driver's Seat?* Buckingham: Open University Press.

Sibbald, B., Gravelle, H. and Bojke, C. (2001) *General Practitioner Job Satisfaction*, Manchester: National Primary Care Research and Development Centre.

Somerset, M., Faulkner, A., Shaw, A., Dunn, L. and Sharp, D. (1999) 'Obstacles on the path to a primary care led NHS', *Social Science and Medicine*, 48: 213–25.

Taylor, D. and Bury, M. (2007) 'Chronic illness, expert patients and care transition', *Sociology of Health and Illness*, 29: 127–45.

Wainwright, D. (1998) 'Disenchantment, ambivalence and the precautionary principle: the becalming of British health policy', *International Journal of Health Services*, 28: 407–26.

Wainwright, D. and Calnan, M. (2002) *Work Stress: the making of a modern epidemic*, Buckingham: Open University Press.

Weiss, M. and Fitzpatrick, R. (1997) 'Challenges to medicine: the case of prescribing', *Sociology of Health and Illness*, 19: 297–327.

Whalley, D., Bojke, C., Gravelle, H. and Sibbald, B. (2006) 'GP job satisfaction in view of contract reform: a national survey', *British Journal of General Practice*, 56: 87–92.

4 Visions of privatization

New Labour and the reconstruction of the NHS

John Mohan

Introduction

As the UK National Health Service (NHS) passes the sixtieth anniversary of its establishment, it is worth recalling Aneurin Bevan's trenchant statement that 'a free health service is a triumphant example of the superiority of collective action and public initiative applied to a segment of society where commercial principles are seen at their worst (Bevan 1952: 109). In many respects, that principle has been retained, though it is coming under increasing challenge. The recent debate at the British Medical Association's annual meeting (July 2008) suggests there is now a wafer-thin line in the medical profession between those who favour top-up fees, or co-payments, for drugs not available on the NHS, and those who oppose it. However, public attitudes reveal little evidence of substantial public support for an extension of charging for health care; partisan accounts such as those of Pollard (2008) are characterized by double counting and exaggeration of the population covered by private health insurance and/or paying privately for some of their health care (for further discussion of this, see Mohan 2008).

Furthermore, although the British private sector in health care has grown steadily, it has never lived up to some of the more optimistic projections made in the early 1980s, when one Conservative minister envisaged 25 per cent of the population having private insurance coverage. The main features of the 'moving frontier' between public and private provision (Finlayson 1994), comparing the patterns evident now with those discussed in my contribution to the previous edition of this book (Mohan 1991), have been a steady expansion in private health insurance and health cash plan coverage, such that circa 12 per cent of the population now has private medical insurance cover coverage compared to 8 per cent twenty years ago and the substantial social and spatial divisions in coverage remain (Foubister *et al.* 2006; King and Mossialos 2005; Laing and Buisson various dates; Gorsky *et al.* 2006: chapter 9). The private acute hospital sector continues a long-term trend towards commercial ownership noted by Rayner (1986, 1987). However, these developments must be set against a background of rapid growth in NHS resources. Moreover, the traffic is not all in one direction: the NHS has bought private facilities at knockdown prices such as the London Heart Hospital, while recent trends suggest that the numbers paying directly for private medical treatment (rather than taking out insurance) are down (Timmins 2005). In an international context, British health care is still exceptional in terms of being funded predominantly by direct taxation and offering universal coverage (Bambra 2005). On this evidence there has not yet been a decisive shift in the public–private boundary and this is consistent with the kind of argument advanced in a series of papers on the theme of 'granny's footsteps' by Martin Powell (1996, 1999); in other words, describing very small and incremental shifts in the moving frontier between the public and private. Such analyses led Powell to conclude that the principles of the NHS had always been compromised to a greater or lesser degree but that those principles were coming under increasing strain at the margins. Nevertheless, the private sector was still relatively small, and the inference was that it was consequently of marginal significance.

If that is still the case, is there anything novel about contemporary developments in the private health sector in Britain or in the relationship between public and private sectors? I argue that there is, and that it lies in the growing significance of private interests in the commissioning and provision of publicly funded health care. While the private health sector is relatively small in the UK, the processes of privatization and commercialization seem set to become of much greater significance to the future character of health care and of the NHS. Consideration of these processes requires that we look not just at the extent of the private sector, but at the relationships between it and the NHS, and at the effects on the NHS of policies designed to pluralize the supply side and to create a contestable market.

The structure of the chapter is as follows. First, I present some cautionary remarks about interpreting shifts in the boundary between the public and private sectors. The principal substantive discussion is then divided into two sections designed to contrast two different visions of privatization. I focus on two key developments: the expansion of the private sector's role in the finance and delivery of health care through the Private Finance Initiative (PFI), Independent Sector Treatment Centres (ISTCs) and new forms of provision of primary care; and the government's attempt to put a social gloss on its policies through new forms of social ownership such as social enterprise and foundation trusts. We might see the NHS as poised between two visions of privatization. One view sees the service as being opened up to the full play of market forces. Indifference to the importance of public provision – or, even worse, a pro-market orientation in which corporate enterprise is enlisted as the solution to social problems – leads towards the commercialization and break-up of the NHS. The other is a much more benign version, in which public enterprise is replaced by new mutuals, social enterprises and cooperatives. While all these might compete to attract contracts, they will be local, democratic, community-controlled, and innovative, developing novel solutions (especially at the interface between health and social care). Both versions have attractions, flaws and vigorous defenders. I should finally point out that the emphasis in this chapter is on the supply side; of course, markets require both supply and demand and in relation to the latter the government's emphasis on choice by individual patients is highly relevant but is covered elsewhere in this volume (see Chapter 8, this volume, by Milewa) and in other published work (e.g. Clarke 2004; Needham 2003).

Moving frontiers, slippery slopes and system dynamics

The boundary between public and private sectors has, of course, been the subject of previous discussion, in which critics have argued that the idea of mixed economies or moving frontiers has its limitations – we need some theoretically informed grounds to provide the basis for assessing change. These arguments are still relevant today. Ruane's (1997) critique of Powell (1996) made the point very well; Davies' (1987) response to Klein's (1984) analysis of developments under the first-term Thatcher government is an earlier illustration. Ruane argued that while Powell presented useful evidence on the changing boundaries between the public and private, his approach lacked theoretical depth so that he was recognizing change without having good reasons for doing so. In an earlier exchange, Davies (1987) challenged Klein's (1984) assertion that no real 'breaks of slope' could be detected and suggested that he was presenting a Panglossian view which failed to consider key changes in the internal dynamics of the NHS under the Conservative government. In her view, absence of malice did not equate to benevolence. Both arguments are, in a sense, debates about *what sort of foundational principles* we should look at. Powell focused on various criteria (comprehensiveness, universality, equity, accountability, charging and so on) which could be identified and checked off against the 'facts'. Minor and incremental departures from these, or steady progression along a slope, did not signify very much. The problem with that kind of analysis is how one might discern when a fundamental change has taken place. Ruane (1997: 54) starts, instead, from an alternative conceptualization of foundational principles, couched in a different vocabulary. The essential nature of the NHS comprises 'collectivism of funding and provision, accompanied by planning and based on the devalorisation of labour'. The crucial defining factor in the organization of these services was the decommodification of labour. The activities of those professionals and workers providing the service were not subject to the extraction of surplus value; market criteria in any shape or form did not interfere with the delivery of public health care. Ruane therefore argued that the fundamental principles of the NHS lay in the organization of the labour process and the degree of decommodification of the provision of care. She contends that we should be seeking a historical perspective on moves away from collectivism and the devalorization of labour, and that apparently unrelated developments can, over time, have substantial cumulative effects that constitute rather more than just a 'break of slope'. Similar points were made by Paton (1997, 2006), on the changes to the labour process within the health service, and by Tudor Hart (2006), who emphasized the uniqueness of the NHS as 'a distinct, unified, nationwide economy independent of business, designed to meet social needs rather than to maximise profit' (see also Leys 2001 and Pollock 2004).

Crucially, Ruane argued that the 'ambiguous status' of some groups in the NHS gave some contemporary developments the potential to effect substantial transformation. Her argument was that reforms up to the mid-1990s had encouraged an entrepreneurial, small business ethos within the NHS, especially among GPs, dentists and ophthalmologists. Arguably, this ethos is now being extended to social enterprises. Managerial reforms, apparently innocuous in themselves, have led to the acquisition of commercial skills and, as a result, effected a transformation in attitudes and values which 'can move the boundaries between the do-able and the unthinkable' (Ruane 1997: 68). The new managerialism, against a background of tight financial constraints and governments supportive of entrepreneurialism, 'pushes managers . . . [towards] methods which entail the valorisation of labour'. The net result was a 'new set of meanings' around health and health care: a narrower definition of health care; changing perceptions of entitlements; a redefinition of accountability in terms of financial and corporate objectives; an undermining of 'lateral solidarities' between users and workers. This is evident, for example, in cultural shifts in the attitudes of managers (Ruane 2002). Ruane's work now looks prescient in the light of recent changes which serve to unbundle and fragment the provision of health care, to extend and deepen market relationships and processes, and to draw into the service large international corporations, some with track records in providing health care (albeit in the USA) and others without it (e.g. the (reputed) involvement of Virgin Healthcare in primary care). Ruane's work also highlights the continuing relevance of political economy approaches to the analysis of health care systems although, as noted by Seale (2008), such approaches have been largely absent from the sociological literature on British health care in recent years.

Analytically, therefore, as Mackintosh and Koivusalo (2005) suggest, we should 'replace the "mix" concept with a model of different paths of institutional change in health care' and focus, instead, on the trajectories and dynamics of health care systems, of which Mackintosh and Koivusalo identify several, including corporatization and segmentation in hospital provision, and globalization in input supply (e.g. medical technologies and equipment) and in labour markets. The primary empirical focus of their work is low-income countries, but at least the second and third of the trajectories and dynamics they identify are both highly relevant to the UK. This emphasis on trajectories is consistent with Salmon's (1995) analysis, in which he commented that the implications of profit maximizing go well beyond the 'presence, size and growth of investor-owned entities'. This is because of the effects of the external environment in which providers of health care operate. Regardless of whether a provider is not-for-profit, for-profit, or public, the degree of competition and the nature of the regulatory environment produce isomorphism (DiMaggio and Powell 1983), such that there is little to distinguish different types of provider in competitive health care markets.

In summary, we need to think about forces and processes as much as boundaries and mixes. The public–private mix is shifting but there are greater changes affecting the overall dynamics and trajectory of the system, with implications for access, equity, employment, and control. These questions assume greater urgency because of the acceptance by the current Labour government of a substantially expanded role for the private sector and for market mechanisms in the delivery of health care.

Commercialization and corporatization

On the eve of the 1997 general election, New Labour gave the voters 24 hours to save the NHS: they had pledged to reconstruct the service if elected. Yet, having rejected Conservative pro-market policies while in opposition, New Labour moved steadily to expand private provision once in office. Pessimistic observers believe that the result will be fragmentation of the NHS and a cherry-picking of profitable parts of the service by commercial organizations, notably multinationals. Kearney (2002) has argued (adopting a form of analysis derived from Polanyi (2001)) that these developments represent the 'privatisation of the commons' – that is, the establishment of property rights in assets that were formerly held by the whole community. There are three consequences, of greater or lesser novelty in a British context, associated with this: commercialization, corporatization and globalization.

The first of these is defined by Mackintosh and Koivusalo (2005: 3–4) as: the provision of health care services through market relationships to those able to pay; investment in, and production of, those services, and of inputs to them, for cash income or profit; and health care finance derived from individual payments and private insurance. An objection to this argument might be that the British health care system is not based on individual pay-ments and private insurance, and that the provision of health care services through market relationships is not something that goes on within the NHS. I agree with the former point but not with the latter: there is substantial evidence that market relationships are developing and being extended and deepened in relation to the provision of NHS care.

The second development is corporatization: the growing significance of large-scale, for-profit enterprises and/or the adoption, by non-profits, of quasi-commercial management structures and behaviours. Salmon (1995) introduced the term to heath care analysis in his work on the corporate transformation of health care. He wrote that 'in 1964, [American] health care was not called an industry' (Salmon 1995: 11), but the injection of Medicare and Medicaid funding made it a highly profitable one, to the point where Whitfield (2001) now speaks of a medical–industrial complex. The risk attendant on corporatization is the effects of the economic power of large commercial entities on the character and delivery of health care and particularly their power to exclude high risks.

The third potentially dangerous consequence is globalization, used in its economic sense, that is, integration of national economies into the international economy through trade, foreign direct investment, capital flows, migration and the spread of technology. As Harrington (2007: 81) puts it, the risk here is that 'economic globalisation, driven by the relentless quest for profit of corporations in the developed countries and enforced by international economic law, *acts inevitably to decompose the bounded and solidaristic bases of national health care systems*' (emphases added).

Major recent British developments which comprise elements of commercialization, corporatization and globalization include: the Private Finance Initiative (PFI), the development of Independent Sector Treatment Centres (ISTCs), the expansion of patient choice to include private providers, the development of alternative providers of primary care, as well as steady processes of outsourcing of support services. The PFI is a mechanism for funding capital investment whereby private companies design, build, own and operate facilities in return for an annual availability payment over an extended period (most attention has focused on hospital provision, but there are similar mechanisms (local improvement finance trusts – LIFTs) in primary care (Aldred 2007, 2008). ISTCs are a vehicle for expanding private sector involvement in routine NHS work; in order to attract investment, they have been backed by guarantees as to long-term contracts; they are treatment centres which specialize in delivering a high volume of a very small range of routine caseload. Alternative providers of medical services (APMS) represent new contractual arrangements for delivery of primary care; in this case, GPs are under contract to private companies, not the state, and the contractors have a duty to manage services required by those patients registered with them (see also Chapter 3, this volume, by Calnan and Gabe). In a further step towards a market-based system, restrictions on the sale of goodwill in the provision of non-essential GP services have been abandoned, leading Pollock (2004) to suggest that this will encourage GPs or contractors to select patients so as to increase the profitability of non-essential services. The government has also pressed NHS authorities to contract-out the commissioning of health services to private companies, brought in for their expertise in managing demand. This would potentially be of far-reaching significance, if companies were able to limit the scope of what will be covered in the manner characteristic of American Health Maintenance Organizations (see the debate between Feachem *et al.* 2002 and Talbot-Smith *et al.* 2004).

These are developments which go well beyond what might have been envisaged of a government committed to rebuilding the NHS as a public service. They have been criticized not only on financial grounds but also on their merits in terms of health policy. Themes of service quality and integration are important here. First, however, in terms of cost, the controversial expansion of the PFI has been heavily criticized. Such data as are publicly available suggest that the capital cost of the PFI schemes to which the NHS is already committed is £10 billion, but over the lifetime of the contracts the NHS will pay £63 billion to the private consortia that have built them.[1] Substantial debt has been created, which is traded as a commodity on the financial markets, such that some companies involved in PFI have made very substantial windfall profits. Claims by the government that PFI entails a transfer of risk from the taxpayer to the private sector appear to have been unfounded while there is profound suspicion about the value-for-money criteria used to assess capital investments. On these points, the government's promised reply to critics of the PFI has never materialized. The central criticism, and one which resonates with Bevan's critique of private interests in health care, is that service development is finance-driven (i.e. constrained by what can be made to work as a profitable private investment) rather than needs-driven (what is necessary for the local population). And it is transparently clear that notwithstanding the government's own obsession with choice, the NHS has had little alternative but to go down the private sector route. PFI was widely referred to as 'the only game in town' as far as new hospital investment was concerned (Ruane 2000). This is also true of the ISTC programme: the government had been prepared to guarantee revenues so as to entice new investment even in circumstances where the ISTCs threatened the viability of existing hospitals (Player and Leys 2008). This is at best debatable in terms of value for money since it generates windfall profits for private companies who are paid whether or not they carry out the number of operations envisaged in the contracts. Hence the comment by Player and Leys (2008) that ISTCs represent a 'hugely expensive and ring fenced bridgehead for private providers, at the expense of NHS trusts'. Furthermore, far from the expansion of private provision solving capacity problems for the NHS, the NHS effectively solves cash-flow problems for the private sector, giving corporations access to substantial public revenue streams.

Second, there have been criticisms of the health policy effects and, in particular, about the adequacy and integration of services. In relation to PFI, there have been questions about the adequacy of hospital capacity, unrealistic throughput targets, effects on staff working within the service, and lack of integration of services (Gaffney *et al.* 1999a, 1999b, 1999c; Gaffney and Pollock 1999; Pollock *et al.* 2002). Despite the expense of PFI developments, they have resulted in above-trend reductions in hospital capacity (Dunnigan and Pollock 2003). The development of ISTCs has also been criticized for a lack of integration. These have been imposed on what are now termed local health economies, often in the teeth of resistance on the grounds of the implications for other local hospitals; for example, the redirection of some elements of workload towards ISTCs means that hospitals can no longer provide the full range of caseloads required for medical training. Criticisms have also been raised by the Healthcare Commission about inadequate standards in such providers of care, with high re-admission and post-operative complication rates associated with reliance on overseas-trained doctors (Healthcare Commission 2007).

A further lack of integration is evident in policies towards primary care. Government ministers have supported the total privatization of commissioning functions by Primary Care Trusts (PCTs), the more entrepreneurial of which organizations would prefer to see the NHS effectively run as a brand, or even a franchise model, with the private sector brought in to deliver the services.[2] The scope for private investment in primary care premises, and the relaxation of restrictions on the sale of goodwill in practices, both open up primary care to profit-making commercial companies. Moves towards practice-based commissioning work against the grain of the population-based planning that distinguished the NHS from insurance-based systems with their potential for cherry picking. New contractual arrangements have been established, not between individual GPs and the State but between individual GPs and the private companies for which they are now able to work. Contractual arrangements between purchasers and APMS (alternative providers of medical services) contain exclusion clauses and do not oblige providers to adopt consistent standards. Management of financial performance by such privately owned providers will be the responsibility of their owners and shareholders, and will not be open to public scrutiny. These open up several possibilities which carry with them the potential to redefine the scope of primary care under the NHS. It might be argued against this that GPs have always been employed as independent contractors, but the crucial difference is that their contract was with the state, not through a commercial body (Pollock and Price 2006; Pollock *et al.* 2007).

Some commentators view these as largely pragmatic and incremental responses which carry no threat to the principle of an NHS free at the point of use. On this view, private ownership is irrelevant, as long as waiting lists come down and health care remains free at the point of use. Indeed, Stevens (2005) argues that the goal is to reduce the demand for private care while Le Grand (2006) suggests that the purpose is to provide a challenge to the NHS's way of doing things. On this view, the NHS was inefficient, bureaucratic and unresponsive, and faced no external threats which would force it to innovate; only the introduction of market disciplines would counteract these tendencies to state failure. Properly designed regulatory frameworks would protect the public interest. Other writers are more sceptical, and they point to the dangers of commercialization. Indeed, some argue that the whole point of recent initiatives is that the government can create a market in health care provision while denying that it is doing so (Player and Leys 2008).

In relation to the themes of this chapter, we have already considered the question of commercialization, but what about corporatization and globalization, and are these matters of concern? In relation to the former, we have not yet witnessed the full corporatization of the service – for all the attention given to the PFI there is still a substantial capital programme not funded privately; ISTC contracts are still only a small portion of total provision; commercial organizations as yet account for only a small number of contracts in primary care, principally to run out-of-hours services. However, the terms on which these entities have been welcomed into the NHS indicate the general trajectory of policy. Indeed, far from the market being the cause of the inverse care law (as Tudor Hart (1971) argued), market forces and capitalist enterprise are now seen as the solution to it, as is demonstrated by the overtures made to private companies to take over primary care in disadvantaged areas. While it is always possible to exaggerate the integration and cohesion of the pre-market NHS, the incorporation of such multinationals is difficult to square with the sense of local identification with individual GPs that has characterized the NHS. External – even international – control of providers of health care matters also sits uneasily with the drive towards local control implicit in NHS foundation trusts and social enterprises. Holden (2005) and Farnsworth (2006) (see also Holden and Farnsworth 2006) place health care in an international context and point out that developments in the NHS have excited the attention of multinational providers. Holden, for example, talks of the internationalization of health care and demonstrates the extent to which it is becoming globalized, while Farnsworth shows how New Labour's pro-business approach inevitably entailed opening up scope in the NHS for private and multinational interests. Collectively they demonstrate how these developments follow from a perception that New Labour had to reposition itself in the eyes of the national and international financial community, which implies being willing to open up to the private sector areas of the public sector that were previously off-limits. Previous analyses of privatization have shown how at first it was confined to marginal, non-clinical areas of health provision but it has gradually shifted centre stage; commencing with ancillary services in the early 1980s – the soft targets of the Thatcher years – but inexorably moving to the core of service provision (for a chronological sequence compare Mohan 1991, 1995; Leys 2001; Pollock 2004).

Official versions of these events have emphasized a range of considerations and constraints which followed from external influences – the perception that insertion into a global economy inevitably entailed restrictions on public expenditure. However, Hay (1998) (see also Hay and Watson 2003) has argued persuasively that, rather than globalization constraining Labour's approach to economic and social policy, in fact Labour's approach to economic and social policy dictated its attitude to globalization and its willingness to open up the public services to private capital. This is novel and contrasts with what Wistow (1989) characterized as the 'naive anti-statism' of the Conservatives during the 1980s.

What about globalization? Of course, the notion that health care is now global and that multinational investments will flow to where the pickings were ripest featured in Griffith *et al.*'s (1987) work on the UK's private health sector twenty years ago, but analyses are now framed with reference to altogether more worrying scenarios. There is an acknowledgement that with declining profitability in manufacturing, international corporations are trying to prise open the public sector as a source of profitable future contracts. Some authors argue that supranational trade regulations – enforced through the provisions of the World Trade Organization's General Agreement on Trade in Services (GATS) – might ultimately undermine the capacity of the NHS to provide comprehensive services. Universal service requirements may be challenged in the courts on the grounds that they are in conflict with the principles of free competition and in fact constitute barriers to trade. Whereas some countries have inserted exemption clauses to services provided in the exercise of government authority, not all have, and this includes the UK government. Pollock and Price (2000, 2003) argue that, through WTO and GATS, welfare entitlements might be redefined in a system driven by multinationals seeking to extract substantial profits. However, an attempt by the European Union (the so-called Bolkestein directive) to introduce liberalization of service provision in the internal market met with opposition, and subsequently public services such as health care were excluded. Whatever the long-term outcome of such discussions, this analysis implies that we have to redefine the focus of our attention towards international entities and regulatory frameworks. Clarke (2004) suggests that we once regarded social policy as taking place primarily within national boundaries. In a longer historical perspective British health care provision has moved from being the domain of local charitable initiatives and of local government, in the pre-NHS era, to the responsibility of nation-states during the Keynesian era. Now, while funding remains a public responsibility, provision seems set to be, to a growing extent, opened up to multinational capital (see Mohan (2002) for the case of hospital policy).

Progressive privatization? Social enterprise, foundation trusts and the new mutualism

If the NHS is to be reconfigured as a competitive market, is it inevitable that it will be one dominated by large-scale commercial providers of care? The government do have an alternative, although it might be described as the iron fist of the market encased in the velvet glove of community ownership. The government's preferred approach is to see the ownership of hospitals returned to local communities through the establishment of NHS foundation trusts, and the emergence of a large number of 'social enterprises' providing health care locally. The justification for these policies arguably originated in the writings of commentators such as Paul Hirst (1994) about associative democracy. Hirst, and others, argued that the 'idea that the welfare systems prior to neoliberalism were a roaring success in terms of delivery and client satisfaction was simply misplaced' (Brown *et al.* 2000: 6). The policy response proposed by Hirst was therefore to decentralize and pluralize the state, and to use competition as a spur to innovation. If, in the process, the outcome were to be a greater degree of inequality in access to services, this trade-off is accepted as a price to be paid for local control (see the debate between Hirst (1999) and Stears (1999)). The creation of stand-alone entities competing with each other for NHS business was part of this agenda and was defended as an element in the move away from allegedly unresponsive one-size-fits-all hierarchical and centralized models of health care provision. The establishment of NHS foundation trusts from 2004 signalled governmental determination to free hospitals from the shackles of centralized chains of accountability, but the government insisted that these did not constitute privatization since there were caps on the commercial activities of foundation trusts. In relation to social enterprise, the 2006 White Paper, *Our Health, Our Care, Our Say* (Department of Health 2006a), articulated the government's vision, particularly in the field of community care. Units to promote social enterprises have been set up in the Department of Health, and the establishment of the cross-departmental Office of the Third Sector signals the government's determination to expand the scope for provision of public services through voluntary bodies and social enterprises. What might be the outcome of these initiatives? For insights we can examine historical precedents, and we can consider contemporary research on the role of non-profits in health care delivery.

On the former point, government spokesmen have insisted that their proposals are consistent with a tradition of pluralist socialism which would have been very familiar to, and endorsed by, the founders of the NHS. Former Health Minister Hazel Blears argued that in the pre-NHS era 'local people had . . . provided the money and support to develop and maintain the hospital. The sense of affiliation felt for their local hospital was developed through a form of funding and governance that provided people with a real local relationship' (Blears 2002: 11). Blears refers here to the hospital contributory schemes, mass subscription schemes of a quasi-insurance kind designed to support individual hospitals or groups of hospitals. The schemes certainly provided a vehicle for voluntarism and citizen involvement, but beyond a relatively small number of activists, most contributors were passive participants, regarding the schemes as 'a tolerable nuisance in default of a better organisation of hospital service' (Gorsky *et al.* 2006: 152). Moreover, the relationship which the schemes had with the hospitals shows that they achieved relatively little in terms of wresting the control of hospitals away from professional elites. So, despite a large-scale membership, the extent to which these enhanced community participation and control was debatable.

Turning to the present day, the early development of foundation trusts does not suggest great enthusiasm for participation (Gorsky 2006; Lewis *et al.* 2006).

Furthermore, the dominant tradition in Labour politics in the 1930s favoured a local government health service, so, historically, it is not strictly accurate to suggest that the party preferred a mixed economy of welfare dominated by mutuals and voluntary organizations. This is to say nothing of the substantial inequalities that existed in a health care system which did not have the capacity for risk-pooling a service funded through direct taxation (Mohan 2003), nor is it to mention the problems of collective action and competition that characterized the voluntary hospitals and their principal funders, the contributory schemes. Any revived mutualism would need to develop strong regulatory structures to avoid the re-emergence of such difficulties. In this context, much will depend on the external competitive environment.

This brings us to the lessons of contemporary research on the role of non-profits in health care delivery. The literature on the role of non-profits in health care delivery reveals some disquieting results. Far from non-profit ownership being a guarantee of the social purpose of an organization, it is clear that, as predicted many years ago by DiMaggio and Powell (1983) institutional isomorphism occurs, so that organizations have to mimic their competitors in order to survive. In a fiercely competitive marketplace, this means that non-profits will adopt strategies that are very hard to distinguish from those of the commercial competitors. The consequence, in relation to health care, has been that non-profits have found it difficult to compete, and that there are few discernible differences between non-profits and commercial entities on questions of outcome or quality of care. If it is the case that social enterprises and non-profits are launched into a market that is red in tooth and claw, consideration must be given to how they will be able to compete successfully. Without protection in the start-up phase, the likelihood is that they will fail. This is particularly so given the strong probability that, according to those already involved in social enterprises, commercial firms are approaching the NHS marketplace with a substantial 'war chest' in order to help them attract new business (Marks and Hunter 2007), while there are already concerns about the ability of GPs to compete with big business (Arie 2006).

However much we might like to believe that the establishment of a plurality of providers will be associated with the revival of a public service ethos, the reality is more likely to be that social enterprises and non-profits will struggle to get established at the margins while large-scale, multinational corporations will cherry pick the most profitable contracts. For historical precedent we need to look only at the fate of the British non-profit hospital sector after 1948, when the growing involvement of American multi-nationals from the 1970s onwards squeezed out the remaining British non-profits (Griffith *et al.* 1987); within the UK voluntary sector the reality at the moment is a concentration of contract funding in larger, established organizations (Reichardt *et al.* 2008).

In short, although many people would argue that such forms of privatization have what David Donnison (1985) regarded as progressive potential, the regulatory environment into which new initiatives will be born will allow limited space for their growth and development. If individual patient choice is the driver of innovation and efficiency, it is difficult to reconcile this with the long-term financial planning that might be thought necessary to allow social enterprise to flourish. A more plausible scenario is therefore one in which established commercial entities cream off possibilities for profit-making while social enterprises struggle to pick up crumbs from the table. The extent to which the government has granted commercial organizations preferred bidder status on very favourable terms for the provision of services such as ISTCs indicates the likely direction of policy. Furthermore, there is also a suspicion that the real aim is the fragmentation of a bloc of support for collectivism by creating a multiplicity of competing, self-interested entities, thereby weakening collective bargaining and union resistance. Although third sector advocacy groups, such as the Association of Chief Executives of Voluntary Organisations (ACEVO), insist that third sector provision is not primarily about cost-cutting, investigations of terms and conditions of service point towards a different conclusion (Davies 2007, 2008).

Whatever the outcome, sociology has to come to terms with a multiplicity of new organizational forms. These rather oxymoronic entities – can something be enterprising if it's social, or social if it's enterprising? – are difficult to categorize and the challenge is in exploring the tensions between the social and the enterprising. On some definitions, an organization can be characterized as a social enterprise if it does not distribute more than 50 per cent of its profits to shareholders, and if it pursues a public purpose such as the delivery of health care. On this definition it is not surprising that Leadbeater (2007) characterizes Nuffield Hospitals as a social enterprise, but this seems debatable, given the fees charged by such private hospital chains. More generally, what are the system-wide implications of these developments? For example, will it be possible to have a genuinely national service provided by this plethora of enterprises, mutuals, co-ops, and multinationals, and what trade-offs are going to be involved? These enterprises will operate in circumstances not of their own choosing, and there is consequently much to be done regarding how they will operate, their organizational structures and the working relationships within them, and the circumstances in which they may or may not flourish.

A second point concerns the question of how far it is possible to expand the capacities of the social enterprise sector beyond a small number of success stories. The literature keeps coming back to a small number of examples of high-profile initiatives. As Mulgan (2006) acknowledged in a commentary on social enterprise research, the literature is anecdotal and hagiographical;

many publications and reports concentrate on individual case studies and success stories, particularly when discussing innovations. To what extent can these be reproduced elsewhere? We need to know more about the conditions in which they get established in the first place and what contributes to their continued success.

Conclusions: fatal remedies

How are we to interpret the developments in the privatization of health care over the past decade? Can we speak of a strategy designed deliberately to shift the NHS in a particular direction, a blueprint or master plan? In this scenario the NHS would become merely a brand, a kite mark for a range of services provided by a mix of public and private organizations. Would this matter? It could certainly be argued that this would lead to fragmentation, and it is ironic that former government strategists such as Chris Ham (2008) now recognize the risks of applying market forces uncritically in health care. Drawing on the insights of economists Coase and Williamson – insights which were available well before the first wave of market-led reforms in Britain in 1991 – Ham has implied that while contestable markets might have their place in planned care, the real challenges the NHS faces are in the treatment of chronic conditions, where a much greater degree of integration is required. He therefore argues for models of integrated care in the latter case, though it is ironic that his source of inspiration on integration is American practice, in the form of Health Maintenance Organizations (HMOs) such as Kaiser Permanente, despite criticisms of the applicability of that particular model of health care in a British context (Talbot-Smith *et al.* 2004). The forms of market segmentation implied in that system are consistent with a market-led division of labour, and therefore can be seen not as a way in which states maintain commitments to welfare, by making the welfare state work more efficiently, but rather as the harbinger of privatization, which shifts the basis of access away from need and towards the ability to pay.

However, alternative scenarios are possible here. Thus, as Fougere (2001) put it, marketization might fuel private sector growth and therefore strip the public sector of the political and economic resources it requires to satisfy its diverse publics; an alternative is a 'boomerang' scenario, in which markets produce such disquiet and complaint that a hierarchical regime is reborn. Despite the distress signals over the effects of market forces, exemplified through the election of anti-hospital closure candidates to councils and even to parliament, or legal challenges to the outsourcing of public services, there is no sign of the rebirth of old-style planning (the recent announcement of a reconsideration of the ISTC programme was swiftly followed by a continued push on the outsourcing of primary care commissioning, for example). A third outcome, and one where I think Fougere is optimistic, concerns the potential of reform for new ways of organization. He drew inspiration from work on regional governance and development which has emphasized progressive models of social organization, based on decentralized innovation and collective learning, processes of mutual comparison and flexible adaptation from the bottom up. However, critics (e.g. Lovering 1999) would argue that such models of the associational economy (Cooke and Morgan 1998) overestimate the extent to which such models of production incorporate egalitarian social relationships and exaggerate the extent to which they can be transported to a UK context. Translated into the NHS this would imply a very optimistic view of the potential of social enterprises; a culture of mutual learning was not, for example, evident in responses from Marks and Hunter's (2007) social enterprise interviewees, who wished to protect their own innovative ideas from emulation for fear of loss of competitive advantage.

There are dangers here, and they are far more significant than minor shifts in the public–private boundary. Some critics believe that an uncritical reliance on market forces and individual choice is not consistent with Labour's social aims of governing for the many, not the few. They also worry that in opening up the NHS to commercial organizations, the government risks pressures from multinational capital to open up the whole process of purchasing health care to the private sector and redefining entitlements. One can detect, for example, rhetoric implying a move away from provision based on need, as in commissioning guidance to primary care trusts, which emphasizes that they should 'bear down on differences in health seeking behaviour' (Department of Health 2006b, quoted in Pollock and Price 2006: 566). It is also possible to envision – as in the contractual arrangements for APMS – a redefinition of the NHS into a 'core service that can be topped up with locally negotiated additional elements provided by corporations (Pollock and Price 2006: 565). In both of these scenarios, the formerly open-ended commitments of the NHS to providing care at the point of need are circumscribed. In summary, New Labour has not made a principled defence of the way in which the NHS has successfully delivered care, that is, in a decommodified form. Instead the government have simply said they are committed to a tax-funded NHS but indifferent to the precise mode of service delivery. Policy adaptations are based not on principled accommodation that leaves space for the pursuit of equality through different means, but rather by an 'acceptance' that necessitates a pre-emptive value shift that is glossed over by a vague commitment to social justice (Page 2007). In this process, the introduction of the remedies of competition, markets and private enterprise may be fatal to the ideals of the NHS.

Acknowledgements

I am grateful to the editors of this volume for their forbearance and suggestions for improvement, and I would particularly like to acknowledge the comments of Sally Ruane on an earlier version of this chapter.

Notes

1 The source for these figures is a list of individual PFI contracts, available at the following (regularly-updated) site: http://www.hm-treasury.gov.uk/ppp_pfi_stats. htm
2 For an example of the possibilities, see the following description of the Heart of Birmingham health trust's 'franchising strategy', which pointed to the lessons to be learned from such private sector exemplars as ASDA, Tesco, Virgin and McDonalds: www.telegraph.co.uk/news/uknews/1569187/GP-surgeries-%27 could-be-run-by-Tesco-or-Virgin%27.html

References

Aldred, R. (2007) 'Closed policy networks, broken chains of communication and the stories behind an "entrepreneurial policy": the case of NHS Local Improvement Finance Trust (NHS LIFT)', Critical Social Policy, 27: 131–51.

Aldred, R. (2008) 'NHS LIFT and the new shape of neo-liberal welfare', Capital and Class, summer.

Arie, S. (2006) 'Can GPs compete with big business?' British Medical Journal, 332, 1172–3.

Bambra, C. (2005) 'Worlds of welfare and the healthcare discrepancy', Social Policy and Society, 4: 31–42.

Bevan, A. (1952) In Place of Fear, London: Heinemann.

Blears, H. (2002) 'Mutualism and the development of the National Health Service', in Hogan, S. (ed.) Making Healthcare Mutual: a publicly funded, locally accountable NHS, London: Mutuo.

Brown, K., Kenny, S. and Turner, B. (2000) Rhetorics of Welfare: uncertainty, choice and voluntary associations, Basingstoke: Palgrave.

Clarke, J. (2004) Changing Welfare, Changing States: new directions in social policy, London: Sage.

Cooke, P. and Morgan, K. (1998) The Associational Economy, Oxford: Oxford University Press.

Davies, C. (1987) 'Things to come: the NHS in the next decade', Sociology of Health and Illness, 9: 302–17.

Davies, S. (2007) Third Sector Provision of Local Government and Health Services, London: UNISON.

Davies, S. (2008) 'Contracting out employment services to the third and private sectors: a critique', Critical Social Policy, 28: 136–64.

Department of Health (2006a) Our Health, Our Care, Our Say: a new direction for community services, London: HMSO.

Department of Health (2006b) 'Supporting practice based commissioning in 2007/08 by determining weighted capitation shares at practice level'. Online: www.dh.gov.uk/en/Publicationsandstatistics/Publications/PublicationsPolicyAnd Guidance/DH_4127155.

DiMaggio, P. and Powell, W. (1983) 'The iron cage revisited: institutional isomorphism and collective rationality in organisational fields', American Sociological Review, 48: 147–60.

Donnison, D. (1985) 'The progressive potential of privatisation', in J. Le Grand and R. Robinson (eds) Privatisation and the Welfare State, London: Allen and Unwin.

Dunnigan M.G. and Pollock, A.M. (2003) 'Downsizing of acute inpatient beds associated with the private finance initiative', *British Medical Journal*, 326: 905–8.

Farnsworth, K. (2006) 'Capital to the rescue? New Labour's business solutions to old welfare problems', *Critical Social Policy*, 26: 817–42.

Feachem, R., Sekhri, N. and White, K. (2002) 'Getting more for their dollar: a comparison of the NHS and California's Kaiser Permanente', *British Medical Journal*, 324: 135–43.

Finlayson, G. (1994) *Citizen, State and Social Welfare in Britain 1830–1990*, Oxford: Clarendon Press.

Foubister, T., Thomson, S., Mossialos, E., and McGuire, A. (2006) *Private Health Insurance in the UK*, Trowbridge: Cromwell Press.

Fougere, G. (2001) 'Transforming health sectors: new logics of organising in the New Zealand health system', *Social Science and Medicine*, 52: 1233–42.

Gaffney, D. and Pollock, A.M. (1999). 'Pump-priming the PFI: why are privately financed hospital schemes being subsidized?' *Public Money and Management*, 19: 55–62

Gaffney D., Pollock, A.M., Price, D. and Shaoul, J. (1999a) 'The politics of the private finance initiative and the new NHS', *British Medical Journal*, 319: 249–53.

Gaffney, D., Pollock, A.M., Price, D. and Shaoul, J. (1999b) 'PFI in the NHS – is there an economic case?' *British Medical Journal*, 319: 116–19.

Gaffney, D., Pollock, A.M., Price, D. and Shaoul, J. (1999c) 'NHS capital expenditure and the private finance initiative – expansion or contraction?' *British Medical Journal*, 319: 48–51.

Gorsky, M. (2006) 'Hospital governments and community involvement in Britain: evidence from before the NHS', *History and Policy*, paper 40. Online: www.historyandpolicy.org/papers/policy-paper-40.html.

Gorsky, M., Mohan, J. and Willis, T. (2006) *Mutualism and Health Care: British hospital contributory schemes during the 20th century*, Manchester: Manchester University Press.

Griffith, B., Iliffe, S. and Rayner, G. (1987) *Banking on Sickness: commercial medicine in Britain and the USA*, London: Lawrence and Wishart.

Ham, C. (2008) 'Competition and integration in the English NHS', *British Medical Journal*, 336: 805–7.

Harrington, J. (2007) 'Law, globalisation and the NHS', *Capital and Class*, 92: 81–106.

Hay, C. (1998) 'Globalisation, welfare retrenchment and "the logic of no alternative"', *Journal of Social Policy*, 27: 525–32.

Hay, C. and Watson, M. (2003) 'The discourse of globalisation and the logic of no alternative: rendering the contingent necessary in the political economy of New Labour', *Policy and Politics*, 31: 289–315.

Healthcare Commission (2007) *Independent Sector Treatment Centres: a review of the quality of care*, London: Healthcare Commission.

Hirst, P. (1994) *Associative Democracy*, Cambridge: Polity.

Hirst, P. (1999) 'Associationalist welfare: a reply to Marc Stears', *Economy and Society*, 28: 590–7.

Holden, C. (2005) 'The internationalisation of corporate healthcare: extent and emerging trends', *Competition and Change*, 9: 201–19.

Holden, C. and Farnsworth, K. (2006) 'The business-social policy nexus: corporate power and corporate inputs into social policy', *Journal of Social Policy*, 35: 473–94.

Kearney, M. (2002) 'Unhealthy accumulation: the globalisation of healthcare privatisation', *Review of Social Economy*, 60: 331–57.

King, D. and Mossialos, E. (2005) 'The determinants of private health insurance prevalence in England, 1997 to 2000', *Health Services Research*, 40: 195–212.

Klein, K. (1984) 'The politics of ideology and the reality of politics: the case of Britain's health service in the 1980s', *Milbank Memorial Fund Quarterly*, 62: 2–109.

Laing and Buisson (various dates) *Laing's Health Care Market Review*, London: Laing and Buisson.

Le Grand, J.(2006) 'A better class of choice', *Public Finance*, 31 March.

Leadbeater, C. (2007) *Social Enterprise and Social Innovation: strategies for the next ten years*, London: Office of the Third Sector.

Lewis, R., Hunt, P. and Carson, D. (2006) *Social Enterprise and Community-based Care: is there a future for mutually-owned organisations in community and primary care?* London: Kings Fund.

Leys, C. (2001) *Market-driven Politics*, London: Verso.

Lovering, J. (1999) 'Theory led by policy: the inadequacies of the "new regionalism"', *International Journal of Urban and Regional Research*, 23: 379–95.

Mackintosh, M. and Koivusalo, M. (2005) 'Health systems and commercialisation: in search of good sense', in M. Mackintosh and M. Koivusalo (eds) *Commercialization of Health Care: global and local dynamics and policy initiatives*, Basingstoke: Palgrave.

Marks, L. and Hunter, D. (2007) *Social Enterprise and the NHS: changing patterns of ownership and accountability*, London: Unison.

Mohan, J. (1991) 'Privatisation in the British health sector: a challenge to the NHS?' in J. Gabe, M. Calnan and M. Bury (eds) *The Sociology of the Health Service*, London: Routledge.

Mohan, J. (1995) *A National Health Service?* London: Macmillan.

Mohan, J. (2002) *Planning, Markets and Hospitals*, London: Routledge.

Mohan, J. (2003) 'Voluntarism, municipalism and welfare: the geography of hospital utilization in England in the 1930s', *Transactions, Institute of British Geographers*, 28: 55–74.

Mohan, J. (2008) *Charging Ahead Regardless? The Labour government, NHS charges, and co-payments for health care*, MS submitted for publication.

Mulgan, G. (2006) 'Cultivating the other invisible hand of social entrepreneurship: comparative advantage, public policy, and future research priorities', in A. Nicholls (ed.) *Social Entrepreneurship: new models of successful social change*, Oxford: Oxford University Press.

Needham, C. (2003) *Citizens and Consumers: New Labour's marketplace democracy*, London: Catalyst.

Page, R. (2007) 'Without a song in their heart: New Labour, the welfare state and the retreat from Democratic Socialism', *Journal of Social Policy*, 36: 19–37.

Paton, C. (1997) 'The politics and economics of health care reform', in C. Altensteter and W. Bjorkman (eds) *Health Policy Reform: national variations and globalisation*, Basingstoke: Macmillan.

Paton, C. (2006) *New Labour's State of Health: political economy, public policy and the NHS*, Aldershot: Ashgate.

Player, S. and Leys, C. (2008) *Confuse and Conceal: the NHS and independent sector treatment centres*, London: Merlin Press.

Polanyi, K. (2001 [1944]) *The Great Transformation: the political and economic origins of our time*, New York: Basic Books.

Pollard, S. (2008) 'Beyond the matron state', *The Guardian*, 3 July. Online www.guardian.co.uk/commentisfree/2008/jul/03/nhs.health.

Pollock, A. (2004) *NHS plc: the privatisation of our health care*, London: Verso.

Pollock, A. and Price, D. (2000) 'Rewriting the regulations: how the World Trade Organisation could accelerate privatisation in healthcare systems', *The Lancet*, 356: 1995–2000.

Pollock, A. and Price, D. (2003) 'The public health implications of world trade negotiations on the General Agreement on Trade in Services and public services', *The Lancet*, 362: 1072–5.

Pollock, A. and Price, D. (2006) 'Privatising primary care', *British Journal of General Practice*, 56: 565–6.

Pollock, A.M., Price, D., Viebrock, E., Miller, E. and Watt, G. (2007) 'The market in primary care', *British Medical Journal*, 335: 475–7.

Pollock, A.M., Shaoul, J. and Vickers, N. (2002) 'PFI and "value for money" in NHS hospitals', *British Medical Journal*, 324: 1205–9.

Powell, M. (1996) 'Granny's footsteps, fractures and the principles of the NHS', *Critical Social Policy*, 16: 27–44.

Powell, M. (1999) 'New labour and the third way in the British NHS', *International Journal of Health Services*, 29: 353–70.

Rayner, G. (1986) 'Health care as a business: the emergence of a commercial hospital sector in Britain', *Policy and Politics*, 14: 439–59.

Rayner, G. (1987) 'Lessons from America? Commercialization and growth of private medicine in Britain', *International Journal of Health Services*, 17: 197–216.

Reichardt, O., Kane, D., Pratten, B. and Wilding, K. (2008) *The UK Civil Society Almanac 2008*, London: NCVO.

Ruane, S. (1997) 'Public-private boundaries and the transformation of the NHS', *Critical Social Policy*, 51: 53–78.

Ruane, S. (2000) 'Acquiescence and opposition: the private finance initiative in the NHS', *Policy and Politics*, 28: 411–24.

Ruane, S. (2002) 'Public-private partnerships – the case of PFI', in C. Glendinning, M. Powell and K. Rummery (eds) *Partnerships, New Labour and the Governance of Welfare*, Bristol: Policy Press.

Salmon, J. (1995) 'A perspective on the corporate transformation of healthcare', *International Journal of Health Services*, 25: 11–42.

Seale, C. (2008) 'Mapping the field of medical sociology: a comparative analysis of journals', *Sociology of Health and Illness*, 30: 677–95.

Stears, M. (1999) 'Needs, welfare and the limits of associationalism', *Economy and Society*, 28: 570–89.

Stevens, S. (2005) 'The NHS works', *Prospect*, 107.

Talbot-Smith A., Gnani, S., Pollock, A.M. and Pereira Gray, D. (2004) 'Questioning the claims from Kaiser', *British Journal of General Practice*, 54: 415–21.

Timmins, N. (2005) 'Challenges of private provision in the NHS', *British Medical Journal*, 331: 1193–5.

Tudor Hart, J. (1971) 'The inverse care law', *The Lancet*, 1: 405–12.

Tudor Hart, J. (2006) *The Political Economy of Health Care: a clinical perspective.* Bristol: Policy Press.

Whitfield, D. (2001) *Public Services or Corporate Welfare: rethinking the nation state in the global economy*, London: Pluto.

Wistow, G. (1989) 'Offloading responsibilities for care', in R. Maxwell (ed.) *Reshaping the NHS*, Oxford–New Brunswick: Transaction Books.

5 The pharmaceutical industry, the state and the NHS

John Abraham

Introduction: core sociological dimensions and terrain

In analysing medicine in the NHS, medical sociologists have typically focused on conventional debates about the proletarianization[1] and de-professionalization[2] of health professionals via managerialism of the capitalist state and consumerism, respectively (Elston 1991). A key concern is the impact of those processes on medical dominance and doctors' clinical autonomy. Yet those discussions are limited to the interactions between the medical profession, patients and NHS managers (Annandale 1998: 223–50; Britten 2001). The wider context that shapes or challenges medical dominance needs to be scrutinized by going beyond the terms of these traditional debates to include the roles of the pharmaceutical industry, the state, the courts, and the media (Gabe and Bury 1996). In this chapter, I hope to demonstrate why medical sociology should break into fresh and exciting areas of theoretical synthesis and empirical enquiry by diversifying away from fixation on medical dominance to consider the relationships between the pharmaceutical industry, state agencies and patient organizations. This is important because such relationships can significantly affect NHS patients and professionals.

I take a comprehensive approach, tracing the relationships between the pharmaceutical industry, the state, and the NHS from the creation of the Health Service to the present as they have grappled with the key issues of pharmaceutical safety, efficacy, cost-effectiveness, pricing, promotion and advertising. To examine these relationships, medical sociology needs to expand its horizons into areas of political economy in order to synthesize a 'political sociology of medicine' that conceptualizes the interactions of the state with various organized interests and is capable of examining how those organized interests are related to ideology and real health interests (Abraham 2002a).

In the first section, I show that from the NHS's inception, its interests diverged from those of the pharmaceutical industry, and that this was well known by the government. I argue that, because the pharmaceutical industry was so important to the post-war UK capitalist economy, these tensions were resolved by establishing a 'corporate bias' permitting the industry privileged access to, and influence over, the state, not afforded to any other interest group. In the next two sections, I explain how such corporate bias has unmistakably manifested itself in the emergence, conceptualization and implementation of drug safety, efficacy and pricing regulation. The industry and the state have recruited medical experts to serve their interests in safety and efficacy regulation, but it is the dominance of industry interests and commercial power, often so coveted by the state and senior medical experts, to the exclusion of public accountability, that commands attention, rather than medical dominance per se. Corporate bias in the negotiation of NHS prices is so extreme that the price-setting system is based on the profitability of the manufacturing firm and is completely insensitive to the therapeutic value of the drug to NHS doctors and patients.

Having discussed regulations ensuring that all NHS drugs are more efficacious than placebo, I turn to the 'rational' and cost-effective prescribing of efficacious drugs. Here, I suggest that the state has at times asserted its own interests, independently of the industry and in conflict with it, especially with the creation of a national cost-effectiveness assessment institute. Doctors' concerns about clinical autonomy have been salient in this context and proletarianization theory may have some purchase. However, the power of the industry to use the courts, gain priviliged access to government, and mobilize alliances of organized groups of patients and health professionals has arguably been more important in frustrating the state's rationalization objectives, and in re-directing them in line with industry interests – what political sociologists call 'regulatory capture' (Abraham 1995a).

Traditionally, medical sociology has developed the concept of 'medical-ization' – the making of the 'social' medical, such as the definition of various behaviours as a medical condition known as attention-deficit-hyperactivity-disorder (ADHD). To complement 'medicalization', in the final section, I introduce the new concept of 'pharmaceuticalization', which I define as the process by which social, behavioural or bodily 'conditions' are treated, or deemed to be in need of treatment, with medical drugs by doctors (or patients). I argue that the response of the state to doctors' apparent irrational prescribing, and to the demands of patients to access new drugs on the NHS has to be understood by reference to pharmaceuticalization and what Sklair (1991) calls the 'culture-ideology of consumerism' that facilitate such prescribing and demands.

A nationalized health service and a private pharmaceutical industry: the early post-war period

With the introduction of the NHS in 1948, health care became nationalized and placed predominantly in the public sector, but the pharmaceutical industry remained in the private sector, for better or worse. Many of the complex relationships between the pharmaceutical industry, the state, and the NHS stem from that initial decision to keep the industry in the private sector. For example, there is the fact that the NHS has to purchase its medicines from an industry that largely controls the direction of drug development, and seeks maximization of prices and profits to meet its commercial objectives. Consequently, the state has had to become involved in the regulation, rather than direction, of the industry with respect to drug safety, efficacy, cost-effectiveness, profits, pricing and advertising.

With the NHS, the benefits of free medical care were extended to the whole population and the government footed the bill (Bruce 1961). Consequently, the number of prescriptions to be paid for by the government trebled (Public Record Office (PRO) 1951). In addition, many companies sought to replicate potent therapeutic breakthroughs such as penicillin, creating a plethora of equally powerful drugs (Mann 1984). Industrial promotion of drugs to doctors intensified with consequent increases in drug prescribing, while the large research-based firms used patents to command high monopoly prices for their drugs (Silverman and Lee 1974: 8–80).

Thus, very soon in the life of the NHS, the cost and value-for-money of drugs purchased by the Service became a significant issue. In 1949 the Ministry of Health (MoH) established the Joint Committee on Prescribing (JCP) to consider restricting NHS doctors from prescribing 'medicines of doubtful value' or 'unnecessarily expensive brands of standard drugs' (HMSO 1950: 4). The Ministry's review of drug legislation found that:

> a major cause of the proprietary [NHS] drug bill is the prescription of duplicate or doubtful medicines following skillful propaganda from the drug firms to the doctors in the service, and in some cases following advertising to the public which in turn results in pressure on the doctor by the patient.
>
> (PRO 1951)

Meanwhile, the MoH issued a circular asking doctors not to prescribe brand name preparations unless 'satisfied that a standard [generic] drug cannot be prescribed with equal effect' (PSGB 1950a). The Association of the British Pharmaceutical Industry (ABPI) was anxious about the Ministry's plans to rationalize drug prescribing because the NHS was the industry's largest customer and too much standardization of the home trade could damage the industry's export capabilities (PSGB 1950b). These were particularly influential arguments because recovery of the post-war UK economy was led by the export boom of the sectors that had done well during the war, including the pharmaceutical industry (Aldcroft 1986: 1–43; PSGB 1956a).

In private meetings and correspondence with the MoH, the ABPI, supported by the government's Board of Trade, argued that it was undesirable for the JCP to publish a report which classified drugs therapeutically because such a list would be used to keep British products out of foreign markets (PRO 1950a, 1950b, 1950c). For the cost-cutting benefit of the

NHS, the JCP lists were published, but discreetly (PRO 1950d). Nonetheless, corporate bias had been established. For the rest of the decade, the industry and its allies in the Board of Trade persuaded the MoH that the export trade of the pharmaceutical industry was so precious that further rationalization of the NHS drug supply should be avoided (PSGB 1954; PSGB 1956b).

Safety and efficacy regulation for NHS drugs: protecting industry interests

For the first twenty-three years of the NHS there was no systematic scientific testing and regulatory oversight of new medicines coming into use by the service, even though, in 1962, government expert advisers estimated that more than half were not correctly clinically tested (PSGB 1962a, 1962b). Drug safety and efficacy regulation was not introduced until 1971 when the 1968 Medicines Act came into effect. A national drug regulatory agency, the Medicines Division within the Department of Health (DoH), with a full-time scientific staff was formed to review the manufacturers' data on new drugs. It was empowered to permit (or deny) approval of those drugs on to the British market according to various techno-scientific criteria. Even under the Medicines Act, initially, 'old' drugs that had entered the market before 1971 could continue to be used in the NHS without meeting such criteria. There were 36,000 medicinal products in this category, of which 4,000 were prescription drugs (Binns 1980). It was not until a 1975 EEC directive requiring all medicines to be reviewed according to modern licensing standards, that the DoH set up a committee to assess the safety and efficacy of these 'old' drugs – a task not completed until 1990, nearly thirty years after the Thalidomide disaster and over forty years into the life of the NHS (Abraham 1995a).

It is often supposed that the Thalidomide disaster provoked the government to step in to protect public safety with the Medicines Act. However, the slowness in the introduction of the Medicines Act – ten years after Thalidomide – indicates many factors other than Thalidomide were at work in the evolution of modern drug regulation (Abraham 1995a: 80–5). That evolution is better understood as the culmination of a long negotiating process between the industry and the state about how best to restore public confidence in drugs and the pharmaceutical industry. Those negotiations reveal that protection of industry interests was paramount in formulating safety and efficacy regulation (PSGB 1962c; Wheeler 1964).

In 1964, the government established the Committee on Safety of Drugs (CSD), who reviewed data submitted to them by pharmaceutical firms, and advised the manufacturers and the government on whether new drugs were safe enough to go on the market. While its members were not employed by the industry, they were permitted to have direct and/or indirect financial interests in pharmaceutical companies, such as shareholdings and/or research grants, respectively (PSGB 1963a). From the outset, the CSD declared that industry data submitted to it and its deliberations about drug safety were confidential. Thus, the CSD was sealed off from public scrutiny and accountability (PSGB 1963b). Simultaneously, the Committee's regulatory review was deliberately rapid (averaging less than three months) so as not to 'exercise a detrimental effect on pharmaceutical research progress by unduly delaying the introduction of a possibly valuable drug or even by preventing its use altogether' (PSGB 1967). Such extensive concern for industry interests was not without impact on the protection of patients, as a former member of the CSD explained:

> Looking back I see only one major error in our performance. We were so aware of the enormous cooperation that we received from the drug industry that the main Committee made every effort it could to see that submissions from firms were handled as rapidly as possible – as a result ... the Adverse Reactions subcommittee and ... the work of that subcommittee suffered.
>
> (Wade 1983)

The CSD served as a prototype for the formalized safety regulation of the 1968 Medicines Act. While the Act went beyond arrangements associated with the CSD, three crucial regulatory principles associated with the CSD continued beyond its demise: close involvement of industry interests; 'light-touch' (i.e. speedy) regulatory review; and *secrecy* of decision making. These reflect the corporate bias endemic to safety and efficacy regulation.

Close involvement of industry interests is illustrated by the fact that many members of CSD's successor, the Committee on Safety of Medicines (CSM), who advised the DoH on the safety and efficacy of all new drugs, and the new Medicines Commission, who advised the government on the membership of the CSM, were permitted to have financial interests in pharmaceutical firms (Collier 1985; Delamothe 1989). Indeed, in May 1969, the pharmaceutical industry was invited to discuss with the DoH the Medicines Commission's functions, structure and membership (ABPI 1970). Regarding regulatory review, the government assured industry that the new regulatory regime under the Medicines Act was to aim for a 'CSD type' speed of administration, and that, with some of its members drawn from industry, it was unlikely that the Medicines Commission would limit the introduction of new products by being unduly exacting (PSGB 1968a, 1968b, 1970). Noting the medical profession's dependence on the industry's well-being, the chairman of the new Medicines Commission warned that laws to assure drug safety and efficacy should not impose unnecessary restraints on the industry's prosperity (PSGB 1968b). Meanwhile, *secrecy* increased. Section 118 of the 1968 Medicines Act made it a criminal offence for the Medicines Division and all expert advisers involved in UK drug regulation to divulge any information about the medicines licensing process to the public without government authorization.

After the Medicines Act, NHS doctors and patients could be confident that new drugs were tested for safety and efficacy (more effectiveness than placebo in controlled trials). In addition, doctors were brought into the regulatory system via the 'yellow card' post-marketing surveillance scheme, which asked doctors to report to the DoH on a voluntary basis all suspected adverse drug reactions (ADRs) they observed in clinical practice. The scheme was supposed to enable the CSM to track ADRs associated with each new drug on the market. It was intended to provide an early warning system about dangerous drugs that had slipped through pre-market testing and regulatory review. However, doctors reported, and continue to report, less than 10 per cent of ADRs (Lumley *et al.* 1986; Medawar and Hardon 2004: 154; Millar 2001; Walker and Lumley 1987). Corporate bias ensured that regulatory interventions which were more effective in protecting public safety (but less favourable to industry interests), such as much more rigorous pre-market regulatory review and restricted release of new drugs on to the market, were dismissed.

Neither the yellow card system nor the pre-market safety testing introduced under the Medicines Act prevented thousands of NHS patients being severely injured or killed by the betablocker, Practolol, and the anti-arthritis drug, Opren – the two largest drug disasters in the UK in the 1970s and 1980s, respectively. Neither of these drugs, which possessed modest efficacy at best, were therapeutic breakthroughs. Furthermore, more rigorous pre-market testing and regulatory assessment could have given much more weight to their toxicity and adverse reactions. For example, US regulators refused to approve Practolol on to their market and the Swedish authorities withheld marketing approval for Opren (Abraham 1995a: 98–178; Abraham and Davis 2006).

Despite these disasters, weak regulation persisted and the pharmaceutical industry continued to press for more rapid (and arguably even weaker) regulatory review throughout the 1980s. This was often accompanied by the threat that ostensibly onerous regulation would cause 'early developmental work on new drugs to go abroad to the detriment of British industry and UK departments of pharmacology' – a perspective eventually adopted by the UK regulators themselves (Griffin and Long 1981). In response, the government decided to take up the pharmaceutical industry's suggestion that manufacturers would pay the cost of regulatory review in exchange for a more 'efficient service', by which was meant more rapid approval (Scrip 1988a). Previously the Medicines Division had been funded 65 per cent by licensing application fees from the pharmaceutical industry and 35 per cent by the government via taxes (Scrip 1988b). Following this review, in 1989, the Medicines Division was abolished and reconstituted as the Medicines Control Agency (MCA), which was to be entirely funded by industry fees – further consolidating corporate bias. In effect, the MCA came to be run as a business selling its regulatory services to the industry and promoting itself as the fastest licensing authority in the world for new drugs (Scrip 1991).

Supporters of this new arrangement argued that it saved taxpayers' money which could be diverted into the NHS, while government and industry claimed that important new drugs would reach NHS patients faster. On the other hand, the drug regulatory agency's complete reliance on pharmaceutical industry fees for its income might compromise its independence, making it vulnerable to industry demands for rapid regulatory review that minimized checks on the safety and efficacy of NHS drugs. The optimistic proposition that comprehensive industry funding would lead to increased access to the new drugs needed by NHS patients has proven to be false. The number of new drug innovations and the number of new drugs offering significant therapeutic advance have both fallen in the decade from the early 1990s (Abraham and Davis 2007; Abraham and Reed 2002). Regarding regulatory checks, until mid-1988, about ten drug product licences were suspended or revoked by the Medicines Division on average per year. Yet over the next three years no drug lost its licence until Upjohn refused to withdraw Halcion (Abraham and Sheppard 1999).

Moreover, major drug safety problems affecting many thousands of NHS patients continued under the funding regime of the MCA and its successor (since 2003), the Medicines and Health-care-products Regulatory Agency (MHRA). Many of these were investigated in an eight-month inquiry by the UK Parliament's House of Commons Health Committee (HCHC) into 'The Influence of the Pharmaceutical Industry' in 2005 – the world's longest and most wide-ranging legislative scrutiny of the pharmaceutical sector ever to take place. Just as the yellow card system failed to warn of safety problems with Practolol in the 1970s, it failed to detect the dangers of the anti-arthritis drug, Vioxx, which was introduced into the NHS in 1999. It is estimated that Vioxx may be associated with tens of thousands of heart attacks and strokes in the US (Topol 2004). However, between 1999 and 2004, when Vioxx was withdrawn worldwide, the yellow card scheme recorded just six heart attacks in 1999, nine in 2000, seven in 2001, five in 2002, seven in 2003, and four in 2004, even though the number of UK prescriptions rose from 162,600 in 1999 to 2,128,600 in 2003 (HCHC 2005: 31).

The HCHC also heard that, since the early 1990s, severe withdrawal reactions and suicidality had occurred among many patients taking anti-depressants, known as selective serotonin re-uptake inhibitors (SSRIs). For ten years, the manufacturers of these drugs and the MCA asserted that it was rare for patients taking them to experience withdrawal reactions. However, in 2003, after an expert working group of the MHRA went public with its more thorough review of the evidence, the manufacturers and the regulators revised their risk estimate upwards from 'rare' to '25 to 30 per cent' (HCHC 2005: 81–8). The MHRA's expert working group also published warnings about the use of SSRIs by children, but only some years after concerns about the association of suicidality with these drugs was first raised (HCHC 2005: 86).

Profiting from the NHS: the price of the state's conflicting objectives

Even adjusting for inflation, the NHS's expenditure on pharmaceuticals has continued to rise. According to the government's Office of Fair Trading (OFT), by 2007 the NHS annual spend had grown to £8 billion on brand name drugs and had an overall drugs bill of £11 billion (OFT 2007: 9). Apart from increases in the number of prescriptions (associated with an ageing population), the main reason for the rising NHS drugs bill is the high prices of pharmaceuticals. The average price of drugs purchased by the NHS has risen annually by between 7 and 13 per cent since 1980, mainly because of newly introduced pharmaceuticals that are very highly priced, heavily promoted and frequently prescribed.

The pharmaceutical industry's influence over NHS drug prices is dominant. The prices of branded medicines are controlled by a voluntary arrangement between the government's DoH and the pharmaceutical industry, known as the Pharmaceutical Price Regulation Scheme (PPRS). It controls prices indirectly by controlling companies' profits, so the price of a new drug at launch is entirely a matter for the company concerned (ABPI 1993). Under the scheme, it is acceptable for companies to be within 40 per cent above or below their annual targets, but profits more than 40 per cent above are deemed excessive and supposed to be corrected either by the company reducing its prices or making a repayment of the excess to the government (HCHC 2005: 34–5). The PPRS was first introduced in 1957 and is renegotiated periodically by the government and by the ABPI (usually every five years). The overall official objectives of the PPRS are to:

- secure the provision of safe and effective medicines for the NHS at reasonable prices;
- promote a strong and profitable pharmaceutical industry capable of sustained R&D expenditure.

As such, regulation of NHS drug prices reflects corporate bias in both conception and negotiation.

The PPRS has been maintained for over fifty years, but its objectives (above) are fundamentally conflicting (Sainsbury Committee 1967: 51). For example, each company is allowed to set drug promotion costs against sales to estimate profits. By claiming large promotion costs, companies can provide estimates of relatively small profits enabling to them to charge high prices to the NHS (HCHC 1994: xvi). Thus, the PPRS encourages companies' drug promotion of new branded drugs, even though such promotion is one of the drivers of the growing NHS drugs bill. Moreover, if a company's profits are more than 40 per cent below the agreed target, it may apply to the government to increase its drug prices. Hence, if the NHS is successful in persuading GPs and hospitals to prescribe more generics instead of expensive brand name drugs, then the manufacturers of the brand name products are entitled to increase the price of their products to the NHS.

Furthermore, the operation of the PPRS relies on companies' estimates of their expenditure on R&D. Yet claims about the average cost of R&D for drugs vary at least five-fold (McIntyre 1999). Transnational pharmaceutical companies may artificially inflate their research costs by pretending to charge themselves a lot for cheap chemicals imported from foreign subsidiaries – a practice known as 'transfer pricing' (Collier 1989: 118–20). In 1983, the government's Comptroller and Auditor General found that the DoH lacked the resources to check on individual companies (Public Accounts Committee 1983). Even if one accepts the PPRS estimates of companies' promotion, R&D and profits, problems of enforcement are extensive. From 1988–91, about two-thirds of the major pharmaceutical suppliers to the NHS made excessive profits, but of these, an average of just one company each year was required to make price reductions (HCHC 1994: xviii).

In the 2004 PPRS renegotiations, the ABPI and DoH agreed a 7 per cent price reduction for branded prescription medicines purchased by the NHS in exchange for favourable incentives for the industry's R&D. The government claimed that this would save the NHS £1.8 billion over five years (BBC News 24 2004). Yet in 2007, the government's Office of Fair Trading (OFT 2007: 2–5) concluded that the NHS was still paying at least £500 million per year too much for brand-name prescription drugs, and some NHS drugs were priced at ten times the cost of equally beneficial alternatives. The OFT (2007) recommended that pharmaceutical pricing should be directly linked to drugs' therapeutic value to NHS patients, rather than to the financial cost of industry research and promotion. In early 2008, the government entered into dialogue with the ABPI with the intention of cutting the NHS drugs bill by a further 10 per cent annually – about £1 billion per year (BBC News 24 2008).

Clinical autonomy, industry influence and the interests of the state: from 'rational' prescribing to cost-effectiveness at NICE

Until the mid-1980s, NHS GPs could prescribe virtually whatever medicines they pleased, confident that the health service would foot the bill. This began to change in 1984 when Kenneth Clarke, the Minister of Health, introduced a Limited List of medicines, which implied that approximately 1,800 preparations would no longer be paid for by the NHS. The List encouraged rational prescribing since nearly all the medicines excluded were therapeutically unimportant. Nevertheless, the pharmaceutical industry, some of whose products would lose a major market, led a fierce campaign against the Limited List, gaining the support of the British Medical Association (BMA) and the Labour Party (Medawar 1992: 176–80). In

1986, the government gave ground by establishing the Selected List – a 'watered down' Limited List.

The 1986 Selected List pertained to just seven therapeutic categories, but in 1992 it was extended to others, including: benzodiazepines; drugs for allergic disorders; drugs for vaginal and vulval conditions; contraceptives; drugs used in anaemia; topical anti-rheumatics; drugs acting on the ear and nose; and drugs acting on the skin. This was of sociological and policy significance because it established the principle that the central state, advised by expert medical scientists, could dictate to doctors which drugs of proven efficacy were prescribable on the NHS. For the first time, therapeutically efficacious drugs could be ineligible for prescription on the NHS because there existed other efficacious drugs with greater cost-effectiveness (HCHC 1994: xxiv–xxv). This was hardly proletarianization of the medical profession, but it was the state asserting its own interests.

For many GPs, this list represented an unacceptable curtailment of their right to exercise unfettered clinical judgement, and might even prevent patients from receiving the most appropriate treatment. As for the industry, it claimed that the list acted as a disincentive to pharmaceutical firms to undertake research within the therapeutic categories covered by the list, thereby undermining the prospect of new treatments for patients with those conditions (HCHC 1994: xxv–xxvi). However, as the government pointed out, there was no evidence that long-established local hospital formularies[3] had had any negative effect on pharmaceutical innovation, and doctors' clinical 'freedom' should not extend to prescribing drugs on the NHS for which there existed more cost-effective alternatives (DoH 1994a). Furthermore, the UK government's Audit Commission reported that more rational prescribing could save the NHS over £400 million per year (Audit Commission 1994).

The government's attempts to control NHS prescribing centrally began to unravel when Secretary of State for Health Frank Dobson tried to limit doctors' prescription of Viagra – the first successful oral treatment for erectile dysfunction. When it was approved onto the US market in March 1998, it was prescribed at a rate of 20,000 per day (Anon. 1998a; Anon. 1998b). With marketing approval in the UK immanent, the NHS faced the implications for public health provision of having to pay for millions of Viagra prescriptions (Anon. 1998c; Anon. 1998d).

Hence, in September 1998, the DoH sent a circular to NHS doctors advising them not to prescribe Viagra 'save in exceptional circumstances' (Anon. 1999a). However, Pfizer, the manufacturers of Viagra, sucessfully challenged the legality of the circular in the courts in May 1999. The judge's verdict demonstrated to the government that the Selected List alone was an insufficient mechanism for achieving cost-effective NHS prescribing because it failed to take account of the possibility that a new therapy could be uniquely clinically effective but very poor value for money. Consequently, in April 1999, the government established the National Institute of Health and Clinical Excellence (NICE), which was to review evidence and make scientifically robust national recommendations to doctors and the NHS about therapeutically efficient and cost-effective prescribing. The DoH let it be known that it expected NICE recommendations to be followed 'to the letter' (Anon. 1999b).

For many medical sociologists, these controversies over the eligibility of drug prescribing on the NHS were part of a 'battleground over clinical autonomy' between the state and NHS doctors (Britten 2001). On this view, at stake is whether such increased managerialism by the state amounts to proletarianization. However, there are clearly other relevant issues worthy of note, such as: the extent to which the state has asserted it own interests in conflict with industry on this particular issue; the fact that it was the power of industry opposition in campaigns and in the courts to deconstruct policies more than any other factor that has driven the state to develop such strong convictions for robust decision making and the establishment of NICE. Seen in this light, sociological understanding of the 'battleground over clinical autonomy' is enriched. The fate of clinical autonomy depends not merely on the managerialist tendencies of the state, but also on a balance and inter-action of interests, especially the extent to which the pharmaceutical industry allies itself with either the medical profession or the state – as recently acknowledged by Britten (2008: 178–81).

NICE: regulatory capture, corporate bias or protecting the NHS?

The formal aims of NICE are: 'to promote clinical excellence and the effec-tive use of available resources in the NHS . . . to promote the appropriate use of those interventions which offer good value to patients and to discour-age the use of those which do not . . . [and] to ensure that, it is sympathetic to the longer term interest of the NHS in encouraging innovation of good value to patients' (NICE 1999). It is vitally important to pharmaceutical companies that NICE recommends their products for use in the NHS because the health service comprises the lion's share of the prescription drug market in the UK.

In October 1999, NICE recommended that GlaxoWellcome's influenza drug Relenza should not be used in the NHS because it was likely to reduce the duration of symptoms by only one day, and there was insufficient evidence about the drug's effects in 'at risk' groups (Anon. 2001a). GlaxoWellcome responded by leading protests in the media and beyond which, joined by other pharmaceutical companies, included threats to move pharmaceutical laboratories out of the UK (BBC online 1999). In November 2000, NICE issued new guidance on Relenza recommending the drug for use in 'at risk' individuals based on new evidence prepared by the manufacturer. However, three months later, the *Drugs and Therapeutics Bulletin* (*D&TB*), a highly respected publication among NHS doctors, questioned whether there had been any change in the scientific evidence-base to support NICE's altered guidance (BBC online 2001). The public controversy over Relenza left many doctors and NHS managers with the impression that 'maybe NICE had made a change in response to major political pressure from the media and the drug industry' (HCHC 2002: 9–11).

In the case of Relenza, the question of whether NICE was undergoing 'regulatory capture' was the salient matter, not clinical autonomy. The government's handling of whether beta-interferon should be prescribed on the NHS for the treatment of multiple sclerosis (MS) raised similar issues. MS is a disabling degenerative neurological disease affecting over 85,000 people in the UK (Crinson 2004). In 1995, just before beta-interferon was licensed in the UK, the DoH was concerned that treatment of all MS patients with the expensive beta-interferon would have cost 10 per cent of the entire NHS drugs budget (New 1996). For this reason, beta-interferon was one of the first drugs to be assessed by NICE, whose preliminary appraisal in July 2000 was that the drug should not be funded by the NHS (Anon. 2001b). On hearing this, the pharmaceutical manufacturers, MS patient groups, consultant neurologists and the Royal College of Nursing appealed against NICE's preliminary assessment (Crinson 2004). Having considered these appeals, in November 2001, NICE reiterated that beta-interferon was not cost-effective for the NHS, though the Institute's final appraisal guidance report was not published until 4 February 2002 (NICE 2002).

Meanwhile, the DoH negotiated a 'risk-sharing scheme' with the pharmaceutical manufacturers (Biogen, Teva-Aventis and Serono) that would see NHS funding for beta interferon prescriptions as if NICE had given a positive recommendation (DoH 2002). The government presented the risk-sharing scheme as clinical research intended to confirm the cost-effectiveness of the drug via post-market monitoring, but it lacked many of the scientific standards of a clinical trial (Sudlow and Counsell 2003). From late 2002, the government's scheme imposed a statutory obligation upon local health authorities and NHS Trusts to fund the prescribing of beta-interferon. In return, the manufacturers agreed to reduce slightly the cost of the drug to the NHS (Crinson 2004). In this case, the established norm of corporate bias within the state reasserted itself as a mechanism for by-passing an institute over-zealous about protecting the interests of the NHS, making the institute more vulnerable to regulatory capture.

Such vulnerability is accentuated because the institute has neither routine access to relevant unpublished data nor the right to make public all the unpublished data it consults (HCHC 2002, 2005). There is no legal requirement on pharmaceutical manufacturers to supply NICE with all the relevant information about drugs under assessment. NICE can readily review all the relevant published data/evidence, but, consistent with corporate bias, its access to unpublished data depends on whether the drug companies and/or the MHRA are willing to provide such data. This was revealed most dramatically in 2003 when NICE concluded that SSRI antidepressants were safe for children from a review of the published evidence, but after reviewing the unpublished data as well, reached the opposite conclusion. Furthermore, even when pharmaceutical firms and/or the MHRA offer unpublished data, it is often supplied in confidence. Consequently, part of the evidence basis for NICE's decisions may lack transparency and accountability to other interests, including NHS doctors and patients.

By 2002, NICE had recommended the vast majority (twenty-eight out of thirty-one) of the treatments and interventions (mostly pharmaceuticals) it had appraised either for routine or selected use with a net financial impact on the NHS of *increased* costs of £135–£155 million (Sadler and Dent 2002). This raises the question of whether NICE's objective to be 'sympathetic to the longer term interest of the NHS in encouraging innovation' may have shaped the institute's priorities in the interests of commercial sponsors of research, such as the pharmaceutical industry, possibly at the expense of its other objectives. In this respect, NICE's efforts to protect the interests of the NHS have been visited by the corporate bias endemic to UK government–industry relations.

Pharmaceuticalization, consumerism and ideology

As the UK government acknowledged as early as 1951 (see above), pharmaceutical advertising and promotion are part of the ideological context that facilitates irrational prescribing and patient demand for drugs (Lexchin 1993). Promotion and advertising are huge and growing, but are, in effect, self-regulated by the industry in the UK (HCHC 2005: 58). Such regulation is entirely responsive and retrospective, rather than preventative. For example, in April 2002, Schering ran a problematic advertisement about its product Yasmin, which the *Drugs and Therapeutic Bulletin* (*D&TB*) publicly declared was misleading in August 2002. Initially, Schering threatened to sue *D&TB*, but withdrew this threat after the Advertising Authority, prompted by *D&TB*'s complaint, found the advertisement to have breached regulations on eleven counts in November 2002. It was not until February 2003 that the company was forced to withdraw the advertisement and publish a corrective statement – 10 months after the product had been on prescription by NHS doctors (HCHC 2005: 62–3).

Probably more influential on NHS doctors, however, are the more subtle aspects of drug promotion involving the integration of senior members of the medical profession and medical science into pharmaceutical marketing strategies. Pharmaceutical companies pay medical experts grants/ consultancies to be involved in the development of their products and then fund them to act as 'opinion leaders', who speak favourably about the drug at medical symposia and edit special supplements of journals reporting positive findings about the drug in collaboration with scientists and 'medical writers' employed by the manufacturer (Abraham 1994a; HCHC 2005: 54–7; Healy 2006). These companies may also hire public relations firms to create an exaggerated, favourable media and professional reception for a research article showing their drug in a positive light, while delaying publication of findings that reveal problems with the drug (Abraham 1994b, 1995b). Frequently, 'negative' findings about drugs are not published at all, leading to a systematic bias in medical literature read by NHS doctors (HCHC 2005: 55–6; Lexchin *et al.* 2003). Pharmaceuticalization is also facilitated by drug companies' strategies to contain criticism. This may involve: withdrawal of funding from institutions that provide platforms for the critics' views; attempts to prevent further publication of critics' data; or using experts supportive of the company to undermine critics' concerns about the product (Abraham 2002b; Abraham and Sheppard 1999; Healy 2004).

Sometimes pharmaceuticalization and medicalization go hand in hand. For example, doctors' prescribing of pharmaceuticals may increase because of widening diagnostic criteria regarding conditions for which new drugs are emerging or for which existing drugs may be 're-packaged' for a new market (Conrad and Potter 2000). Such medicalization by the psychiatry profession partly explains why, between 1993 and 2002, NHS prescriptions in England for SSRIs to treat depression grew from 1,884,571 to 15,500,000, and for Ritalin to treat ADHD grew from 3,500 to 161,800 (American Psychiatric Association 1994; DoH 1994b, 2003). Supporters of such pharmaceuticalization argue that it reflects advances in medical science which enable people 'with' ADHD and depression, who would previously have gone undiagnosed, to be treated (Castellanos 2002; Harding 2001). However, case studies from sociology, and beyond, suggest that pharmaceuticalization, including industry-sponsored 'disease awareness campaigns' aimed at doctors and patients via expert opinion leaders, has exaggerated the benefits and neglected the serious adverse effects of tranquillizers and antidepressants (Abraham and Sheppard 1999; Gabe 1991; Healy 2004; HCHC 2005: 69–70; Medawar 1992; Medawar and Hardon 2004).

Gabe and Bury (1996), however, argue that, regarding drug safety, 'expert systems', such as medical associations and opinion leaders, have become 'chronically contested' by lay publics in the courts and the media. They draw attention to a 'rise in consumerism' and a 'fracturing' of medical expertise in the context of reflexive modernization. While an increase in the critical reflexivity and expertise of consumers is undeniable, it is possible for this to have occurred simultaneously with an even greater increase in homogenization, oligopolization and corporatization of medical expertise within the medical association–industry–government complex – an increase that is in the interests of the pharmaceutical industry, and at the expense of consumer/patient interests (Abraham and Lewis 2002). Insofar as medical expertise is embedded in, and/or recruited in the service of, the interests of the government–industry complex, then it follows that power is not necessarily shifting from medical dominance to consumers/patients, even if there is increasing visibility of some medical experts supporting the interests of consumers/patients. This could explain the meagre success of citizen activism in battles against pharmaceutical companies over safety and drug injury to patients (Abraham 1994b; Abraham and Sheppard 1999; HCHC 2005: 65–6).

In fact, the analysis of Gabe and Bury (1996) seems much more salient to recent cases in which patients and patient groups have campaigned for quicker access to new drugs on the NHS. For example, a few months after a US trial in May 2005 with women suffering from early-stage breast cancer reported promising results with Roche's drug Herceptin, two women with such cancer threatened their NHS Trusts with litigation in the national media because the Trusts would not fund their treatment with the drug. Even though Herceptin had not even been licensed as safe and efficacious by the MHRA, let alone recommended as cost-effective for the NHS by NICE, one of the Trusts backed down after being undermined on television by the secretary of state for health in October 2005, while the other had its decision over-ruled in a high-profile court case in April 2006 (BBC News 24 2006a).[4] Similarly, in March 2005, NICE recommended that four drug treatments licensed for Alzheimer's disease (Aricept, Exelon, Reminyl and Ebixa) should not be funded by the NHS because they were not cost-effective. However, following a high-profile media campaign and a formal appeal involving patient groups, such as the Alzheimer's Society, NICE revised its guidance to allow NHS funding for people with moderate stages of the disease, but not those with early-stage Alzheimer's (BBC News 24 2007). Subsequently, in 2008, contrary to NICE, the courts ruled that it was 'unfair' to deny people with early-stage Alzheimer's access to these drugs on the NHS.

It is significant that all these successful cases of consumer activism have involved patient groups seeking access to drugs, in alliance with pharmaceutical manufacturers. In the case of Herceptin, the activism itself may have been marshalled by Roche who, after publication of the promising US trial, hired a public relations firm to contact some women in the UK with breast cancer to ask them if they would be willing to help to get the drug funded on the NHS before NICE, or even MHRA, approval (BBC News 24 2006b). Regarding the campaign for access to Alzheimer's drugs, the manufacturers were the lead claimants in the court cases and centrally involved in the formal appeal to NICE – as also occurred with the MS Society campaign for access to beta-interferon (BBC News 24 2007). The evidence suggests that the apparent power of patient activism to challenge medical expertise may significantly depend on whether it is supporting or contravening the fundamental interests of the pharmaceutical industry. While patients' demands for new drugs can result from their own independent, real health interests, the sociological significance of the apparent challenges from consumerism, and associated media coverage, should not be over-stated because many such challenges may largely reflect the power of the pharmaceutical industry's ideological devices.

Moreover, many patient organizations that campaign for availability of better treatments for various medical conditions, are increasingly funded by pharmaceutical companies (O'Donovan 2007). These organizations may be very different from the collectivities involved in litigation against drug manufacturers cited by Gabe and Bury (1996) and Abraham and Lewis (2002). Such close associations are clearly important to the industry as an additional pathway, beyond doctors, for creating consumer demand for their products via what the drug firms call 'patient education' (HCHC 2005: 74–6; Herxheimer 2003).

The industry wants to take such 'patient education' further by direct-to-consumer advertising (DTCA) of prescription drugs – a practice currently illegal in the EU, though permitted in the US and New Zealand. In campaigning for DTCA, the industry has used the discourse of the 'expert patient' to characterize patients as consumers able to decide which drugs are best for themselves.[5] Some medical sociologists have accepted this discourse at face value, casting the debate about DTCA in terms of empowerment of lay patients versus expert 'medical dominance' (Fox *et al.* 2005). However, such discussions lack any analysis of the interests involved and, remarkably, ignore the evidence of widespread problems for patients' health and NHS resources posed by misleading advertisements to doctors, let alone patients. The 'expert patient' discourse needs to be put in its proper sociological context by relating it to the interests of those planning to provide the 'information' intended to construct 'patient expertise' and the ideological nature of its emergence. Seen in this light, apparently the industry wishes to use patient groups as a means of de-regulation and market expansion, without regard to wider health interests (Medawar and Hardon 2004: 121).

Perhaps in tune with New Labour's liberal individualist tendencies, the DoH (2001) also adopted the concept of 'expert patient' uncritically as it agreed in 2004 to double the number of drugs to be reclassified from prescription-only medicine (POM) to over-the-counter (OTC) status annually (HCHC 2005: 88–9). This recommendation came not from patients or consumers, but from the government-industry Pharmaceutical Industry Competitiveness Task Force (PICTF), whose overall aim is to ensure that the UK is an attractive location for the pharmaceutical industry. The policy accelerated the pace at which NHS patients could be turned into 'retail' consumers of pharmaceuticals. It is in the interests of the state because OTC medicines are not reimbursed by the NHS; they are out-of-pocket private consumer purchases. Thus, while such 'consumerism' is unlikely to be in the interests of consumers/patients, it helps pharmaceutical manufacturers to market more of their products directly to NHS patients because there is no ban on DTCA for OTC drugs (Abraham 2007).

Conclusion

In its dealings with the pharmaceutical industry, the state has not served the NHS and its patients well. Because of corporate bias, regulation of drug safety, efficacy and pricing have been consistently weak, slow to develop, and subject to repeated cycles of crisis or disaster as a result of an apparent incapacity to learn lessons from the past and reform. This is why, during a period of about half a century, the state has failed to protect NHS patients from 'subsequent Thalidomides', such as Practolol, Opren and Vioxx, and to insist that pharmaceutical prices for the NHS are linked to therapeutic value. The maintenance of the PPRS is testimony to the reluctance of the state to develop a price-control system that better protects the interests of the NHS over and above the trade interests of the pharmaceutical industry.

The state has asserted its own interests in efficient use of NHS resources for drug prescribing. That managerialism has brought it into multi-dimensional conflicts with doctors, patients and the pharmaceutical industry that are not solely about curtailment of clinical autonomy or proletarianization; they are also about industry interests and the capacity of the state to withstand industry power to organize campaigns and court challenges. Much of NICE's work has been forthright in attempting to protect the interests of the NHS, but it has been vulnerable to regulatory capture because of its objective to be sympathetic to industry innovation, its lack of control over unpublished industry data, and corporate bias in other more powerful parts of the state.

Regarding NHS prescribing, pharmaceuticalization, which has been encouraged by many medical professional associations and has expanded doctors' prescribing horizons, may be more significant than medical sociology's traditional preoccupation with curtailment of clinical autonomy (and alleged proletarianization). Moreover, acceptance of the consumerist discourse of 'expert patients' as if a reflection of 'patient demand', runs the risk of mis-identifying pharmaceuticalization as de-professionalization, and of failing to distinguish between strategies of industry/government to advance their interests and the interests of patients and health. If it is to avoid unwitting ideological reproduction, medical sociology needs to recognize the ideological nature of this discourse and to scrutinize how the industry and the state create pharmaceutical consumerism.

The growing activism and media visibility of patients do not necessarily imply a shift of power in their favour in terms of either de-professionalization of doctors or challenges to the medical expert–industry–state complex because of countervailing consolidations of the latter away from the media spotlight. Patient groups have had some success when allied with pharmaceutical companies, but such consumerism is largely limited by patient groups functioning as new marketing strategies putting pressure on regulators to approve products quickly. Consider the fact that the 'expert patient' discourse developed to support DTCA of prescription drugs never once mentioned the need to correct the current situation in which the industry and the state withhold from NHS patients and citizens extensive information about drug safety and efficacy in order to protect the commercial interests of pharmaceutical companies. Evidently, patients' 'expertise' is to be formed from the information that the pharmaceutical industry and the government choose to make available. Thus, it may be that the promotion of 'expert patients' should not be regarded as 'lay empowerment', but rather at least partly as an ideological fusion of corporate bias and consumerism.

Notes

1　According to the proletarianization thesis, the medical profession is gradually being stripped of control over its terms and conditions of work and absorbed into the mass of workers (the proletariat) under the logic of capitalist expansion.
2　Deprofessionalization theory implies that the medical profession's authority and monopoly over knowledge is being eroded by the emergence of a more educated populace.
3　Local hospital formularies are lists recommending which drugs doctors working in the hospital should or should not prescribe.
4　In summer 2006, *Herceptin* was licensed for treatment of early-stage breast cancer by the MHRA and recommended for use in the NHS by NICE (BBC News 24 2006b).
5　The concept 'expert patient' dates back to at least the mid-1980s in US discussions of patient self-care (Taylor and Bury 2007).

References

Abraham, J. (1994a) 'Negotiation and accommodation in expert medical risk assessment and regulation', *Policy Sciences*, 27: 53–76.
Abraham, J. (1994b) 'Bias in science and medical knowledge', *Sociology*, 28: 717–36.
Abraham, J. (1995a) *Science, Politics and the Pharmaceutical Industry*, London: UCL Press.
Abraham, J. (1995b) 'The production and reception of scientific papers in the medical-industrial complex', *British Journal of Sociology*, 46: 167–90.
Abraham, J. (2002a) 'Do we need a political sociology of medicine?', paper presented at British Sociological Association Medical Sociology Conference, York, 8 September.
Abraham, J. (2002b) 'Transnational industrial power, the medical profession and the regulatory state', *Social Science and Medicine*, 55: 1671–90.
Abraham, J. (2007) 'Neo-liberal corporate bias as a framework for understanding UK pharmaceuticals regulation', *Social Theory and Health*, 5: 161–75.
Abraham, J. and Davis, C. (2006) 'Testing times', *Social History of Medicine*, 19: 127–47.
Abraham, J. and Davis, C. (2007) 'Interpellative sociology of pharmaceuticals: problems and challenges for innovation and regulation in the 21st century', *Technological Analysis and Strategic Management*, 19: 387–402.
Abraham, J. and Lewis, G. (2002) 'Citizenship, medical expertise and the capitalist regulatory state in Europe', *Sociology*, 36: 67–88.

Abraham, J. and Reed, T. (2002) 'Progress, innovation and regulatory science', *Social Studies of Science*, 32: 337–69.

Abraham, J. and Sheppard, J. (1999) *The Therapeutic Nightmare*, London: Earthscan.

Aldcroft, D.H. (1986) *The British Economy*, Sussex: Harvester.

American Psychiatric Association (1994) *Diagnostic and Statistical Manual of Mental Disorders*, Arlington: APA.

Annandale, E. (1998) *The Sociology of Health and Medicine*, Cambridge: Polity.

Anon. (1998a) 'Viagra breaks all records in the US', *Scrip*, 2331: 20.

Anon. (1998b) 'US insurers turn down Viagra citing lack of safety data', *Scrip*, 2351: 14.

Anon. (1998c) 'Viagra recommended for EC approval', *Scrip*, 2338/39: 36.

Anon. (1998d) 'No Viagra reimbursement in EU?', *Scrip*, 2351: 3.

Anon. (1999a) 'UK rules DoH Viagra circular unlawful', *Scrip*, 2441: 4.

Anon. (1999b) 'No flexibility in UK NICE advice', *Scrip*, 2439: 6.

Anon. (2001a) 'Why not zanamivir?' *Drugs and Therapeutics Bulletin*, 39: 9–10.

Anon. (2001b) 'Effectiveness, efficiency and NICE', *British Medical Journal*, 322: 934–44.

Association of the British Pharmaceutical Industry (ABPI) (1970) 'Legislation: Medicines Commission', *ABPI Annual Report*, 1969–70: 9.

ABPI (1993) *A Guide to the Pharmaceutical Price Regulation Scheme*, London: ABPI.

Audit Commission (1994) *A Prescription for Improvement*, London: HMSO.

BBC News 24 (2004) 'Billion-pound price cut won for NHS medicine bill', *news.bbc.co.uk*, 3 November (accessed online 20 July 2008).

BBC News 24 (2006a) 'Woman wins Herceptin court fight', *news.bbc.co.uk*, 12 April (accessed online 20 July 2008).

BBC News 24 (2006b) 'Herceptin: was patient power key?' *news.bbc.co.uk*, 9 June 2006 (accessed online 20 July 2008).

BBC News 24 (2007) 'Alzheimer's drugs remain limited', *news.bbc.co.uk*, 10 August (accessed online 20 July 2008).

BBC News 24 (2008) 'Ministers seek to cut NHS drugs budget', *news.bbc.co.uk*, 7 January (accessed online 20 July 2008).

BBC online (1999) 'Drug companies join flu protest', *news.bbc.co.uk*, 6 October (accessed online 20 July 2008).

BBC online (2001) 'Guidance over anti-flu drug "wrong"', *news.bbc.co.uk*, 15 February (accessed online 20 July 2008).

Binns, T.B. (1980) 'The Committee on the Review of Medicines', *British Medical Journal*, 281: 1614–15.

Britten, N. (2001) 'Prescribing and the defence of clinical autonomy', *Sociology of Health and Illness* 23: 478–96.

Britten, N. (2008) *Medicines and Society*, Basingstoke: Palgrave.

Bruce, M. (1961) *The Coming of the Welfare State*, London: Batsford.

Castellanos, X. (2002) 'Development trajectories of brain volume abnormalities in children and adults with ADHD', *Journal of the American Medical Association*, 288: 1740–48.

Collier, J. (1985) 'Licensing and provision of medicines in the UK', *Lancet*, 326: 377–80.

Collier, J. (1989) *The Health Conspiracy*, London: Century.

Conrad, P. and Potter, D. (2000) 'From hyperactive children to ADHD adults', *Social Problems*, 47: 559–82.

Crinson, I. (2004) 'The politics of regulation within the "modernized" NHS', *Critical Social Policy*, 24: 30–49.

Delamothe, T. (1989) 'Drug watchdogs and the drug industry', *British Medical Journal*, 299: 151–52.

Department of Health (DoH) (1994a) *The NHS Drugs Budget Cm2683*, London: HMSO.

DoH (1994b) *Prescription Cost Analysis*, London: Government Statistical Service.

DoH (2002) *Cost Effective Provision of Disease Modifying Therapeis for People with Multiple Sclerosis*, London: TSO.

DoH (2001) *The Expert Patient*, London: HMSO.

DoH (2003) *Prescription Cost Analysis*, London: Government Statistical Service.

Elston, M. (1991) 'The politics of professional power', in J. Gabe, M. Calnan and M. Bury (eds) *The Sociology of the Health Service*, London: Routledge.

Fox, N.J., Ward, K.J. and Rourke, A.J. (2005) 'The "expert patient"', *Social Science and Medicine*, 60: 1299–309.

Gabe, J. (ed.) (1991) *Understanding Tranquilliser Use*, London: Routledge.

Gabe, J. and Bury, M. (1996) 'Halcion nights', *Sociology*, 30: 447–69.

Griffin, J.P. and Long, J.R. (1981) 'New procedures affecting the conduct of clinical trials in the UK', *British Medical Journal*, 283: 481.

Harding, R. (2001) 'Unlocking the brain's secrets', *Family Circle*, 20 November: 10–11.

Healy, D. (2004) *Let Them Eat Prozac*, London: New York University Press.

Healy, D. (2006) 'The new medical oikumene', in A. Petryna, A. Lakoff and A. Kleinman (eds) *Global Pharmaceuticals*, London: Duke University Press.

Herxheimer, A. (2003) Relationships between the pharmaceutical industry and patients' organizations', *British Medical Journal*, 326: 1208–10.

HMSO (1950) *The Second Interim Report of the Joint Committee on Prescribing*, London: HMSO.

House of Commons Health Committee (HCHC) (1994) *The NHS Drugs Budget*, London: HMSO.

HCHC (2002) *National Institute for Clinical Excellence*, London: TSO.

HCHC (2005) *The Influence of the Pharmaceutical Industry*, London: TSO.

Lexchin, J. (1993) 'Interactions between physicians and the pharmaceutical industry', *Journal of the Canadian Medical Association*, 149: 1401–7.

Lexchin, J., Bero, L.A., Djulbegovic, B. and Clark, O. (2003) 'Pharmaceutical industry sponsorship and research outcomes and quality', *British Medical Journal*, 326: 1167–70.

Lumley, C.E., Walker, S.R. and Hall, G.C. (1986) 'The under-reporting of adverse drug reactions seen in general practice', *Pharmaceutical Medicine*, 1: 205–12.

Mann, R.D. (1984) *Modern Drug Use*, Lancaster: MTP Press.

McIntyre, A. (1999) *Key Issues in the Pharmaceutical Industry*, Chichester: John Wiley.

Medawar, C. (1992) *Power and Dependence*, London: Social Audit.

Medawar, C. and Hardon, A. (2004) *Medicines out of Control?* Amsterdam: Askant.

Millar, J.S. (2001) 'Consultations owing to adverse drug reactions in a single practice', *British Journal of General Practice*, 51: 130–1.

New, B. (1996) 'The rationing agenda in the NHS', *British Medical Journal*, 312: 1593–601.

NICE (1999) *National Institute for Clinical Excellence: Framework Document*, London: DoH.

NICE (2002) *Beta Interferon and Glatiramer Acetate for the Treatment of Multiple Sclerosis*, London: DoH.

O'Donovan, O. (2007) 'Corporate colonization of health activism?' *International Journal of Health Services*, 37: 711–33.

Office of Fair Trading (2007) *The Pharmaceutical Price Regulation Scheme: an OFT market study*, London: OFT.

Pharmaceutical Society of Great Britain (PSGB) (1950a) 'Annual report of the ABPI', *Pharmaceutical Journal*, 164: 301.

PSGB (1950b) 'Pharmaceutical industry and export drive', *Pharmaceutical Journal*, 164: 11.

PSGB (1954) 'ABPI annual dinner', *Pharmaceutical Journal*, 172: 312.

PSGB (1956a) 'Recruitment by the industry', *Pharmaceutical Journal*, 176: 1.

PSGB (1956b) 'British pharmaceutical industry', *Pharmaceutical Journal*, 176: 239.

PSGB (1962a) 'Clinical trials of drugs', *Pharmaceutical Journal*, 188: 429.

PSGB (1962b) 'Drug toxicity', *Pharmaceutical Journal*, 189: 523–4.

PSGB (1962c) '"Magnificent" export performance', *Pharmaceutical Journal*, 189: 445.

PSGB (1963a) 'Committee on Safety of Drugs: members and terms of reference', *Pharmaceutical Journal*, 190: 534.

PSGB (1963b) 'Committee on Safety of Drugs: memo to manufacturers and importers', *Pharmaceutical Journal*, 191: 433.

PSGB (1967) 'Safety of drugs', *Pharmaceutical Journal*, 199: 59–60.

PSGB (1968a) 'The Medicines Bill in committee', *Pharmaceutical Journal*, 200: 334–45.

PSGB (1968b) 'Medicines Bill', *Pharmaceutical Journal*, 200: 368–89.

PSGB (1970) 'Medicines Act reassurance for manufacturers', *Pharmaceutical Journal*, 204: 48.

Public Accounts Committee (1983) *Dispensing of Drugs in the NHS*, London: HMSO.

Public Records Office (PRO) (1950a) MH133/76 Note of discussion on 8 June between MoH and ABPI.

PRO (1950b) MH133/76 Memorandum from J.S. Walmsley, Secretary of the PAGB to the MoH regarding the Second Interim Report of the JCP, 14 June.

PRO (1950c) MH133/76 Letter from Sir J.H. Woods, Board of Trade, to Sir William Douglas, MoH, 20 July.

PRO (1950d) MH133/76 Letter, Sir William Douglas to Sir J. Woods, Board of Trade, 28 July.

PRO (1951) MH58/688 Review of Drug Legislation.

Sadler and Dent (2002) 'From guidance to practice – why NICE is not enough', *British Medical Journal*, 324: 842–5.

Sainsbury Committee (1967) *Report of the Committee of Enquiry into the Relationship of the Pharmaceutical Industry with the National Health Service*, Cmnd 3410, London: HMSO.

Scrip (1988a) *World Pharmaceutical News*, 1279: 3.

Scrip (1988b) *World Pharmaceutical News*, 1270: 24.

Scrip (1991) *World Pharmaceutical News*, 1635: 2.

Silverman, M. and Lee, P.R. (1974) *Pills, Profits and Politics*, Berkeley: California U.P.

Sklair, L. (1991) *Sociology of the Global System*, London: Harvester.

Sudlow, C. and Counsell, C. (2003) 'Problems with UK government's risk sharing scheme for assessing drugs for multiple sclerosis', *British Medical Journal*, 326: 388–92.

Taylor, D. and Bury, M. (2007) 'Chronic illness, expert patients and care transition', *Sociology of Health and Illness*, 29: 27–45.

Topol, E.J. (2004) 'Failing the public health – rofecoxib, Merck, and the FDA', *New England Journal of Medicine*, 351: 1707–9.

Wade, O.L. (1983) 'Achievements, problems and limitations of regulatory bodies', in D. Farrell (ed.) *Medicines Review Worldwide*, London: British Institute of Regulatory Affairs.

Walker, S.R. and Lumley, C.E. (1987) 'Reporting and under-reporting'. in R.D. Mann (ed.) *Adverse Drug Reactions*, Carnforth: Parthenon.

Wheeler, D.E. (1964) 'President's statement', *ABPI Annual Report*, (1963–64): 2–3.

6 Evidence-based practice in UK health policy

Stephen Harrison and Kath Checkland

Introduction

The belief that medical practice ought in some way to be based on 'evidence' is by no means new. However, widespread acceptance of the explicit doctrine that daily clinical practice should be based on sound and systematically assembled research evidence about the effectiveness of each therapeutic procedure ('intervention' hereafter) employed has grown only over the last forty years and has been a formal component of UK health policy only since the early 1990s. The principle has been extended to other clinical professions, including nursing, midwifery, dentistry and physiotherapy, so that more generic expressions such as 'evidence-based practice' and 'evidence-based health care' are now current. Similar reasoning has also been employed in sectors other than health, especially in education, criminal justice and social work (Davies *et al.* 2000). Evidence-based medicine (EBM) and its derivatives is usually presented by its proponents in the language of science, and there is clearly some justification for this; currently dominant ideas are certainly based on the notion of applying scientific research findings to clinical practice. But EBM is also a political phenomenon, in at least two senses. First, there is more than one conception of what constitutes EBM, so that contemporary orthodoxy represents the dominance of one set of ideas, and their exponents, over another. Second, this orthodoxy has become a core element of UK public policy.

The first and second sections of this chapter sketch some different conceptions of EBM as the means of introducing the main dimensions of disagreement about EBM, along with some elements of the history of relevant concepts (for fuller historical accounts, see Oakley 2000; Daly 2005). The third section covers the more recent history of how EBM became a central element of National Health Service (NHS) policy, whilst the fourth assesses its broad impact within UK medicine and elsewhere. The final section suggests ways in which EBM might be viewed sociologically.

Evidence in medicine: concepts and histories

References to 'evidence' in the context of clinical care imply a concern with cause and effect, that is, the impact of interventions on relevant health outcomes. However, there is more than one view about how valid causal relationships are to be found. For brevity, we might represent the alternative possibilities as poles of a spectrum. One pole represents the primacy of the participants' own experience, reflection upon it and peer discussion as the source of valid knowledge about the effectiveness of health care. In this model, 'evidence' is, as it were, internal to the clinician. The opposite pole represents the primacy of accumulated, externally generated, published research findings. This latter view, which places great emphasis on the adequacy of research methods in generating valid knowledge, has a long history, though it is perhaps only since the early 1990s that it has become widely reflected in clinical medical discourse. It seems to contain three key elements: systematic comparison, randomization of research subjects to comparison groups, and aggregation of research findings from multiple studies.

First, the idea of establishing the validity of causal inferences in health care through systematic clinical comparison is perhaps best symbolized historically in the now-famous experiment of citrus fruit as treatment for the debilitating disease of scurvy, frequently suffered by sailors, conducted in 1747 by James Lind, a British naval surgeon. Lind identified twelve similarly diseased sailors whom he divided into six groups, each of which received a different treatment. The pair who received oranges and lemons regained their fitness in six days, whereas the other ten did not (Porter 1997: 295). This is now regarded as probably the world's first controlled clinical trial, though Lind's theory about why citrus fruits were effective was mistaken, and it was another fifty years before his findings were generally adopted on British ships. Other early attempts to employ systematic comparisons were those of the Parisian school of physicians of the early nineteenth century, one of whom, Pierre Louis, employed a 'numerical method' to evaluate whether the outcome for what we now assume to be pneumonia was better if blindly selected groups of patients were 'bled' early or late in the course of their disease, and if large or small amounts of blood were removed (Lilienfield and Lilienfield 1979). This approach was subsequently advocated by Florence Nightingale in relation to both assessing the effectiveness of interventions and measuring the performance of hospitals (Oakley 2000: 117).

Second, by the late nineteenth century concern about possible bias in making such comparisons and consequent bias in the research findings led to ideas about alternation and randomization of research subjects to control and intervention groups. The Danish medical researcher Fibiger was employing alternation (allocating the first patient to one group, the second to another, and so on) in the 1890s when studying an anti-diphtheria serum (Oakley 2000: 146). It was still being employed in clinical trials fifty years later (Chalmers 2002). In the early twentieth century, the prominent statistician R.A. Fisher (whose work on inferential statistics is still highly influential in medicine and more generally) advocated randomization on the grounds that valid inferences about causality could only be drawn where experimental subjects had an equal chance of being selected for each of the treatments and control groups in the study, and that randomization would equalize the distribution of 'confounders' (factors that, though unknown to the researcher, might affect experimental results) between the groups (Marks 1997: 144). However, subsequent advocates of randomization tended to rely more on pragmatic considerations such as the known variability of human disease (implying that individual case reports are not a valid basis for generalization) and the possibility that clinicians' optimism about new treatments might bias allocation to study groups or bias the interpretation of results. This was the justification for the approach adopted in the UK Medical Research Council's 1948 trial of the then new antibiotic streptomycin for pulmonary tuberculosis (TB) (Porter 1997: 529). This was apparently the world's first randomized controlled trial (RCT) of a medical intervention and was paralleled by an American trial. The rationale for the RCT approach is that the validity of research findings is ensured by systematic comparisons between patients receiving the intervention being researched and 'control' groups, that is, patients receiving placebos, no treatment, and/or existing conventional treatment, as the case may be. In addition, random allocation of patients to these groups is held to minimize any bias arising from pre-existing differences between them (for a detailed account of RCT method, see Elwood 1988: 96–101). The UK streptomycin trial was designed by A.B. Hill and imitated the approach employed by Fisher in his agricultural experiments. The patient allocation method was originally planned as alternation, but was modified to randomization as the means of avoiding special pleading by clinicians in the difficult ethical context of an almost certainly fatal disease and a drug in short supply. The streptomycin trial has come to be regarded as a pivotal moment in the history of contemporary medical science; the *British Medical Journal* devoted an entire issue to celebrating its fiftieth anniversary (Yoshioka 1998). However, the most UK prominent proselytizer of the notion that randomization is crucial in avoiding bias in biomedical outcomes research dates was A.L. Cochrane, whose book *Effectiveness and Efficiency: Random Reflections on Health Services* (Cochrane 1972) advocated RCTs as rigorous evaluations of medical interventions.

Third, Cochrane and his sympathizers also supported the concept of systematically reviewing trials of a particular clinical intervention so as to provide an up-to-date statement of contemporary knowledge on that topic. In the mid-1970s, special quantitative methods, described as 'meta-analysis', were developed independently in the social sciences and medicine in order to aggregate the results of multiple controlled studies (Hunt 1997; Daly 2005). Some of the intellectual developments behind EBM, as it was to become institutionalized in the UK in the 1990s, developed in Canada (Daly 2005). Indeed, the term 'evidence-based medicine' seems to have been coined in Canada, originally as a label for teaching medical students based on research evidence (Evidence-Based Medicine Working Group 1992: 2420–5), but very quickly afterwards as a philosophy of clinical practice (Guyatt and Rennie 1993). All three of these elements can be seen as crystallized in the so-called 'hierarchy of evidence' (Sackett *et al.* 2000: 173–7), sometimes traced to a review of the research evidence about the value of periodic health examinations for children (Canadian Task Force 1979). This 'hierarchy' is widely cited as an authoritative definition of the soundness of scientific research purporting to demonstrate the effectiveness of clinical interventions. RCTs and systematic reviews of RCTs occupy the pinnacle of the hierarchy. Other methods are ranked lower in the hierarchy, with other types of controlled study second to the RCT and uncontrolled methods a poor third. Advocates of RCTs often regard uncontrolled (non-experimental) methods as suitable only for feasibility testing and/or hypothesis-building with a view to an eventual controlled study.

Applied models of EBM

EBM is not simply a question of how medical knowledge is generated, but also raises questions how it should be implemented. Alternative ways of thinking about this can also be represented by two poles of a spectrum. One pole implies that it is largely individual clinicians who internalize and apply knowledge, so that the application of EBM is primarily a matter of the internal motivation of professionals, perhaps supported by information systems that provide easy access to advice or to published research evidence. On this view, clinical professionals can largely be relied upon to integrate valid evidence into their daily practice, with few or no organizational implications. In contrast, the other pole implies that professional motivation is insufficient, so that managerial and/or organizational effort is required in order to implement EBM. Such external means of distillation and promulgation of knowledge might take the form of rules such as 'clinical guidelines' or 'protocols' (Berg 1997a), which are essentially algorithmic, that is, they guide their user to courses of clinical action, dependent upon stated prior conditions: 'if . . . then' logic. Such guidelines may be accompanied by incentives and/or sanctions to adhere to them.

Figure 6.1 combines the two spectra that we have been discussing as axes of a matrix; the vertical axis concerns the source of valid knowledge, whilst the horizontal axis concerns how it is put into practice. The four cells of the matrix each provide a basic model of EBM. Model 1 may be called reflective practice; it centres on the notions that individual clinicians should be constantly self-critical of their own practice, that such a critique can be facilitated by regular audit of the outcomes of practice, and that both the audit itself and remedial action based on it are best facilitated by an open

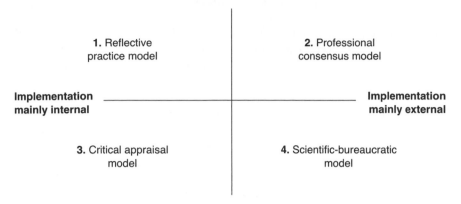

Figure 6.1 Four models of 'evidence-based practice'.

Source: S. Harrison (2002) 'New Labour, modernisation and the medical labour process', *Journal of Social Policy*, 31(3): 465–85.

and non-defensive, collegiate approach involving other clinicians as peers (Argyris and Schon 1977: 90–1). Model 2 is built on the generation of professional consensus, initially by bringing together professional elites to 'consensus conferences' to discuss published evidence and personal experience of a particular clinical topic, with the aim of producing a 'consensus statement' to guide the behaviour of the professional rank and file. The key feature of such a model is the generation of consensus, and the participants may be carefully selected to this end (Lancet 1992).

Model 3 may be called critical appraisal after its preferred approach to the interrogation of published research findings. It rejects one of the central assumptions of Models 1 and 2, that personal experience, even if critically examined, is the main source of valid knowledge. It substitutes the view (expressed in the 'hierarchy of evidence') that only RCTs provide clearly valid inferences about the effects of interventions, and that the appropriate means of aggregating the findings of several trials is meta-analysis or other forms of systematic review. Most of the development of the hierarchy of evidence originates from proponents of critical appraisal. Its preference for the formal aggregation of published research evidence therefore implicitly downgrades the type of personal experience upon which Models 1 and 2 are based. Nevertheless, critical appraisal assumes that neither academic research nor clinical guidelines can be applied unproblematically and hence practitioners should be trained to study research reports and assess their validity and applicability for themselves, also taking care to consider the relevance and value of interventions to individual patients. The approach has been described by proponents as 'the integration of best research evidence with clinical expertise and patient values' (Sackett *et al.* 2000: 1). Model 4 may be called scientific-bureaucratic medicine (Harrison 2002); like critical appraisal, it centres on the assumption that valid knowledge is mainly to be obtained from the accumulation of research conducted by experts according to the scientific criteria expressed in the 'hierarchy of evidence'. It further assumes that working clinicians are likely to be both too busy and insufficiently skilled to interpret and apply such knowledge for themselves, so that clinical practice should be influenced through the systematic aggregation by experts of research findings on a particular topic, and the distillation of such findings into protocols or guidelines which may then be communicated to practitioners with the expectation that practice will be influenced accordingly. As we shall see below, scientific-bureaucratic medicine seems to be the currently dominant model of EBM in the UK. Clinical guidelines can therefore be seen as a species of bureaucratic rule, hence the label for Model 4. Although they do not claim either to be applicable to all patients or to determine clinical action completely, the prevailing assumption is that they will normally be followed and exceptions will be both rare and carefully documented.

This last point is the nub of the difference between critical appraisal and scientific-bureaucratic medicine. Although both share the same concept of evidence, and although the concepts of critical appraisal are often cited in justification of guideline adherence, these models differ in respect of their attitudes to guidelines. As the leading exponent of critical appraisal has put it:

> Evidence based medicine is not 'cookbook' medicine. Because it requires a bottom up approach that integrates the best external evidence with individual clinical expertise and patients' choice, it cannot result in slavish, cookbook approaches to individual patient care. External clinical evidence can inform, but can never replace, individual clinical expertise, and it is this expertise that decides whether the external evidence applies to the individual patient at all and, if so, how it should be integrated into a clinical decision. Similarly, any external guideline must be integrated with individual clinical expertise in deciding whether and how it matches the patient's clinical state, predicament, and preferences, and thus whether it should be applied.
>
> (Sackett *et al.* 1996: 72)

EBM as UK health policy

The adoption of EBM as UK policy can be seen in two phases: first under the Conservative governments of the early and mid-1990s, and subsequently after the election of New Labour in 1997. Following recommendations from a parliamentary committee (House of Lords 1988), the Conservative government created a national research and development strategy for the NHS in 1991, involving the appointment of national and regional research directors, the establishment of national and local research budgets to be the object of competitive bidding, and reorganization of the flow of research funds through NHS hospitals (Baker and Kirk 1996). The central objective of this programme became the assessment of the effectiveness of both new and previously unevaluated health care interventions. A range of specialist institutions was publicly funded as the means of reviewing, collating and disseminating the findings of effectiveness research to the NHS, including the NHS Centre for Reviews and Dissemination (CRD) (NHS Executive 1996a), the Cochrane Centre (www.cochrane.co.uk), and the latter's international collaborations that conduct systematic reviews and aim to set methodological standards for judging clinical research. Throughout this period, it steadily became the conventional academic and policy wisdom that valid evidence of the effectiveness of clinical interventions should be defined by the 'hierarchy of evidence'. The dominance of this approach to evaluating evidence is illustrated by the treatment of CRD's published rules for undertaking systematic reviews (Centre for Reviews and Dissemination 1996) as authoritative, and the difficulty for researchers in obtaining NHS national research funds for health technology studies based on other methodological assumptions. The value of clinical guidelines became official received wisdom (NHS Executive 1996b), and it became officially recognized that research could guide NHS resource allocation decisions:

> The overall purpose of the NHS is to secure, through the resources available, the greatest possible improvement in the physical and mental health of the people . . . In order to achieve this, we need to ensure that decisions about the provision and delivery of clinical services are driven increasingly by evidence of clinical and cost-effectiveness, coupled with the systematic assessment of actual health outcomes.
>
> (NHS Executive 1996a: 6)

These developments coincided with the so-called 'internal market' in the NHS, under which its institutions were divided into 'providers' of care (such as hospitals) and 'purchasers' whose role was to commission services from providers and pay for the care for defined geographical populations (Robinson and Le Grand 1993). The consequent need for purchasers to develop criteria for their commissioning priorities and decisions led to increasing interest in health economics, specifically the microeconomic analysis of the cost-effectiveness of clinical interventions. Such analyses required research data about the effectiveness of interventions and generally adopted the 'hierarchy of evidence' as their criterion of validity.

Despite all this, the Conservative government made relatively few efforts to implement EBM in clinical practice. It could therefore be said that they had legitimized the 'scientific' element of scientific–bureaucratic medicine, but it was to fall to their New Labour successors to institutionalize the bureaucratic element. This post-1997 institutionalization occurred through three main routes. First, the results of health technology assessment and associated microeconomic analysis (in the form of costs per quality-adjusted life year) are employed by the National Institute for Health and Clinical Excellence (NICE) to make recommendations about what interventions should be made available to patients by the NHS. NICE was established in 1999 and by 2005 had reported on 117 topics (Raftery 2006; for more details of NICE's operation, see Rawlins and Culyer 2004; Syrett 2003). Since 2003 the NHS has been legally required to implement most positive NICE recommendations. Second, clinical guidelines have become ubiquitous, alongside increasing managerial and organizational pressures to ensure that they implemented. At national level, NICE commissions the production of evidence-based guidelines on specific topics by groups of experts (www.nice.org.uk/aboutnice/about_nice.jsp (accessed December 2007)), and it is expected that such approved guidelines will normally be followed. In addition, the NHS has numerous local guidelines and guideline implementation programmes, alongside the central specification of *service* models defined in 'National Service Frameworks' (NSFs) (www.dh.gov.uk/en/Policy andguidance/Healthandsocialcaretopics/DH_4070951 (accessed December 2008)) for such topics as coronary heart disease, mental health, cancer, services for older people, services for children, and diabetes. NSFs are written by so-called 'reference groups': groups of experts convened by the Department of Health. They are significantly evidence-based, though the breadth of their subject matter and their concern with service organization means that this does not apply to the whole of their content. Nevertheless, compliance is a dimension of NHS performance management administered by the Healthcare Commission (the 'arms length' agency responsible for inspecting and accrediting all providers of health care in the UK, see http://www.healthcarecommission.org.uk/homepage.cfm, (accessed August 2008), www.dh.gov.uk/en/Publicationsandstatistics/Publications/PublicationsPolicy AndGuidance/DH_4086665 (accessed November 2007)).

Third, the 2004 general practice contract and its associated Quality and Outcomes Framework (QOF) offer general medical practices substantial additional financial rewards in return for meeting specified performance requirements in relation to the management of chronic diseases in their patients. The rhetoric of EBM was prominent in the documentation issued to GPs as the contract was implemented (NHS Confederation/ BMA 2003), and most of the 'quality markers' that attract such payments are in some way 'evidence-based' (Roland 2004). Taken together, these developments suggest that EBM in the UK has come increasingly to resemble the ideal type of 'scientific-bureaucratic medicine' as characterized in Model 4 of Figure 6.1.

EBM: the impact on medicine

Despite the intellectual dominance of EBM in academic medicine and the prominence of its institutions within the NHS, the impact on medicine during its first decade was limited. This can be examined in relation both to the activities of NICE and to the process of implementing clinical guidelines more generally. Since its creation in 1999, NICE on several occasions found that its negative recommendations did not carry political legitimacy (see also Abraham, Chapter 5, this volume). Disputes about recommendations began early in its career with the recommendation in relation to the anti-influenza drug Relenza. Initial guidance from NICE that Relenza should not be provided on the NHS generated an outraged reaction from the manufacturers, GlaxoSmithKline, including a threat to take the company's research function outside the UK. NICE subsequently modified its ruling, declaring that Relenza should be available to at-risk adults in a restricted set of circumstances (Smith 2000). However, this legitimacy deficit was perhaps best illustrated by the example of the drug Interferon Beta (manufactured under various brand names), a treatment for relapsing-remitting multiple sclerosis (for a fuller account, see Harrison and McDonald 2007). Although clinical trials had shown the drug to reduce the frequency and perhaps the duration of relapse, economic evaluations had suggested low levels of cost-effectiveness (Forbes *et al.* 1998). Following launch of the drug in 1996, a number of NHS purchasing authorities took decisions not to fund treatment, but in 1997 the courts ruled against this decision by one authority (Dyer 1997). Interferon Beta was one of the first technologies to be appraised by NICE, which in mid-2000 announced its intention to recommend that the drug should not in future be available on the NHS, on the grounds that modest clinical benefits were considered to be outweighed by very high costs. Critical media coverage followed and appeals against the NICE decision were received from patient groups and various professional associations and pharmaceutical companies. NICE's appeal panel upheld some aspects of these appeals, and resolved to commission further economic modelling and to seek new data from the manufacturers. In mid-2001 NICE announced its decision that Interferon Beta should not be available on the NHS. However, the Department of Health indicated that it had entered into a 'risk-sharing scheme' with the pharmaceutical companies concerned, under which it would fund prescribing of the drug for an agreed period during which an assessment would be made to establish its cost-effectiveness. If the drug reached NICE's usual cost-effectiveness threshold, it would continue to be purchased at the price agreed at the outset of the scheme, but if the cost-effectiveness ratio transpired to be higher, the price would be accordingly reduced. NICE had apparently no previous knowledge of this scheme, and proceeded to issue its final decision recommending against the NHS use of Interferon Beta in early 2002. Although the cost-sharing scheme would not have been possible without NICE's analyses of cost-utility, it is difficult to see the incident as anything other than an illustration of political weakness on the part of NICE.

Subsequent developments provided further evidence of government preparedness to sidestep NICE. Shortly after the Interferon Beta case, the Department of Health pre-empted any recommendation on the drug Glivec for chronic myeloid leukaemia by writing to the NHS suggesting that funds should be made available for the drug despite the fact that NICE's appraisal was not expected for some time (Barbour 2001). A further example occurred in 2005 when, faced with a fierce news media debate (Lancet 2005), the secretary of state for health instructed the NHS to fund the drug Herceptin for patients with early-stage breast cancer of the HER2 positive type; although it was expensive, trial evidence had suggested only modest benefits (Barrett *et al.* 2006) and it had not yet been considered by NICE. As a result, NICE undertook a fast-track appraisal, issuing favourable guidance in 2006 (Barrett *et al.* 2006). NICE has in general continued to face strong opposition from patients, clinicians and drug manufacturers whenever it has attempted to reach unfavourable determinations; for example, NICE's reversal in 2006 of earlier approvals of drugs such as Aricept for patients in the early stages of dementia (Dyer 2006).

This initially limited impact of NICE at national level was paralleled in relation to the implementation of guidelines at a clinical level. Early guideline enthusiasts assumed that simply producing an 'authoritative' guideline would lead to its adoption. However, this proved not to be the case (Harrison 1994), and a research industry developed that sought the 'magic bullet' required to implement guidelines in practice, extrapolating the idea of the 'hierarchy of evidence' from clinical trials to trials of organizational interventions to change clinical practice (Freemantle *et al.* 1999; Gerstein *et al.* 1999). So saturated has this field become that the development of systematic reviews of the evidence (again, mirroring the logic of EBM) was superseded by 'overviews' of systematic reviews (Effective Health Care 1999; Grimshaw *et al.* 2001). These 'overviews' typically reference more than a hundred individual reviews, each of which may cite hundreds of studies, but generally concluding that some interventions are effective in some situations, and that context is important in determining success (Grimshaw *et al.* 2001; Harrison *et al.* 2003). Attention subsequently shifted to removing the organizational 'barriers' to change (Foy *et al.* 2001; for a critique, see Checkland *et al.* 2007), but this has not been shown to bring about change (Shaw *et al.* 2005). Physicians often maintained a sceptical discourse about the appropriateness of EBM in the context of medicine as an 'art' concerned with individual patients rather than populations (Pope 2003; Harrison and Dowswell 2002)

Despite the persistence over a number of years of EBM's limited impact on medicine, by about 2005 there were signs of change in relation to both the authority of NICE and the impact of clinical guidelines. Whilst the pharmaceutical industry continues to resist many of NICE's negative recommendations, and indeed NICE remains cautious in its approach to these (for example, postponing full guidance on the use of drugs to treat macular degeneration in response to criticism arising from the initial consultation document), there have been no further government interventions as in the cases of Herceptin and Interferon Beta, and the recommendation that drugs to treat Alzheimer's disease should only be used in limited circumstances has stood in spite of the criticism and legal challenge it received (Dyer 2007). Furthermore, supporters of NICE have recently become more confident, especially regarding its role in what might be called 'rationing' expensive treatments, with several health economists calling for NICE to lower the economic threshold of effectiveness that drugs and other interventions must achieve to be declared 'cost effective' (Appleby *et al.* 2007; O'Dowd 2007).

Whilst there remains no good evidence of wholesale adoption of clinical guidelines in hospital clinical practice, there is some evidence that doctors see it as their role, in part at least, to persuade patients to accept 'evidence-based' treatments, regardless of their previous experiences of these drugs or worries about side effects (Sanders *et al.* 2008). However, in primary care, financial incentives to follow clinical guidelines seem to have had an effect. General practices were predicted to achieve 700–750 (from a maximum of 1050) points in total in the first year of QOF, but mean achievement for 2004–05 was some 950, yielding some 20 per cent of mean practice income (Cole 2005). Further, this seems to be associated with changes of perception about medicine so that QOF may have been internalized by GPs as the definition of primary care quality (McDonald *et al.* 2007) and the way in which 'cases' ought to be conceptualized and treated (Checkland *et al.* 2008).

Finally, it would seem that commissioners of care are also developing confidence in using EBM to rationalize and defend their decisions with respect to limiting access to certain treatments. Primary Care Trusts (PCTs) are responsible for commissioning services from secondary care providers, and it is increasingly common for them to set thresholds and limits on treatments over and above those recommended nationally by NICE, using the rhetoric of EBM to justify these decisions. For example, a document setting out one PCT's strategy for 2007/08 states:

> Commissioning will get the best from public money: it will buy *clinically effective, cost effective* and safe services; a greater proportion of the commissioning spend will be committed to schemes that improve the health of the population not just paying for the treatment of ill health; but at the same time it will ensure all investments in public health and health promotion *are evidence based* . . . The PCT will manage surgical thresholds by reducing the number of some operations it is willing to

pay for . . . The PCT will use *protocol based prior approval schemes,*
utilisation reviews and customer satisfaction surveys to bring benefits to
patients and providers alike.

> (www.derbyshirecountypct.nhs.uk/content/PCT%20Strategy%
> 2007-09%20Final%20Version.pdf (accessed November 2007,
> emphases added))

The 'prior approval schemes' mentioned here are effectively lists of treatments which will either not be funded or which will only be funded in very
limited circumstances; it seems highly unlikely that, prior to the rise of EBM,
a PCT would have been self-confident enough to state explicitly that access
to some treatments was to be limited. More generally, a discourse has
developed along the lines that RCTs constitute *'the* gold standard' (authors'
emphasis) for research (Eccles *et al.* 2003) to be applied in any situation,
with one medical journalist describing EBM as 'beautiful, elegant, clever and
important', going on to claim that:

> You could do a randomised, controlled trial on almost any intervention
> you wanted to assess: comparing two teaching methods, or two forms
> of psychotherapy, or two plant-growth boosters – literally anything.
>
> (Goldacre 2007)

Possibly as a result of this prevailing orthodoxy, those opposed to the use of
Complementary and Alternative Medicines (CAMs) under the auspices of
the NHS seem to have gained in confidence, using the lack of RCT evidence
as a stick with which to beat their opponents (Colquhoun 2007) (see also
Cant, Chapter 9, this volume). As intellectual and political commitment to
EBM has spread, other health professions have sought to emulate medicine,
with nurses shifting their claims to professional identity away from a rhetoric
of caring towards one of 'science' and evidence-based practice (Traynor
1999; Nursing and Midwifery Council 2005). Beyond the field of medicine,
the Campbell Collaboration advocates RCT evidence in fields such as criminal justice and education (www.campbellcollaboration.org/), explicitly
modelling its methods on those developed by the Cochrane Collaborations.

Despite the expansion of the EBM discourse and the increasing impact
on medicine of EBM in the last few years, it is by no means certain that
the immediate future consists of more of the same. At the beginning of
this chapter, we suggested that EBM as visualized by its original proponents
sought through 'critical appraisal' to marry the best insights from research
evidence with the unique needs and desires of individual patients, but
that policy has led to the dominance of a 'scientific bureaucratic medicine'
paradigm, under which population evidence is applied to individuals via
bureaucratic rules. One of the foundation stones of EBM is that its use of
'valid', 'reliable' and 'reproducible' evidence from large-scale RCTs makes
it a superior means of defining effective care to the use of professional

consensus, what Greenhalgh (2006: 6) describes as the GOBSAT ('Good Old Boys Sat Around a Table') approach. Ironically, however, it may be that as the language of EBM becomes ever more embedded in medical practice, and as bureaucratic rules become the accepted way to implement 'the best' evidence, its requirements for evidence are quietly attenuated in favour of an emphasis on rules. Thus, for example, in 2004 the government announced that, by December 2008, no one on the UK would wait more than 18 weeks for any kind of hospital treatment (Department of Health 2004). The chosen delivery vehicle is 'patient pathways'. These are centrally determined 'best practice' guidelines, which use the rhetoric of EBM to justify their use. The pathways available on the policy's dedicated website www.18weeks.nhs.uk/ Content.aspx?path=/ (accessed May 2008), are detailed documents specifying, for example, exactly which investigations patients should receive for a given set of symptoms. It is expected that these pathways (covering a wide range of specialties from cardiology to oral medicine) will be used to determine patient care throughout the NHS. What is significant for the topic of this chapter is that these pathways are not purely based upon RCT evidence. Indeed, they cannot be so, because in addition to specifying evidence-based treatments (such as aspirin for patients with angina), they also specify models of service delivery for which RCT evidence does not exist. In order to overcome this evidence deficit, the 18 week delivery programme has convened a series of 'consensus events', aiming to 'allow for discussion on the content of the pathways including clarity of the models and, where appropriate, alternative models of care' and to 'reach consensus' on the pathways (Department of Health 2007). Thus, the final pathways are based not upon evidence but upon the supposedly outmoded mechanism of 'professional consensus', presumably an outcome somewhat distant from that originally envisaged by the EBM movement. Of course it remains to be seen how far this new bureaucratic form will become institutionalized in UK health policy or internalized by the medical profession.

Sociological perspectives on EBM

In this final section we suggest three broad perspectives from which EBM might be viewed in sociological terms, though our selection is neither exhaustive nor mutually exclusive. We have not defined these perspectives in theoretical terms, though we suggest some theoretical approaches that are relevant to each.

EBM *as state politics*

From this perspective, EBM may be seen as a component or extension of state or government attempts to increase political control over the practice of medicine (and other professions) through increased regulation and management. In theoretical terms, either neo-Marxist political economy or

Foucauldian 'governmentality' might serve as starting points for analysis. In brief, the neo-Marxist argument distinguishes between basic types of state welfare expenditure (O'Connor 1973). 'Social investment' increases labour productivity through the provision of physical infrastructure such as roads and utilities that no single capitalist could afford. 'Social consumption' reduces the reproduction costs of labour through such programmes as education and basic health services. 'Social expenses' maintain social harmony and legitimate capitalism, thereby discouraging potential social unrest. The British NHS was intended to ensure a healthy workforce, thereby both helping to pay for itself and providing a legitimate response to political demands at the end of a major war (Watkin 1975). However, under economic pressures, state institutions face a contradiction. On the one hand, there is pressure from capitalists to reduce taxation, and on the other, pressure from the public to extend the welfare state, or at least acquiesce in the rising costs of benefits. If government expenditure rises, a 'fiscal crisis' occurs; if the welfare state is cut, a 'legitimacy crisis' is risked. One way of understanding EBM, therefore, is as a means of displacing 'wasteful', 'ineffective' medical interventions, thereby helping to control the high and rising costs of health care in the UK (Harrison 1998). The 'scientific' basis of EBM can be seen as an important contributor to the legitimation of such a strategy. Moreover, the requirement of EBM that medical interventions be narrowly defined has facilitated the regime of 'payment by results' (Dixon 2004), which requires that medical episodes (whether surgical procedures or other forms of care) be categorized and assigned a standardized label (Harrison forthcoming). Such a conceptualization of health care as a largely standardized commodity also facilitates the provision of NHS care by corporate private providers, thereby offering some material benefits back to capitalists.

Foucault's (1991) notion of 'governmentality' implies a very different view of the state, not as an external force, but rather as a collection of institutions, processes, analyses and tactics through which government is achieved, with a habitually obedient, self-regulating population: the 'conduct of conduct'. In this view, the professions, including medicine, are part of this regulatory apparatus (Hindess 2001) but, paradoxically, are also themselves increasingly regulated by governmental agencies and systems of audit. Hence, Johnson (1995: 19–20) sees the increasing regulation of medicine as a result of cost pressures from such factors as an increasingly elderly population. In Flynn's (2002) view, this regulation takes the form of the co-option of medicine into alignment with managerial views of the world, a form of 'soft bureaucracy' where 'processes of flexibility and decentralization co-exist with more rigid constraints and structures of domination' (Courpasson 2000: 57). Again, EBM can be understood as an aspect of this more general approach, with the use of clinical guidelines promoted as much through a discourse of treatment needing to be 'evidence-based' as through explicit incentives or disciplinary measures. The internalization by GPs of QOF targets as a definition of health care 'quality' can be seen as an example of self-surveillance and habitual obedience to government policy.

EBM and medicine as a profession

Most analysts of the concept of 'profession' have argued that 'autonomy' is an important component (for a review, see Harrison and McDonald 2008: ch 2). From this perspective, it makes sense to examine the relationship between EBM and doctors' professional autonomy. In particular, if 'clinical guidelines' are seen as a species of bureaucratic rule, their heavy emphasis in the implementation of EBM ('scientific–bureaucratic medicine') in the UK raises questions about the possible undercutting of medicine's status as a profession. Perhaps the bleakest account (from medicine's point of view) is that of McKinlay and colleagues (McKinlay and Arches 1985; McKinlay and Stoeckle 1988), who saw increasing corporate and managerial control over physicians as 'proletarianization'. Whilst this is hyperbolic (doctors' work is not like that of car assembly workers or call centre operatives), it is nevertheless arguable that EBM has led to an important shift in what Jamous and Peloille (1970) termed the 'indetermination/ technicality [I/T] ratio', that is, an increase in the proportion of elements within medical work that can be clearly specified, with a corresponding reduction in the proportion that must be left to the judgement of the doctor. Thus EBM threatens to undercut long-standing medical and sociological assumptions about uncertainty and indeterminacy in medical work (Armstrong 2007). Of course, the spread of bureaucratically driven modes of production and service is a much more widespread global phenomenon (Ritzer 2000).

A more optimistic (from medicine's point of view) interpretation of new forms of regulation such as EBM is that they represent a new form of stratification *within* medicine rather than overall decline (Freidson 1988). Such 'restratification' (Coburn *et al.* 1997) can be seen as having produced three main strata within the profession. Writing about the United States, Freidson identified an 'administrative elite' of physicians responsible for supervising other fully qualified doctors and a 'knowledge elite' composed of university medical researchers and physicians who also provide professional advice on health policy (Freidson 1984). Both elites may be in conflict with rank-and-file practitioners, since the 'administrative elite' creates a 'less collegial and more superordinate relationship' with rank-and-file professionals, whilst the 'knowledge elite' may produce rules that are impractical for everyday clinical situations. Freidson concludes that, contrary to allegations of proletarianization, professional restratification is a means of maintaining medical power, since both the administrative and the knowledge elites remain within the profession, and sees little evidence that the overall social or intellectual place of medicine has been eroded (Freidson 1984). In the UK context, the EBM movement can be seen as a knowledge elite, though the identity of Freidson's 'administrative elite' is less clear, since relatively few NHS managers are medically qualified. However, recent research in primary care does show that a new strata of local medical elites has emerged, and that such elites have a role in controlling the work of other doctors (McDonald *et al.* 2007; Checkland *et al.* 2008) (see also Chapter 3, this volume, by Calnan and Gabe). Whether or not one concurs with Freidson's broader analysis, it seems clear that in the UK the autonomy of the rank-and-file individual practitioner is being eroded (Armstrong 2002).

EBM *as a social phenomenon*

It is evident from our brief historical account that EBM is a social as much as a technical phenomenon (see Daly 2005 for a detailed account of the personalities and alliances). Indeed, both proponents of EBM and academic analysts have seen it as a 'social movement' (Pope 2003; Daly 2005: 76). As distinct from pressure groups, such social movements are broader and held together by identity as much as interest (Bucher and Stelling 1969; Dalton and Kuechler 1990; Byrne 1997). Pope's (2003) study of the development of EBM draws on Blumer's (1951) analysis of the processes entailed in the formation of a social movement. Thus the work of Cochrane can be seen as 'agitation', whilst a sense of team spirit, self-belief and rectitude was formed through the self-identification of members of the movement as 'clinical epidemiologists' and the appropriation of the term 'evidence-based medicine'. The members also had a clear ideology: to find and appraise evidence about medical interventions and to have it incorporated into clinical practice. Finally, the movement had a strategy for the pursuit of its goals, exemplified in the Cochrane reviews and collaborations referred to above (Pope 2003: 269–72). A variation on this approach might see the proponents of EBM as an 'epistemic community', defined as a (possibly informal) network of professionals with recognized expertise and competence in a particular domain and an authoritative claim to policy-relevant knowledge within that domain or issue area (Haas 1992). According to this literature, an epistemic community shares causal beliefs, normative beliefs, notions of validity, and a policy enterprise, all of which are identifiable in the case of EBM, stretching across North America and northern Europe. From this perspective, a central question would be the process by which EBM became public policy.

Since it constructs knowledge and how it is validated in particular ways which then become regarded as authoritative, EBM is also interesting in relation to the sociologies of knowledge and science (Berg 1997b; Mol 1999). But EBM is not just knowledge, it also entails relationships between such knowledge, the technologies through which it is codified and disseminated (such as systematic reviews and the Cochrane websites) and practised (such as medical interventions) and the humans engaged in the EBM project. These characteristics suggest that Actor Network Theory

(Latour 2005) might provide another lens through which EBM could be viewed sociologically. EBM might be seen as a network into which ideas, technologies and humans are 'enrolled', but which has to be constantly sustained through continued 'performance' of their interrelationships. From this perspective, an important focus would be on how the network is created and sustained.

Concluding remarks

In this chapter we have summarized the development of EBM in the UK, and explained how it has been bureaucratized and institutionalized within the NHS as 'scientific–bureaucratic medicine'. We have discussed its impact on medicine, and suggested that, in spite of initial failures to bring about change, there are some signs that that impact is increasing. Finally, we have suggested some sociological perspectives from which these changes might be profitably considered. The above possibilities are by no means exhaustive, and there are numerous others. It is, for instance, possible to see EBM negatively in primarily normative terms, as 'colonization' of the 'life-world' of informal understandings and practices by bureaucratic rationality (Habermas 1987: 119ff), as ideology (Miles and Loughlin 2006), or as a denial of the individuality of patients (Frankford 1994). Mykhalovskiy and Weir (2004) suggest a range of other Foucauldian approaches that might be adopted. Moreover, we have not sought to adjudicate between the merits of the various perspectives or theories outlined above. Rather, our purpose is to establish that EBM is sociologically interesting and to suggest conceptual directions from which it might be approached.

References

Appleby, J., Devlin, N. and Parkin, D. (2007) 'NICE's cost effectiveness threshold', *British Medical Journal*, 335: 358–59.

Argyris, C. and Schon, D.A. (1977) *Theory in Practice: increasing professional effectiveness*, San Francisco: Jossey-Bass.

Armstrong, D. (2002) 'Clinical autonomy, individual and collective: the problem of changing doctors' behaviour', *Social Science and Medicine*, 55: 1771–7.

Armstrong, D. (2007) 'Professionalism, indeterminacy and the EBM project', *BioSocieties*, 2: 73–84.

Baker, M.R. and Kirk, S. (eds) (1996) *Research and Development for the NHS: evidence, evaluation and effectiveness*, Oxford: Radcliffe Medical Press.

Barbour, V. (2001) 'Imatinib for chronic myeloid leukaemia: a NICE mess', *Lancet*, 358: 1478.

Barrett, A., Roques, T., Small, M. and Smith, R.D. (2006) 'How much will Herceptin really cost?' *British Medical Journal*, 333: 1118–20.

Berg, M. (1997a) 'Problems and promises of the protocol', *Social Science and Medicine*, 44: 1081–8.

Berg, M. (1997b) *Rationalising Medical Work: decision support techniques and medical practices*, Cambridge, MA: MIT Press.

138   *Stephen Harrison and Kath Checkland*

Blumer, H. (1951) 'Collective behaviour', in A.M. Lee (ed.) *New Outline of the Principles of Sociology*, New York: Barnes and Noble.

Bucher, R. and Stelling, J. (1969) 'Characteristics of professional organisations', *Journal of Health and Social Behaviour*, 10: 3–15.

Byrne, P. (1997) *Social Movements in Britain*, London: Routledge.

Canadian Taskforce on the Periodic Health Examination (1979) 'Taskforce Report: the Periodic Health Examination', *Canadian Medical Association Journal*, 121: 1139–254.

Centre for Reviews and Dissemination (1996) *Undertaking Systematic Reviews on Effectiveness*. Report no. 4, York: University of York.

Chalmers, I. (2002) 'MRC Therapeutic Trials Committee's report on serum treatment of lobar pneumonia, *British Medical Journal* 1934', in The James Lind Library. Online: www.jameslindlibrary.org (accessed May 2008).

Checkland, K., Harrison, S. and Marshall, M. (2007) 'Is the metaphor of "barriers to change" useful in understanding implementation? Evidence from general medical practice', *Journal of Health Services Research and Policy*, 12: 95–100.

Checkland, K., Harrison, S., McDonald, R., Grant, S., Campbell, S. and Guthrie, B. (2008) 'Biomedicine, holism and general medical practice: responses to the 2004 General Practitioner contract', *Sociology of Health and Illness*, 30: 788–803.

Coburn, D., Rapport, S. and Bourgeault, I. (1997) 'Decline vs retention of medical power through restratification: an examination of the Ontario case', *Sociology of Health and Illness*, 19: 1–22.

Cochrane, A.L. (1972) *Effectiveness and Efficiency: random reflections on health services*, London: Nuffield Provincial Hospitals Trust.

Cole, A. (2005) 'UK GP activity exceeds expectations', *British Medical Journal*, 331: 536.

Colquhoun, D. (2007) 'Should NICE evaluate complementary and alternative medicines?' *British Medical Journal*, 334: 507.

Courpasson, D. (2000) 'Managerial strategies of domination: power in soft bureaucracies', *Organization Studies*, 21: 141–61.

Dalton, R.J. and Kuechler, M. (eds) (1990) *Challenging the Political Order: new social and political movements in Western democracies*, Cambridge: Polity Press.

Daly, J. (2005) *Evidence-based Medicine and the Search for a Science of Clinical Care*, Berkeley, CA: University of California Press.

Davies, H.T.O., Nutley, S. and Smith, P.C. (eds) (2000) *What Works? Evidence-based policy and practice in public services*, Bristol: Policy Press.

Department of Health (2004) *The NHS Improvement Plan: putting people at the heart of public services*, London: The Stationery Office.

Department of Health (2007) *The Pathways Story: developing the 18 week commissioning pathways*, London: The Stationery Office. Online: www.18weeks.nhs.uk/content.aspx?path=/achieve-and-sustain/Commissioning-pathways (accessed May 2008).

Dixon, J. (2004) 'Payment by results – new financial flows in the NHS', *British Medical Journal*, 328: 969–70.

Dyer, C. (1997) 'Ruling on interferon beta will hit all health authorities', *British Medical Journal*, 315: 143–8.

Dyer, C. (2006) 'NICE faces legal challenge over restriction on dementia drugs', *British Medical Journal*, 333: 1085.

Dyer, O. (2007) 'High Court upholds NICE decision to limit treatments for Alzheimer's disease', *British Medical Journal*, 335: 319.

Eccles, M., Grimshaw, J., Campbell, M. and Ramsay, C. (2003) 'Research designs for studies evaluating the effectiveness of change and improvement strategies', *Quality and Safety in Health Care*, 12: 47–52.

Effective Health Care (1999) *Getting Evidence into Practice*, York: University of York Centre for Reviews and Dissemination.

Elwood, J.M. (1988) *Causal Relationships in Medicine: a practical system for critical appraisal*, Oxford: Oxford University Press.

Evidence-Based Medicine Working Group (1992) 'Evidence-based medicine; a new approach to teaching the practice of medicine', *Journal of the American Medical Association*, 268: 2420–5.

Flynn, R. (2002) 'Clinical governance and governmentality', *Health, Risk and Society*, 4: 155–73.

Forbes, R.B., Lees, A., Waugh, N. and Swingler, R.J. (1998) 'Population-based cost-utility study of interferon-beta 1b in secondary progressive multiple sclerosis', *British Medical Journal*, 319: 1529–33.

Foucault, M. (1991) 'Governmentality', translated by R. Braidotti, revised by C. Gordon, in G. Burchell, C. Gordon and P. Miller (eds) *The Foucault Effect: studies in governmentality*, Chicago: University of Chicago Press (originally published in French, 1978).

Foy, R., Walker, A. and Penney, G.. (2001) 'Barriers to clinical guidelines: the need for concerted action', *British Journal of Clinical Governance*, 6: 166–74.

Frankford, D. (1994) 'Scientism and economics in the regulation of health care', *Journal of Health Politics, Policy and Law*, 19: 773–99.

Freemantle, N., Eccles, M., Wood, J., Mason, J., Nazareth, I., Duggan, C., Young, P., Haines, A., Drummond, M., Russell, I. and Walley, T. (1999) 'A randomized trial of Evidence-based OutReach (EBOR): rationale and design', *Controlled Clinical Trials*, 20: 479–92.

Freidson, E. (1984) 'The changing nature of professional control', *Annual Review of Sociology*, 10: 1–20.

Freidson, E. (1988) *Profession of Medicine: a study of the sociology of applied knowledge*, second edition, Chicago: University of Chicago Press.

Gerstein, H.C., Reddy, S.S.K., Dawson, K.G., Yale, J.F., Shannon, S. and Norman, G. (1999) 'A controlled evaluation of a national continuing medical education programme designed to improve family physicians' implementation of diabetes-specific practice guidelines', *Diabetes Medicine*, 16: 964–9.

Goldacre, B. (2007) 'A kind of magic', *The Guardian*, 16 November. Online: www.guardian.co.uk/science/2007/nov/16/sciencenews.g2.

Greenhalgh, T. (2006) *How to Read a Paper*, Malden, MA: Blackwell Publishing.

Grimshaw, J., Shirran, L., Thomas, R., Mowatt, G., Fraser, C., Bero, L., Grilli, R., Harvey, E., Oxman, A. and O'Brien, M.A. (2001) 'Changing provider behaviour. An overview of systematic reviews of interventions', *Medical Care*, 39 (suppl.2): 2–45.

Guyatt, G.H. and Rennie, D. (1993) 'Users' guide to the medical literature', *Journal of the American Medical Association*, 270: 2096–7.

Haas, P.M. (1992) 'Epistemic communities and international policy co-ordination', *International Organisation*, 46: 1–35.

Habermas, J. (1987) *The Theory of Communicative Action: the critique of functionalist reason*, Oxford: Polity Press.

Harrison, S. (1994) 'Knowledge into practice: what's the problem?' *Journal of Management in Medicine*, 8: 9–16.

Harrison, S. (1998) 'The politics of evidence-based medicine in the UK', *Policy and Politics*, 26: 15–31.

Harrison, S. (2002) 'New Labour, modernisation and the medical labour process', *Journal of Social Policy*, 31: 465–85.

Harrison, S. (forthcoming) 'Co-option, commodification and the medical model: Governing UK medicine since 1991', *Public Administration*.

Harrison, S. and McDonald, R. (2007) 'Fixing legitimacy? The case of NICE and the National Health Service', in A. Hann (ed.) *Health Policy and Politics*, Aldershot: Ashgate.

Harrison, S. and McDonald, R. (2008) *The Politics of Healthcare in Britain*, London: Sage.

Harrison, S. and Dowswell, G. (2002) 'Autonomy and bureaucratic accountability in primary care: what English general practitioners say', *Sociology of Health and Illness*, 24: 208–26.

Harrison, S., Dowswell, G., Wright, J. and Russell, I. (2003) 'General practitioners' uptake of clinical guidelines: a qualitative study', *Journal of Health Services Research and Policy*, 8: 142–7.

Hindess, B. (2001) 'Power, government, politics', in K. Nash and A. Scott (eds) *The Blackwell Companion to Political Sociology*, Oxford: Blackwell.

House of Lords Select Committee on Science and Technology (1988) *Third Report: priorities in medical research*, HL Paper 54–1, London: HMSO.

Hunt, M. (1997) *How Science Takes Stock: the story of meta-analysis*, New York: Sage.

Jamous, H. and Peloille, B. (1970) 'Changes in the French university-hospital system', in J.A. Jackson (ed.) *Professions and Professionalisation*, Cambridge: Cambridge University Press.

Johnson, T.J. (1995) 'Governmentality and the institutionalisation of expertise', in T.J. Johnson, G. Larkin and M. Saks (eds) *Health Professions and the State in Europe*, London: Routledge.

Lancet (1992) 'Guidelines for doctors in the new world', *The Lancet*, 339: 1197.

Lancet (2005) 'Herceptin and early breast cancer: a moment for caution', *The Lancet*, 366: 1673.

Latour, B. (2005) *Reassembling the Social: an introduction to actor-network theory*, Oxford: Oxford University Press.

Lilienfield, A.M. and Lilienfield, D.E. (1979) 'A century of case-controlled studies: progress?' *Journal of Chronic Diseases*, 32: 5–13.

McDonald, R., Harrison, S., Checkland, K., Campbell, S.M. and Roland, M. (2007) 'Impact of financial incentives on clinical autonomy and internal motivation in primary care: ethnographic study', *British Medical Journal*, 334: 1357–63.

McKinlay, J.B. and Stoeckle, J. (1988) 'Corporatisation and the social transformation of doctoring', *International Journal of Health Services*, 18: 191–205.

McKinlay, J.B. and Arches, J. (1985) 'Towards the proletarianisation of physicians', *International Journal of Health Services*, 15: 161–95.

Marks, H.M. (1997) *The Progress of Experiment: science and therapeutic reform in the United States, 1900–1990*, Cambridge: Cambridge University Press.

Miles, A. and Loughlin, M. (2006) 'Continuing the evidence-based health care debate in 2006. The progress and price of EBM', *Journal of Evaluation in Clinical Practice*, 12: 385–98.

Mol, A. (1999) 'Ontological politics: a word and some questions', in J. Law and J. Hassard (eds) *Actor Network Theory and After*, Oxford: Blackwell.

Mykhalovskiy, E. and Weir, L. (2004) 'The problem of evidence-based medicine: directions for social science', *Social Science and Medicine*, 59: 1059–69.

NHS Confederation/British Medical Association (2003) *The New GMS contract 2003 – Investing in General Practice*, London: NHS Confederation.

NHS Executive (1996a) *Promoting Clinical Effectiveness: a framework for action in and through the NHS*, London: Department of Health.

NHS Executive (1996b) *Clinical Guidelines: using clinical guidelines to improve patient care within the NHS*, London: Department of Health.

Nursing and Midwifery Council (2005) *Code of Professional Conduct*, London: NMC.

Oakley, A. (2000) *Experiments in Knowing: gender and method in the social sciences*, Cambridge: Polity Press.

O'Connor, J. (1973) *The Fiscal Crisis of the State*, New York: St Martin's Press.

O'Dowd, A. (2007) 'Economist says NICE should approve fewer costly drugs', *British Medical Journal*, 335: 11.

Pope, C. (2003) 'Resisting evidence: the study of evidence-based medicine as a contemporary social movement', *Health: an Interdisciplinary Journal for the Study of Health, Illness and Medicine*, 7: 267–82.

Porter, R. (1997) *The Greatest Benefit to Mankind: a medical history of humanity from antiquity to the present*, London: Harper Collins.

Raftery, J. (2006) 'Review of NICE's recommendations, 1999–2005', *British Medical Journal*, 332: 1266–8.

Rawlins, M.D. and Culyer, A.J. (2004) 'National Institute for Clinical Excellence and its value judgements', *British Medical Journal*, 329: 224–7.

Ritzer, G. (2000) *The McDonaldisation of Society*, Thousand Oaks CA: Pine Forge Press.

Robinson, R. and Le Grand, J. (eds) (1993) *Evaluating the NHS Reforms*, London: King's Fund.

Roland, M. (2004) 'Linking physician pay to quality of care: a major experiment in the UK', *New England Journal of Medicine*, 351: 1488–54.

Sackett, D.L., Rosenberg, W., Gray, J.A., Haynes, R.B. and Richardson, W.S. (1996) 'Evidence-based medicine: what it is and what it isn't', *British Medical Journal*, 312: 71–2.

Sackett, D.L., Straus, S., Richardson, W.S., Rosenberg, W. and Haynes, R.B. (2000) *Evidence-based Medicine: how to practise and teach EBM*, second edition, Edinburgh: Churchill Livingstone.

Sanders, T., Harrison, S. and Checkland, K. (2008) 'Evidence-based medicine and patient choice: the case of heart failure care', *Journal of Health Services Research and Policy*, 13: 103–8.

Shaw, B., Cheater, F., Baker, R., Gillies, C., Hearnshaw, H., Flottorp, S. and Robertson, N. (2005) 'Tailored interventions to overcome identified barriers to change: effects on professional practice and health care outcomes', *The Cochrane Database of Systematic Reviews*, 3.

Smith, R. (2000) 'The failings of NICE', *British Medical Journal*, 321: 1363–4.

Syrett, K. (2003) 'A technocratic fix to the "legitimacy" problem? The Blair government and health care rationing in the United Kingdom', *Journal of Health Politics, Policy and Law*, 28: 715–46.

Traynor, M. (1999) *Managerialism and Nursing: beyond oppression and profession*, London: Routledge.

Watkin, B. (1975) *Documents on Health and Social Services: 1834 to the present day*, London: Methuen.

Yoshioka, A. (1998) 'Use of randomisation in the Medical Research Council's clinical trial of streptomycin for pulmonary tuberculosis in the 1940s', *British Medical Journal*, 317: 1220–3.

7 Innovation and implementation in health technology

Normalizing telemedicine

Carl May

Introduction

Understanding how and why new technologies become embedded in health services, and how they shape – and are shaped by – the social contexts in which they are enacted has become an important focus of recent sociological writing about health and medicine. Crucial to the emergence of this body of literature have been theories of 'social shaping' which are largely drawn from Science and Technology Studies (STS) that focus on the reciprocal relations between society and technology, and argue that technologies, the actors that employ them, and the conditions in which they are employed are socially constructed (Fox 1996; MacKenzie 1998;Wajcman 2002). While much important research in sociology has focused on the construction, trajectory and forms of innovation in science and technology, other work has pointed to their implementation in practice as a core problem (Linton 2002; Greenhalgh *et al.* 2004). It is implementation, as well as innovation, that is the focus of this chapter.

How to make innovation and modernization central to UK health policy, and technological advances integral to this, are key concerns of government (Wanless 2004). In a speech to the 2002 London E-Summit, the then British prime minister, Tony Blair, outlined the commitments that underpinned current policy:

> The fundamental challenge is to create a knowledge-driven economy that serves our long-term goals of first-class public services and economic prosperity for all. To do so we need to innovate. We need to use ideas and intelligence in new ways that create higher value added products and better quality services. The opportunity to develop the knowledge-driven economy is vastly increased by the digital age. Our ability to find and use information, to share ideas across geographic boundaries, is enhanced immensely by the revolution in communications and computing.
>
> (Blair 2002)

But at the same time, policy makers have struggled to explain what they see as failures in innovation and integration in the British National Health Service (NHS). In March 2005 the House of Commons Health Committee met for a formal inquiry into *The Use of New Medical Technologies within the National Health Service* (House of Commons 2005a, 2005b). In particular, the committee was concerned with the difficulties that the NHS seems to experience in adopting and implementing innovative health technologies. The chairman of the committee, David Hinchcliffe MP, began the session by contrasting the National Health Service with health services in other countries, asking why it seemed so difficult for the service to innovate and incorporate new technologies in clinical practice (House of Commons 2005b). He pointed to:

> [t]he way that we have been slow to adapt to those new technologies, and we have had figures showing that we are more or less at the bottom of the European league on percentage of health care spent on new technologies. Why is this when we have some brilliant ideas – some of the people I meet, some good companies in the forefront of world technology advancing ideas – that we as a country are so slow to take advantage of these innovations?
>
> (House of Commons 2005b)

In posing his question, Mr Hinchcliffe placed the committee's deliberations at a macro-level, focusing on the NHS as a system, and on its organizational deploying of the most advanced techniques and technologies. In its report, the committee argued that the problem had two dimensions: the need for new methods of rapidly and sensitively proving the effectiveness of new health technologies, and the need for new mechanisms to rapidly diffuse innovations through the health service and to encourage professionals and managers to adopt them.

In its report, the committee conceived of new technologies as being inextricably linked to advance and progress – when this is not always the case. The perspective offered here involves suspending the notion that equates technological advance with social progress, and the equally common assumption that technological change determines and drives other social changes – the kind of determinist assumption embedded in naïve accounts of future policy and practice (Kendall 2001). Instead, as Grint and Woolgar (1997) have argued, we need to see that technologies and technological changes,

> are not transparent; their character is not given; and they do not contain an essence independent of the nexus of social actions of which they are a part. They do not 'by themselves' tell us what they are capable of. Instead, capabilities – what, for example, a machine will do – are

attributed to the machine by humans. Our knowledge of technology is essentially social.

(1997: 10)

This chapter seeks to apply some lessons of recent sociological research to a core problem for health care organizations – how to routinely embed new technologies in the everyday practices of health professionals and the people they care for. To do this, I will focus on telemedicine systems in practice. These systems use specialized video-conferencing and data transfer equipment and software to allow professionals and patients to interact remotely, in real time. For example, a nurse can examine a patient with chronic lung disease 'remotely' using devices that measure vital signs and blood chemistry, and may provide advice to the patient, or call an ambulance if she or he needs urgent help (Mair *et al.* 2008).

Telemedicine systems seem to fit well with the policy impetus for innovation. Indeed, for more than thirty years, they have been advocated as a means to secure rapid and responsive access to health care for populations that are under-served by specialist services because of structural or spatial inequalities in service provision (Sinha 2000) and, in the UK, to modernize existing services and make them more responsive to both policy and patients (May *et al.* 2005). But these systems also present a problem. Despite significant support from clinicians, health service managers and policy makers in many countries, telemedicine services seem to have failed to become routinely embedded, or normalized (May 2006), in everyday service provision and neither effort invested in innovation nor implementation seem to have been enough to sustain it as a field of professional practice. Looking at telemedicine systems, then, enables us to examine a mundane real-world problem rather than a novel future. It also poses a question: how can we explain why telemedicine is in some senses a 'failed' innovation – and what would need to happen to make it into a 'successful' one that can be embedded into everyday health care? In this chapter, I am going to approach the problem from the perspective of Normalization Process Theory (May and Finch, in press), and examine four domains of the work that needs to be done to embed telemedicine systems in practice.

- **Coherence:** Work that at a macro-level defines and organizes telemedicine systems as *coherent* systems of practice, and that at a micro-level specifies practices that ultimately ensure their *contextual integration* with health care systems and services.
- **Cognitive participation:** The work that defines and organizes the allocation and performance of tasks through telemedicine systems, and that defines their *skill-set workability* within formal and informal divisions of health care labour.
- **Collective action:** Work that defines and organizes the enacting of

telemedicine as a set of clinical practices, and which makes these practices *interactionally workable* within everyday social contexts.

- **Reflexive monitoring**: Work that defines and organizes mechanisms for social accountability and confidence in the professional knowledge that circulates around telemedicine systems, and that makes possible the *relational integration* of this knowledge with clinical practice.

The point here is to consider the work that goes into making telemedicine systems workable and integrated in everyday clinical practice. Such an approach focuses not on what makes them novel and different, but on how they are like other ways of working and their effects on their users. In this context, to understand the problem posed by the perceived 'failure' of telemedicine, this chapter focuses on the processes by which they might (but have not) become normalized across the health care sector.

Coherence: networks and contingencies

Health 'technologies' are more than the sum of their parts – they are systemic and contingent. That is, like all technologies, they consist not only of artefacts and objects (machines and software that are fabricated and consumed), but also of the knowledge and practice that configure their users and characterize their use. It is these patterns of knowledge and practice that link them to others (Bloomfield and Vurdubakis 1994). Importantly, relations between these elements are reciprocal – technological changes frame patterns of social relationships, while changes in social relations are formed through technological changes. The wider STS literature contains many finely grained and specific studies (Brown and Webster 2004; Webster 2007) that remind us that there is no such thing as *a* technology. Instead, there are complex and contingent matrices of knowledge, artefacts, and practices, and networks of human and non-human actors, engaged in reciprocal social relations through which each shapes the other.

Complexity and emergence are important properties of the operationalization of telemedicine systems. The struggle faced by their users is to make sense of them as coherent sets of practices. Coherence is crucial, as we can see when attempts are made to implement new technologies in existing health services. Nicolini (2006) has pointed to the misalignment of 'technological scripts' (the ways that people who design, build and operationalize a new technology) and 'practices' (the ways that people configure and are configured by the use of that technology) in a telemonitoring service for people with heart problems. Nicolini observes that:

A large part of the designer's work is that of inscribing a vision of . . . the world in the technical content of the new objects. During the design process, the designers work out a scenario for how the system will be used. This scenario is inscribed into the system. The inscription includes programs of action for the users and defines roles to be played by users and the system. . . . however, the patterns of use inscribed in the artefact by the designers only come to life in the context of the daily activity of the users.

(2006: 2757)

The important lesson from studies such as Nicolini's is that the encounter between new technologies and their users is an encounter with patterns of more or less coherent work practices. These contingencies can radically change the distribution of work and the knowledge required to conduct it. But they are often unanticipated by designers and managers, and even by professionals and patients. The configurations and reconfigurations can be highly complex – and they frame 'technology' as a particular kind of problem. Such a view leads us to consider the ways that:

technological change is itself shaped by the social circumstances within which it takes place. The 'new sociology of technology' set out to demonstrate that technological artefacts are socially shaped, not just in their usage, but especially with respect to their design and technical content. Crucially, it rejects the notion that technology is simply the product of rational technical imperatives; that a particular technology will triumph because it is intrinsically the best. Technical reasons are vitally important. But we need to ask why a technical reason was found to be compelling, when it could have been challenged, and what counts as technical superiority in specific circumstances. . . . In this way, technology is a socio-technical product, patterned by the conditions of its creation and use.

(Wajcman 2002: 351)

Technology, then, is not a thing on its own. It involves a complex set of relations between humans and non-humans, artefacts and processes, knowledge and practice, organizations and institutions. But the workability of new technologies depends on their coherence too. For example, according to Finch (2008), the objectives and features of telemedicine systems must be specified in a way that renders them comprehensible to their users and differentiates them from others. Their users must also be clear about the specific contributions that are required of them and these, in turn, must be consistent with the communal specifications or norms that underpin practice. In this context a social shaping perspective, informed by Actor Network or similar theories, reminds us that the production of new technologies can be shaped by notions about the desirability of particular kinds of social relations; for example, simulating 'normal' patterns of doctor–patient interaction in telemedicine systems.

Cognitive participation and communicating innovation

STS perspectives on technology begin with the problem of contingency, and the sense that neither the future nor the present are certain – as Wajcman (2002) puts it – because technologies are patterned and configured by the conditions of their creation and use. The demands of policy are, of course, quite different from those of practice. In this context, the business of understanding barriers to the delivery and integration of new ways of delivering and organizing health care is important because their elimination is seen as a necessary precondition of their successful implementation. This is particularly important in structured evaluations of new technologies; for example, in clinical trials where the problem of integration refers not only to embedding a new treatment modality or other health technology into a health care system, but also embedding the techniques and technologies required for evaluation (Finch *et al.* 2003). Increasingly, such problems are understood in terms of implementation processes and change management:

> Implementation of a new process begins when an innovation has been adopted and ends when the innovation becomes routine or is abandoned. Consequently, implementation involves all activities that occur between making an adoption commitment and the time that an innovation either becomes part of the organizational routine, ceases to be new, or is abandoned . . . behaviour, of organizational members, over time evolves from avoidance or non-use, through unenthusiastic or compliant use, to skilled or consistent use.
>
> (Linton 2002: 65)

As this sets the problem out, implementation is about innovation – especially technological innovation. It need not be. Implementation may be conservative and focus on standardization and the regulation of practices according to specific criteria of adequacy, focusing on holding them in place. Approaches to implementation as a technical problem of practice are formed around an intimate connection with individual behaviour change, and especially with psychological models drawn from cognitive theory. For example, Gagnon *et al.* (2003) and Chau and Hu (2001) have applied individual behaviour models to the adoption of telemedicine systems by physicians in Canada and Hong Kong respectively. Their studies showed how professional motivations to use telemedicine have a complex relationship with what people actually do. This question of cognitive participation represents a crucial – and underexplored – element of accounting for the implementation of new health technologies. While Nicolini (2006) found that a trade-off between remedial and active professional work seemed to determine poor responses to telemedicine systems, Gagnon *et al.* found that positive beliefs about the technological advantages offered by telemedicine were not transferred into personal commitments to these systems in practice.

And, just as telemedicine systems design carries assumptions about what the work is, so too does it carry assumptions about the character of those who do it. In a study of a new Teledermatology service (Mort *et al.* 2003), these assumptions became problematic for all, as this extract from an interview with a specialist nurse suggests:

> Nurse: I don't know what our role is, whether to say 'no we can't give you a diagnosis', that I don't know what they want out of us. . . . I suppose that as the project goes on, the confidence in each other, the doctor and who ever is doing the clinic will grow, so they trust what you're saying. If you think it is X and I agree with you why not tell the patients the diagnosis? But then it defeats the object of using the camera if the nurse can go out and diagnose.

Understanding how new knowledge and practice are 'transmitted' through social networks and organizational clusters is also an important focus of technology studies, and work in this area has drawn extensively on Rogers' Diffusion of Innovations Theory (Rogers 1995; Wejnert 2002). Diffusion of Innovations Theory also places special emphasis on the rationality and intentions of individuals – in particular the 'early adopters' and 'product champions' who engage with the 'new' (Strang and Meyer 1993). But 'diffusion' also implies institutionally shaped patterns of communication (Carter *et al.* 2001) between corporate members of networks.

Telemedicine is an interesting case because it is a technology that has been conventionally presented as an innovation whose time has come, and that is assumed to offer efficiency benefits and to offer major advances in the delivery of care, when in fact this is by no means always true. In this context it is like other health technologies that reconfigure work and redistribute workload through the intensification of labour, steadily adding to the organizational load of work, and to the interactional demands that it makes (Johnstone 2005). Here, the common assumption that new technologies and service innovations diffuse through health care systems through the influence of 'adopters' and 'product champions' is also a problem. In the US, Whitten and Collins (1997) have emphasized the communicative aspects of diffusion. They argue that the diffusion of telemedicine depends on particular kinds of conversations between users and groups of users; importantly they also emphasize that these conversations need not be focused on the contingent technologies themselves but are often about the problems that they are intended to solve. Thus telemedicine is constructed as an a priori solution to policy problems of inequalities, of time and space, of control over groups of its users, and as a solution to problems of quality in practice. This shifts attention onto the problem of professional resistance – who it is often claimed fails to utilize a solution effectively (May *et al.* 2005) – rather than onto problems of integrating new ways of working into existing patterns of practice. The focus of these corporate conversations also changes, so that 'telemedicine' as a field of practice is continually reinvented. Importantly, Whitten and Collins see this telemedicine diffusion network as decentralized:

> In the decentralized system inherent in the diffusion of telemedicine, however, it is unclear who is playing the role of adopter. Is it the physician who sees patients by interactive video? Is it the patient who agrees to be treated by a physician hundreds of miles away? Or is it the insurance company who agrees to reimburse a physician who never actually examined or saw a patient? . . . The jury is still out concerning issues of adoption, as is evidenced through the monitoring of usage rates. A definitive understanding of actual adoption proves to be an almost impossible task for such a decentralized context.
>
> (1997: 32)

This describes an important obstacle to the implementation of telemedicine, and connects it to much wider questions of policy. From the perspective of policy makers, the very complexity of new technologies often seems to be an obstacle to the production of practically workable evaluations and conceptual models to understand them. This is a real problem in the UK. The NHS in England is a federal system composed of more than 750 service providers (NHS Trusts); a very large number of for-profit service providers and suppliers that sell products and services to both the NHS and its patients; and many different policy and regulatory agencies. All are subject to frequent reorganization and changes in policy direction, and are composed of multiple professional groups with diverse contractual relationships and political interests – and so the politics of service provision itself is highly complex and always contentious.

Collective action: why is it so hard to 'implement' telemedicine systems?

So far we have examined two key problems in understanding how and why new technologies become embedded in health care practice: their coherence – how a 'technology' is bound to assumptions about its users and ideas about practice; and their associated processes of cognitive participation – the social processes of enrolment and engagement that draw groups of users into its field.

These perspectives can help us because they focus attention on motivation and agency – the voluntary engagement of users of a technology. But these are only part of the story. Indeed McLaughlin and colleagues (1999) have pointed to the ways that in such contexts the 'boundaries between the development, diffusion and implementation of a technology blur' (1999: 51), and have pointed to the regulation and constraints that follow from attempts to embed new technologies in the fabric of organizational structures. This means that implementation is not only a matter of individual behaviour change and the communication of innovations, but also about complex group processes and accomplishments in contexts where technological change is mandatory.

Continuing to take a 'social shaping' perspective, and acknowledging these caveats, we can now focus on the processes and accomplishments of collective action in which attempts to embed telemedicine systems in clinical practice have been framed. This approach focuses attention on the social relations, processes and practices that relate to the work of implementation and operationalization. In this context, and like proponents of all new technologies incorporated in health care settings, proponents of telemedicine systems face four key challenges as they seek to normalize them in clinical practice (May *et al.* 2007). We will work through these challenges: interactional workability, relational integration, skill-set workability and contextual integration, in turn.

Telemedicine systems raise questions about the interactional workability of a new technology – and ask, how does a new technology affect interactions between people and practices? In the case of telemedicine we can start with the interaction itself. There are strong social norms and conventions that govern ideas about what can legitimately be dealt with in a clinical encounter, what the form of the work is, what the role of each participant is, how the work is to be completed in the time and space available, and the formal and informal rules that govern the verbal and non-verbal conduct of an interaction (Strong 1979; Heritage and Maynard 2006). A psychiatrist in a British study (May *et al.* 2001) explains how video-conferenced clinical encounters changed her practice:

> I found that you have to maintain eye contact in what I think is a slightly artificial way and that was partly because of the problems with the sound. If you both spoke at the same time the picture froze and therefore you couldn't look away and just throw in the odd remark. So I think that makes a slight difference to face to face communication. And also I was sitting – I suspect you can probably set this up in another way – but the way we had it the patient was clearly sitting straight in front, and I was sitting straight in front [of each other] and I don't interview people face to face like that. . . . It definitely wasn't as relaxing as it could have been, you know, how you sit back and move your chair. . . . It would remind me of old fashioned psychiatry. I remember when I started, the psychiatrist sat behind a desk, and the patient was on the other side. But we don't communicate that way now. . . .

The problematic form and conduct of electronically mediated clinical encounters is a consistent feature of critical studies of telemedicine, which reconfigures professional–patient relations. It introduces non-human intermediaries (Mort *et al.* 2003), new and 'artificial' forms of interactional conduct and clinical practices (May *et al.* 2001; Nicolini 2007), and changes the ways in which agreement about the outcomes of interactions are negotiated and organized (Miller 2001; Finch *et al.* 2007b).

Telemedicine systems raise problems of relational integration which prompts us to ask – how does a new technology relate to existing knowledge and relationships? Here, analysis is concerned with the knowledge and practice of those enacting telemedicine as a set of enacted practices. In particular, we need to focus on social patterns of accountability – what knowledge is required to operationalize this knowledge and who possesses this knowledge and is permitted to employ it – and what are the formal and informal rules that govern its distribution within networks (May *et al.* 2006b). Similarly, we need to consider the problem of confidence – how users of a technology come to agree the practical utility and reliability of the knowledge and practice mediated by other participants in telemedicine services and encounters. The question of diagnostic safety has always been an important but limiting focus of professional and policy debate about telemedicine, when empirical studies have revealed more complex questions and negotiations about what the knowledge imparted and lost in tele-medicine is (Mort *et al.* 2003; Finch *et al.* 2005). An important Canadian study by Lehoux *et al.* (2002) points to the ways that accountability and confidence are constructed in practice.

> Except for medical internists in the most remote hospital, respondents thought there was nothing wrong with their existing means of communication. They did not feel it was difficult to obtain advice from an expert, nor did they experience trouble in having their patients seen by a consultant. The very idea that the technology could institute a process by which a consultant formulates an opinion without directly examining a patient was received with scepticism by all neurologists, as well as several cardiologists and pulmonary medicine specialists. While most of them agreed that it would be nice to assist an isolated colleague fraught with a complex case, they recognised that those cases are complex for tertiary care specialists too. The more complex a case is, the more likely the consultant will want to 'start from scratch', e.g., to personally gather all the relevant clinical information and avoid the 'interpretation' of the referring physician.
>
> (2002: 897)

Telemedicine systems in this study were conceived of by their suppliers as technologies that opened up communications and subtracted problems of time and space. It was supposed that they would add efficiency to health services, but in fact, in this Canadian case – as in the Italian service described by Nicolini (2006, 2007), and the telepsychiatry service discussed above (May *et al.* 2001) – these new systems added more work aimed at inter-actional management and assessing the credibility of knowledge, with little perceived pay-off in the form of benefits for practitioners and patients.

Problems of interactional workability and relational integration focus attention on the point of contact between professionals and their patients, and on the networks of knowledge and practice in which they are located. These are immediate aspects of the clinical practices in which health technologies such as telemedicine systems come to be located, and we have seen that they both tell us something about how, and why, it has proved difficult to 'implement' telemedicine systems. One way in which policy makers have explained this is to claim that 'professional resistance' is the problem – and that doctors, especially, resist attempts to modernize services and make them more accessible and responsive to patients (May *et al.* 2005). It is true that in the UK there has been a series of collisions between the profession and the New Labour government after 1997 that have focused on conditions of service, workload and service organization. But telemedicine systems offer an interesting corrective to this view: internationally, doctors seem eager to use them (Gagnon *et al.* 2003; Whitten and Mackert 2005; MacFarlane *et al.* 2006) but find them hard to integrate with existing modes of clinical practice. Resistance may be a local issue, but as we have seen, this does not explain wider problems of integration and workability. To fully explain these, we have to take a step beyond the micro-contexts of the clinical encounter and its social networks, and consider factors that relate to the structural contexts in which telemedicine systems are operationalized.

Although the costs of labour and problems of training are often the focus of interest in new technologies (Lansisalmi *et al.* 2006), questions about skill-set workability are less common – but how the division of labour in a health care system is affected by a new technology is of central importance in understanding its implementation. Indeed, conflicts and contests about the impact of new technologies on the allocation and performance of work are of primary importance across a range of industries (Edgerton 2006). Telemedicine systems radically change divisions of labour because they draw into question the roles and expectations of participants. Changes in role lead to changes in the allocation of work. In teledermatology, especially, this has involved using specialist nurses to do the work of interacting with patients to collect diagnostic and management data – a task formerly undertaken by doctors (Mallett 2003; Finch *et al.* 2007a). This corresponds to a more general trend to shift specialist work to nurses, using protocols that give structure and focus to their practice (Hanlon *et al.* 2005). These moves are not always welcomed – for example, mental health professionals involved in a telepsychiatry service were concerned about losing control of their therapeutic interactions with patients (May *et al.* 2001), as were specialist nurses delivering a remote monitoring service for people with obstructive airways disease (Mair *et al.* 2005). But as Finch and her co-authors have shown (Finch *et al.* 2007a), renegotiating and re-engineering professional roles – even within a very limited field of action – is vital. In this context, radical changes to the division of labour are still underpinned by medical dominance. Nicolini observes that:

In a ward, because of the intense regime of interaction, it is not unusual for non-medical [i.e. nursing] staff to carry out medical duties. This however, presupposes a regime of proximity in which there is always a doctor nearby . . . All this changes when distance is introduced in the equation.

(2007: 907)

Nicolini argues that responses to distance involve performative remedial strategies. She draws out several that have also been observed in other studies. These include: practices that 'downplay' the interpretive work of nurses and 'linking' practices that articulate nursing work to medical decisions (Mort *et al.* 2003). They also include symbolic work that affirms the subordination of nursing knowledge and practices through protocols. The latter shift the subjective judgement of professionals to an 'objective' textual authority (May *et al.* 2006).

Formal divisions of labour, within health services, are not the only ones that may be radically changed by telemedicine. Simple devices that transmit information about blood sugar levels (for people with diabetes) or blood oxygenation (for people with congestive heart disease) bring patients themselves into the realm of allocated clinical work and the performance of technical competencies, as the burden of health care data collection is shifted to them. Indeed, a constant refrain in policy over the past decade has been a new kind of patient – activated, resourceful and engaged (Coulter 2001; Kendall 2001) – who uses technologies knowledgeably for self-care (Kennedy *et al.* 2003). In this context, telemedicine systems blur the boundaries between formal and informal health care provision in new and interesting ways.

The increasingly blurred boundaries between formal and informal health care systems, and the complicating effects of new technologies on professional (and lay) divisions of labour are reflected, too, in their contextual integration. This raises the question, how does a complex intervention relate to the organization in which it is set? There is now a substantial body of work that explores the execution of health technologies. This work focuses on the production and organization of knowledge and practice and the distribution of resources, costs and risks within organizations (Currie and Guah, 2006), managerial decision-making regarding the adoption of the intervention, and formal and informal mechanisms for its evaluation (Lansisalmi *et al.* 2006). Managing investment and controlling costs are a problem in telemedicine – and most NHS services have been supported through R&D funding streams. The problem of funding and managing costs appears regularly in the international literature too (Obstfelder *et al.* 2007). Managing the money is central to integrating telemedicine in the decision-making processes of any health care agency. But integration means rather more than that, and it also refers to the ways that new systems of practice are linked, organizationally, to other already existing forms of work in an organization – perhaps as responsibility for a procedure moves from one professional group to another – or as negotiations proceed to modify existing practices to make new ones possible, minimising the disruption and risk associated with change, and how new resources are obtained and used in practice (Finch *et al.* 2007a).

Reflexive monitoring

A key feature of contemporary medicine is that it is subject to large-scale, institutional modes of reflexive monitoring. Formal practices of evaluation are routinely embedded in the fabric of health care provision, and technologies of evaluation – randomized controlled trials, systematic reviews, qualitative process evaluations, health technology assessments and cost effectiveness studies – are woven into the process of technological change. These institutionalized forms of reflexivity are focused through new regulatory sciences, in particular, through health technology assessment (Faulkner 1997; Lehoux 2006). These provide formal means of integrating technological and political domains – linking 'gold standard' methods to secure policy and spending decisions (see Chapter 6, this volume, by Harrison and Checkland).

Knowledge produced by these methods is conceived of as evidence, and is assumed to be both highly transportable and methodologically generalizable. In fact, this kind of institutional reflexivity is both arguable and argued about – because it is mainly about the outcomes of evaluations, and tells us little about the processes by which these outcomes are achieved (May 2006a). The House of Commons Health Committee's Inquiry, discussed in the introduction to this chapter, was an exercise in institutional reflexivity that called clinicians, system manufacturers and researchers to account – and which attempted to argue for alternatives to large clinical trials that included a better understanding of the processes of making technologies such as telemedicine workable and integrating them in everyday health care provision. In an ethnography of policy makers working on the business of making and using evidence, a senior NHS manager asserted:

> Really, we need to identify *who* needs evidence, and *what* sort of evidence they need. It's important because telecare is a link between different policy areas and evidence is the glue that can hold them together. We need to draw on a range of evidence – and there's a lot of frustration about the definition of proper evidence. We need to work on what you might call qualitative evidence because that's much more suited to this task.
>
> (May 2006a: 526)

Reflexivity of this kind is not confined to large-scale, institutional modes of evaluation. The patient satisfaction survey, and the consultation exercise, are ubiquitous techniques for providing post-hoc support for changes in service provision, and – at the same time – for holding the staff who provide them in a relationship that disciplines and constrains their practice (Williams *et al.* 2003). Yet they often tell us little about what users really think or feel about technological change (Mair and Whitten 2000).

Implementation processes have been characterized in this chapter as the result of cognitive participation in a set of relations (framed by norms and conventions that include shared beliefs about action, rules about appropriate forms of behavior, and so forth), and collective action (framed by patterns of conduct, the distribution of knowledge and practice, divisions of labour, and the availability of material and symbolic resources). Reflexive monitoring is thus embedded in the engagement of technology users. But the reflexivity of participating (or observing) actors also means that their beliefs about the process and its outcomes are themselves important components of the blurred constructions of development, diffusion and use described by McLaughlin *et al.* (1999), and there is no automatic connection between evidence of effectiveness and beliefs about the necessity of implementation (Dopson *et al.* 2003). The process by which knowledge is constructed and beliefs framed by actors – reflexive monitoring – is therefore central to the ways that they make sense of a practice and project it into the future.

Conclusion

This chapter began with an acknowledgement of the great complexity of the socio-technical networks that are implicated in technological change, and it has proceeded through a discussion of explanations for the problems of telemedicine development and implementation. In particular, I have been concerned to develop a line of argument about the normalization and routine embedding of telemedicine systems in health services, by reference not only to my own research but also to international studies. In doing this, I have sought to make the point that the proponents of telemedicine services face fundamental problems of individual cognitive participation, collective action, and institutional reflexive monitoring. In this context I have sought to simplify the complexities of socio-technical networks by focusing on a conceptual model that focuses primarily on the work that people do to operationalize a new technology in interactional, relational, skill-set and contextual domains. None of these networks represents simple linear processes, they are messy, difficult, contingent and unpredictable.

Telemedicine systems are useful vehicles to consider these problems precisely because they are so unstable in clinical practice, and are the focus of conflicts and contests between different groups of professionals, health care managers and policy makers. But we also need to keep the problematic political quality of 'implementation' in sight. Langstrup (2008) has argued that the notion of implementation is often deployed in ways that assume the 'organizational setting and its actors as pre-givens, thus making the critical task the creation of a fit between technology and organization'. Sociological understanding of the implementation of telemedicine need not be founded on this political assumption. Instead, it can begin with the question: what is the system of practice? In other words, to focus on what the work is, and how work is interactionally shaped and how it is institutionally framed.

Acknowledgements

I gladly acknowledge the contribution of Tracy Finch, Frances Mair, Maggie Mort and Elizabeth Murray in the genesis of the ideas presented here, and thank them, and Catherine Exley, for their comments on this chapter. Parts of this chapter are drawn from, May, C. 'A rational model for assessing and evaluating complex interventions in health care', published under a creative commons licence in *BMC Health Services Research*, 2006, 6, article 86.

References

Blair, A. (2002) 'Speech to e-summit'. Online: www.numberten.gov.uk/output/Page 1734.asp (accessed 16 May 2007).

Bloomfield, B.P. and Vurdubakis, T. (1994) 'Boundary disputes: negotiating the boundary between the technical and the social in the development of IT systems', *Information Technology and People*, 7: 9–24.

Brown, N. and Webster, A. (2004) *New Medical Technologies and Society: reordering life*, Cambridge: Polity.

Carter, F.J., Jambulingam, T., Gupta, V.K. and Melone, N. (2001) 'Technological innovations: a framework for communicating diffusion effects', *Information and Management*, 38: 277–87.

Chau, P.Y.K. and Hu, P.J.H. (2001) 'Information technology acceptance by individual professionals: a model comparison approach', *Decision Sciences*, 32: 699–719.

Coulter, A. (2001) *The Autonomous Patient*, Oxford: Oxford University Press.

Currie, W.L. and Guah, M.W. (2006) 'IT-enabled healthcare delivery: The UK National Health Service', *Information Systems Management*, 23: 7–22.

Dopson, S., Locock, L., Gabbay, J., Ferlie, E. and Fitzgerald, L. (2003) 'Evidence-based medicine and the implementation gap', *Health*, 7: 311–30.

Edgerton, D. (2006) *The Shock of the Old: technology and global history since 1900*, London: Profile.

Faulkner, A. (1997) '"Strange bedfellows" in the laboratory of the NHS? An analysis of the new science of health technology assessment in the United Kingdom', in M.A. Elston (ed.) *The Sociology of Medical Science and Technology*, Oxford: Blackwell.

Finch, T. (2008) 'Teledermatology for chronic disease management: coherence and normalization', *Chronic Illness*, 4: 127–34.

Finch, T.L., Mair, F.S. and May, C.R. (2007a) 'Teledermatology in the UK: lessons in service innovation', *British Journal of Dermatology*, 156: 521–7.

Finch, T., May, C., Mort, M. and Mair, F. (2005) 'Telemedicine, telecare, and the future patient: innovation, risk and governance', in A. Webster and S. Wyatt (eds) *Innovative Health Technologies: meaning, context and change*, Basingstoke: Palgrave.

Finch, T.L., Mort, M., Mair, F.S. and May, C.R. (2007b) 'Telehealthcare and future patients: Configuring "the patient"', *Health and Social Care in the Community*, 16: 86–95.

Finch, T., May, C., Mair, F., Mort, M. and Gask, L. (2003) 'Integrating service development with evaluation in telehealthcare: an ethnographic study', *British Medical Journal*, 327: 1205–9.

Fox, R. (ed.) (1996) *Technological Change*, Amsterdam: Harwood Academic.

Gagnon, M.P., Godin, G., Gagne, C., Fortin, J.P., Lamothe, L., Reinharz, D. and Cloutier, A. (2003) 'An adaptation of the theory of interpersonal behaviour to the study of telemedicine adoption by physicians', *International Journal of Medical Informatics*, 71: 103–15.

Greenhalgh, T., Robert, G., Macfarlane, F., Bate, P. and Kyriakidou, O. (2004) 'Diffusion of innovations in service organizations: Systematic review and recommendations', *Milbank Quarterly*, 82: 581–629.

Grint, K. and Woolgar, S. (1997) *The Machine at Work: technology, work and organization*, Oxford: Blackwell Publishers Ltd.

Hanlon, G., Strangleman, T., Goode, J., Luff, D., O'Cathain, A. and Greatbatch, D. (2005) 'Knowledge, technology and nursing: the case of NHS direct', *Human Relations*, 58: 147–171.

Heritage, J. and Maynard, D.W. (2006) 'Problems and prospects in the study of physician-patient interaction: 30 years of research', *Annual Review of Sociology*, 32: 351–74.

House of Commons (2005a) *House of Commons Health Committee: the use of new medical technologies within the NHS, Volume 1*. London: The Stationery Office.

House of Commons (2005b) *House of Commons Health Committee: the use of new medical technologies within the NHS, Volume 2: Oral and Written Evidence*. London: The Stationery Office.

Johnstone, P.L. (2005) 'Technology-related factors contributing to labour intensification of surgical production', *Prometheus*, 23: 27–46.

Kendall, L. (2001) *The Future Patient*, London: Institute of Public Policy Research.

Kennedy, A., Gately, C. and Rogers, A. (2003) *National Evaluation of the Expert Patient Programme: assessing the process of embedding the EPP in the NHS*, Manchester: NPCRDC.

Langstrup, H. (2008) 'Making connections through online asthma monitoring', *Chronic Illness*, 4: 118–26.

Lansisalmi, H., Kivimaki, M., Aalto, P. and Ruoranen, R. (2006) 'Innovation in healthcare: a systematic review of recent research', *Nursing Science Quarterly*, 19: 66–72.

Lehoux, P. (2006) *The Problem of Health Technology: policy implications for modern health care systems*, London: Routledge.

Lehoux, P., Sicotte, C., Denis, J.L., Berg, M. and Lacroix, A. (2002) 'The theory of use behind telemedicine: how compatible with physicians' clinical routines?' *Social Science and Medicine*, 54: 889–904.

Linton, J.D. (2002) 'Implementation research: state of the art and future directions', *Technovation*, 22: 65–79.

MacFarlane, A., Murphy, A.W. and Clerkin, P. (2006) 'Telemedicine services in the Republic of Ireland: an evolving policy context', *Health Policy*, 76: 245–58.

MacKenzie, D. (1998) *Knowing Machines: essays on technical change*, London: The Massachusetts Institute of Technology Press.

Mair, F. and Whitten, P. (2000) 'Systematic review of studies of patient satisfaction with telemedicine', *British Medical Journal*, 320: 1517–20.

Mair, F.S., Goldstein, P., May, C., Angus, R., Shiels, C., Hibbert, D., O'Connor, J., Boland, A., Roberts, C., Haycox, A. and Capewell, S. (2005) 'Patient and provider perspectives on home telecare: preliminary results from a randomized controlled trial', *Journal of Telemedicine and Telecare*, 11: 95–7.

Mair, F.S., Hiscock, J. and Beaton, S.C. (2008) 'Understanding factors that inhibit or promote the utilization of telecare in chronic lung disease', *Chronic Illness*, 4: 110–17.

Mallett, R.B. (2003) 'Teledermatology in practice', *Clinical and Experimental Dermatology*, 28: 356–9.

May, C. (2006a) 'Mobilizing modern facts: Health Technology Assessment and the politics of evidence', *Sociology of Health and Illness*, 28: 513–32.

May, C. (2006b) 'A rational model for assessing and evaluating complex interventions in health care', *BMC Health Services Research*, 6: 86.

May, C. and Finch, T. (forthcoming) 'Implementation, embedding, and integration: an outline of Normalization Process Theory', *Sociology*.

May, C., Finch, T., Mair, F. and Mort, M. (2005) 'Towards a wireless patient: chronic illness, scarce care and technological innovation in the United Kingdom', *Social Science and Medicine*, 61: 1485–94.

May, C., Finch, T., Mair, F.S., Ballini, L., Dowrick, C., Eccles, M., Gask, L., MacFarlane, A., Murray, E., Rapley, T., Rogers, A., Treweek, S. and Wallace, P. (2007) 'Understanding the implementation of complex interventions in health care: the Normalization Process Model', *BMC Health Services Research*, 7: 148.

May, C., Gask, L., Atkinson, T., Ellis, N.T., Mair, F. and Esmail, A. (2001) 'Resisting and promoting new technologies in clinical practice: the case of telepsychiatry', *Social Science and Medicine*, 52: 1889–901.

May, C., Rapley, T., Moreira, T., Finch, T. and Heaven, B. (2006) 'Technogovernance: evidence, subjectivity, and the clinical encounter in primary care medicine', *Social Science and Medicine*, 62: 1022–30.

McLaughlin, J., Rosen, P., Skinner, D. and Webster, A. (1999) *Valuing Technology: organisations, culture and change*, London: Routledge.

Miller, E.A. (2001) 'Telemedicine and doctor-patient comunication: an analytical survey of the literature', *Journal of Telemedicine and Telecare*, 7: 1–17.

Mort, M., May, C.R. and Williams, T. (2003) 'Remote doctors and absent patients: acting at a distance in telemedicine?' *Science, Technology and Human Values*, 28: 274–95.

Nicolini, D. (2006) 'The work to make telemedicine work: a social and articulative view', *Social Science and Medicine*, 62: 2754–67.

Nicolini, D. (2007) 'Stretching out and expanding work practices in time and space: the case of telemedicine', *Human Relations*, 60: 889–920.

Obstfelder, A., Engeseth, K.H. and Wynn, R. (2007) 'Characteristics of successfully implemented telemedical applications', *Implementation Science*, 2. Online: www.implementationscience.com/content/2/1/25.

Rogers, E.M. (1995) *The Diffusion of Innovation*, fourth edition, New York: Free Press.

Sinha, A. (2000) 'An overview of telemedicine: the virtual gaze of health care in the next century', *Medical Anthropology Quarterly*, 14: 291–309.

Strang, D. and Meyer, J.W. (1993) 'Institutional conditions for diffusion', *Theory and Society*, 22: 487–511.

Strong, P. (1979) *The Ceremonial Order of the Clinic: patients, doctors and medical bureaucracies*, London: Routledge.

Wajcman, J. (2002) 'Addressing technological change: the challenge to social theory', *Current Sociology*, 50: 347–63.

Wanless, D. (2004) *Securing our Future Health: taking a long-term view*, Final Report, London: The Stationery Office.

Webster, A. (2007) *Health, Technology and Society: a sociological critique*, Basingstoke: Palgrave Macmillan.

Wejnert, B. (2002) 'Integrating models of diffusion of innovations: a conceptual framework', *Annual Review of Sociology*, 28: 297–326.

Whitten, P. and Collins, B. (1997) 'The diffusion of telemedicine: communicating an innovation', *Science Communication*, 19: 21–40.

Whitten, P.S. and Mackert, M.S. (2005) 'Addressing telehealth's foremost barrier: provider as initial gatekeeper', *International Journal of Technology Assessment in Health Care*, 21: 517–21.

Williams, T., May, C., Mair, F., Mort, M. and Gask, L. (2003) 'Normative models of health technology assessment and the social production of evidence about telehealthcare', *Health Policy*, 64: 39–54.

8   Health care, consumerism and the politics of identity

Timothy Milewa

Introduction

Tensions around service quality, levels of provision, management, the rights of patients and the role of the market raise questions about the identity of health service users. Are they simply patients in receipt of more or less adequate care, citizens exercising their social right to 'free' health care, discerning consumers or are such identities fluid and hybrid? This chapter focuses on the meaning and impact of 'consumer' identities in British health care by addressing three questions. First, has there been radical change in the portrayal of health service users within the narratives of policy since the early days of the National Health Service in terms of ascribed, possibly contested, identities? In a second respect, what evidence is there to suggest an accentuated 'consumer' consciousness on the part of health service users? And in a third regard, how might such change be explained and evaluated from a sociological perspective? An overview of relevant policies and examination of trends in relation to areas that include patient choice, complaints and litigation suggest that 'consumerist' aspects of the health service user can only be understood with reference to wider social perceptions and motivations around ideas such as trust, obligation and responsibility.

Health service users and the crafting of identities

Significant state involvement in health care entails tensions that centre on more than just issues of regulation, funding and access. Even within a 'universal' system of health care, factors such as age, location, medical condition and the ability to access private provision may influence the 'identities' of health service users in relation to health care. Patients can – according to specific aspects of policy, political discourse, provision and self-labelling – be cast, for example, as citizens exercising their right to health care; marginalized groups in need of assistance; stakeholders with an interest in a particular service or policy or discriminating consumers to whose preferences service providers should attempt to cater (Barnes *et al.* 2007: 9). Accordingly, this section of the chapter examines the portrayal of health service users in aspects of policy. A brief contextual overview is followed by a focus upon 'consumer-oriented' strands of health policy concerned with patient choice, the 'expert patient', patient safety and changes in arrangements for patient and public involvement in aspects of health service planning.

In terms of context, the role and influence of health service users received little sustained official attention in health policy before 1974 when Community Health Councils were established in England and Wales to represent the interests of the public in the NHS. The latter were designed to act as a source of information for local residents, as a means to help aggrieved patients pursue complaints and as a focal point for liaison with corresponding health authorities over issues of local concern (Gerrard 2006). But the election of a Conservative government in 1979 began, to a limited extent, to introduce a discourse of consumerism with regard to health service users. A political concern with enhanced efficiency and fostering business-like practices in the public sector prompted the NHS (Griffiths) Management Inquiry in 1983 – an investigation that underpinned the development of an extensive professional management function in the NHS from 1985. The associated political and managerial vocabulary of responsiveness, quality improvement and performance targets entailed an implicit concern with the needs of health service 'consumers'. The latter were not akin, however, to 'customers'. After 1990 health authorities and a limited number of general practitioners were required to plan and then commission health services from providers while taking into account, in a thorough-going manner, 'advice' from local health service users (Milewa *et al.* 1998). At the same time the *Patients' Charter* made explicit certain standards that could be expected in the health service but, again, these did not portray patients as customers. National standards included the continued right to choose a general practitioner; maximum waiting times for surgery; more information on the nature and location of health services; the continued right to complain and, with certain restrictions, the ability to access medical records (Carr 1992). This quasi-consumerist portrayal of health service users became, however, more nuanced after the election of the New Labour government in 1997. The party's period out of office between 1979 and 1997 had prompted a search for policy rationales that sought to move beyond both the discredited orthodoxies of post-war social democratic intervention and the neo-liberal individualism associated with aspects of Conservative party policy in the 1980s and 1990s. The approach adopted was premised on a 'Third way' of running the NHS – 'a system based on partnership and driven by performance' (Department of Health 1997: par. 2.2). Subsequent interventions thus reiterated elements of a consumerist discourse but also encouraged more inclusive, socially cohering approaches to patient and public involvement together with ongoing, deliberative methods of gauging the views and preferences of health service users (Parkinson 2004).

Policies and identities

More specifically, turning first to aspects of a 'consumerist' policy discourse, one of the more prominent emphases in New Labour health policy was on 'choice'. Pilot schemes in 2002 gave some patients who had waited over six months for elective surgery the right to opt for another provider. And in 2006 patients referred to hospitals for treatment were given a choice of at least four hospitals from lists compiled by corresponding Primary Care Trusts – lists supplemented in the same year by a national 'menu' of Foundation Trusts (hospitals granted enhanced autonomy by the government on the basis of their performance) and privately owned or managed Independent Sector Treatment Centres (Department of Health 2007). Moreover, in June 2008 it was announced that a new system would be piloted in 2009 whereby patients with selected chronic illnesses would be given control of significant personal budgets that could be used to 'purchase' care. The wording was, however, very cautious: 'The budget itself may well be held on the patient's behalf, but we will pilot direct payments where this makes most sense for particular patients in certain circumstances' (Department of Health 2008: 42).

But did this concern with choice (casting patients in the role of consumers to a limited extent) chime with the wishes of health service users? Approximately 59 per cent of 'lay' adults aged 16 and over in a survey in 2003 indicated that they would, hypothetically, want a degree of choice between hospitals were they to require surgery (this was an interview-based survey of 2057 people – data were weighted to the general population's profile). About 40 per cent would want to participate in the choice of surgeon for their operation, 45 per cent would want to be involved in choosing specific medications or treatments and 42 per cent would prefer choice in relation to complementary and alternative treatments (such as acupuncture) (MORI 2003). And in more concrete terms, in one of the earlier initiatives in patient choice, 50 per cent of coronary heart disease patients who had been waiting for surgery for six months opted for treatment at an alternative hospital to that originally intended rather than wait any longer (Bate and Robert 2006: 669).

More reflectively, however, the meaning of 'patient choice' is itself contestable. Choice can encompass the selection of secondary care providers (as implied by the government) as well as decisions on the type of treatment administered, preferences for associated social care packages, the determination of health care practitioner, recourse to private sector provision and the use of self-treatments (Appleby *et al.* 2003: 47; Winters 2006). Choice is also something that can be (and is) exercised on behalf of patients by general practitioners and health service organizations (Pickard *et al.* 2006). In short, if the reality of choice is linked to ideas of an accentuated consumerist identity on the part of health service users, we need to be very clear about whose understanding of choice is being employed, in what circumstances and the degree to which it reflects consensus on the part of the government, health service providers and patients.

Similar points might be made in relation to a government-sponsored programme of training opportunities and information resources for patients with selected chronic conditions (such as arthritis, asthma, diabetes and epilepsy). The Expert Patients Programme, launched in 2002, was designed to help patients communicate better with clinicians, engage more effectively with treatment regimes and to develop a pro-active, goal-centred approach to coping with medical conditions (Department of Health 2001a). But, as with choice, the rationale for the Expert Patient Programme and thus the identity of the 'expert patient' is not clear-cut. There is, suggest Taylor and Bury (2007), little evidence to suggest that patient-led education programmes generate better health outcomes than those led by 'professionals'. Similarly, the degree to which feelings of self-efficacy rather than education influence health outcomes is uncertain. And in a third respect, projects such as the Expert Patients Programme run the risk of 'blaming' patients for their own plight while ignoring wider determinants of health and illness. On the other hand, as Kelleher (1994) observes, conceptions of the 'lay expert' and the activities of self-help groups can represent a conscious attempt by patients and carers to wrest control of health care from a sometimes remote and rarefied medical profession and health care system. This trend is perhaps evident in the growth of the internet as a medium of communication between health service users (Seale 2006). As Gillett (2003) indicates in relation to AIDS/HIV, internet sites and discussion groups can focus on the provision of 'expert' advice by patients to patients, the recounting of personal experiences and also criticisms of particular approaches to treatment. The contrasting perspectives offered by Taylor and Bury and Kelleher thus serve to emphasize the malleability of the idea of the expert patient in relation to issues such as responsibility and empowerment.

Caution should also be exercised when interpreting policy interventions around the issue of patient safety. This topic generated considerable media, public and patient concern in the 1990s and 2000s in relation to topics that ranged from infections acquired in hospitals to the monitoring of doctors to safeguard health service users. In terms, for example, of concerns expressed by patients, only 53 per cent of hospital inpatients who participated in a postal questionnaire survey in 2006 thought that their ward or room was clean – a slight decrease from 56 per cent in 2002 (Richards and Coulter 2007: 11). And with regard to monitoring doctors, an inquiry into how an English general practitioner, Harold Shipman, was able to murder scores of his patients between 1974 and 1998 without detection not only generated public concern and government action but also accentuated apparent self-reflection on the part of the medical profession itself. Reports by the Chief Medical Officer for England – *Supporting Doctors, Protecting Patients in 1999* and *Assuring the Quality of Medical Practice in 2001* – led to the foundation of the National Clinical Assessment Authority in

2001 (renamed the National Clinical Assessment Service in 2005). The service acts in an advisory role to NHS organizations when the latter refer cases about the performance or skills of individual doctors or dentists. This role can encompass general advice but also very detailed reviews of individual professional performance (Baker 2004; National Patient Safety Agency 2007).

But, as with the idea of patient choice and the expert patient, these interventions can be linked to more than one pressure for change and a less than clear-cut idea of which 'identity' is being addressed in relation to health service users. From the state's perspective, the economic rationale for addressing patient safety is pressing. A Department of Health report in 2000, *An Organisation with a Memory*, suggested that 10 per cent of admissions to NHS hospitals were followed by 'adverse events' that caused harm to patients and that these cost at least £2 billion per year (Gubb 2007: 1; Davis *et al.* 2007). Enhancing patient safety thus became a primary goal for the NHS in 2001 when the National Patient Safety Agency was established to monitor and address patient safety issues (Department of Health 2001b). But were health service users here being portrayed just as patients in need of protection or as cost-conscious taxpayers as well? Similarly, Waring (2007) makes the point that enhanced regulation of medicine may not simply reflect public disquiet and an attempt by the state to safeguard patients. In the face of an increasing emphasis upon evidence-based practice (*cf.* Timmermans and Berg 2003), clinical governance and systems of surveillance, the medical profession perhaps has an interest in ensuring that its 'practice, culture and discourse' subsume new regulatory procedures rather than have them imposed from without – an extension of the medical demesne within which, perhaps, health service users remain patients rather than become 'consumers' (Waring 2007: 176).

Health service users and the 'new' spaces of collaboration

But health policies do not focus solely on the individual experience of health care. The New Labour government became associated between 1997 and 2008 with attempts to imbue patient and public involvement strategies with a normative conception of the responsibilities that attend health care as a 'right' of citizenship. Politicians such as Tony Blair, David Blunkett, John Prescott and Jack Straw argued – episodically – for a quasi-communitarian activism whereby 'stakeholder' groups (such as patient advocacy bodies and community associations) should play a major part in making decisions and formulating policies (Milewa 2004). Some indication of what this meant was given by Prime Minister Gordon Brown in 2007 when he disparaged 'old models of consultation' and 'commands from Whitehall'. He went on to argue that solutions to problems in areas of policy such as health would not come from 'a narrow debate between what states do and what markets do' but would necessitate 'new ways and means to bring together citizens to discuss both specific challenges that need addressing, and concrete proposals that we can discuss for change' (Office of the Prime Minister 2007).

This 'deliberative turn' was implicit, episodically, through an emphasis upon creating or facilitating new spaces of dialogue and negotiation. At a national level, for example, the Cabinet Office helped to establish the People's Panel (based on a pool of over 5000 people). Between 1998 and 2002 questionnaires, interview surveys and citizens' juries were used to gauge views on issues such as out-of-hours health services, transport, local democracy and housing (Davies *et al.* 2006: 24). The government also funded a national debate, GM Nation?, that used nine stakeholder work-shops and 675 open meetings across the country to gauge views on the acceptability of genetically modified food (Heller 2003: 64). Similarly in 2006 ScienceWise (a government initiative designed to encourage public engagement in debates around science and technology) funded a project in which a broad range of participants attended twenty-seven workshops to discuss the use of drugs in mental health treatment, policy towards drugs designed to enhance cognition and approaches to recreational drugs (Department for Innovation, Universities and Skills 2008). Another ini-tiative, 'Your Health, Your Care, Your Say', was marked by its explicit link to a planned white paper on health and social care. More than 250 people, drawn from a wide range of backgrounds, attended four regional workshops in 2005 and nearly 1000 were present at a corresponding Citizens' Summit in Birmingham. In each case participants received written information on relevant issues of health policy and health service delivery in advance. At the events they were seated in groups of ten and, with the aid of a facil-itator, encouraged to discuss each of the topics about which they had been briefed – discussions accompanied by occasional polling and the chance to raise issues not on the agenda. A Citizens' Advisory Panel, based on those thought able to influence wider constituencies, reviewed findings from these events with the secretary of state for health and civil servants prior to the drafting of the white paper. The role of the national initiative in shaping the contents of the document was then outlined at a conference in March 2006 (Warburton 2006: 13–14).

This apparent concern to foster deliberative decision making was also evident, more uncertainly, at a local level through a change in emphasis from static structures of patient and public involvement to facilitated 'spaces' of engagement. The Community Health Councils in England (encompassing over 80 per cent of the United Kingdom's population) had initially been replaced in 2003 by 572 Patient and Public Involvement Forums ('Patient Forums') – one for each primary care and hospital trust. But these bodies, which numbered 394 by the end of 2007, were abolished in 2008 (Stationery Office 2007). One reason offered by the Department of Health was that the forums had not capitalized sufficiently on the experience of those involved previously with Community Health Councils (House of Commons Health Committee 2007: 27–8). The forums were thus replaced in 2008 by

105 Local Involvement Networks (LINks) in England – bodies designed to be more flexible in engaging local stakeholders. Each LINk would be based on an (elected) local authority jurisdiction rather than correspond to an NHS Trust. Local authorities would sub-contract the management of the LINks to third party organizations, such as voluntary associations, with a view to the latter providing a flexible means through which local residents and voluntary sector organizations could become engaged in order to address issues of concern with local authorities and health and social care organizations (Department of Health 2006).

The framing of patients and citizens

Emphases on choice, patient expertise and safety can be seen as examples of a consumerist discourse but might also be interpreted with reference to other agendas (such as the medical profession's posited attempt to 'colonize' the issue of patient safety, the idea of the expert patient as a means to individualize responsibility for care and the link drawn between patient and public involvement and 'active' citizens). Accordingly, although the changing policy narratives discussed above often constituted considerably more than rhetoric, they accentuated rather than diminished the uncertainties and tensions around the identities of health service users.

Patients, citizens and 'consumerism'

An emphasis upon the discourse of policy and attendant reforms tells us little, however, about how health service users have engaged with these identities or indeed constructed their own. This section of the chapter examines evidence of 'consumerist' pro-activism on the part of patients and citizens on two levels. The first is that of the individual consumer. What do data pertaining to levels of trust on the part of health service users, recourse to private medical insurance, complaints and litigation suggest with regard to attitudes to health care provision? The second focus is upon independent collective mobilizations in and around health care and health policy on the part of patients and carers.

In terms of 'trust' on the part of health service users, results from a series of postal questionnaire surveys (in the years 2004, 2005 and 2006) indicate that, on average, 76 per cent of informants had 'complete confidence and trust' in their NHS general practitioners. The corresponding figures for hospital doctors remained at approximately 80 per cent in each of these three years and those for nurses at about 74 per cent (Richards and Coulter 2007: 10, 29). These figures echo results from a postal survey to a random sample of 1187 adults aged 18 years and over in England and Wales. The survey indicated that 83 per cent of respondents would, always or most of the time, trust general practitioners to put the interests of patients above the 'convenience' of the organizations in which they worked. The corresponding figure for general practice nurses was 87 per cent and that for NHS hospital doctors was 76 per cent (Calnan and Rowe 2004: 21). But levels of trust vary markedly between different aspects of health care. In terms of *mistrust*, Calnan and Sanford (2004), drawing on the same data as Calnan and Rowe, report that 17 per cent of respondents had little or no trust in the idea, for example, that considerable care would be taken to keep their medical records confidential, and that 63 per cent were similarly sceptical that doctors spend enough time with their patients (Calnan and Sanford 2004: 93). Similarly, although only 29 per cent of respondents reported a great or fair amount of confidence in health service managers, the figure in relation to general practitioners was almost 90 per cent (Calnan and Rowe 2004: 21).

But what of some of the choices exercised by health care users that might reflect a 'consumerist' outlook? Turning first to private medical insurance, data tend not to be conclusive. Expenditure on private medical insurance was equivalent in 2000 to just over 5 per cent of the budget devoted to the NHS. And although 11.5 per cent of the population were covered by private medical insurance, two-thirds of subscribers were in schemes financed entirely by their employers (King and Mossialos 2005: 196). And analysis of the British Household Panel Survey between 1996 and 2000, encompassing 8529 individuals in the final year, suggests that possession of private medical insurance is associated more with the individual characteristics of subscribers than misgivings about collectively funded health care (such as the waiting times for inpatient and outpatient care). Beyond the impact of education and higher status employment, one of the strongest influences on the use of private medical insurance appeared to be general political orientation. Those who tended to vote for centre-right political parties were over three times as likely as those who did not to purchase medical insurance on an individual basis. They were also twice as likely to make use of such cover as a benefit of employment (King and Mossialos 2005: 204). Overall, however, these data (particularly the small percentage of people who purchase health insurance privately) do not contradict earlier research findings to the effect that, in the United Kingdom, possession of private health insurance is not indicative of a major social cleavage, founded on distinct groups of 'consumers' and 'non-consumers', in the manner of fundamental social divisions sometimes associated with class or ethnicity (Busfield 1990; Calnan *et al.* 1993).

Other potential indicators of a consumerist outlook on the part of health service users include complaints. In England, Scotland and Wales (encompassing over 95 per cent of the United Kingdom's population), the number of complaints in connection with family health services (such as general practitioners), community health services and hospitals grew from 142,189 in 1997–98 to 150,793 in 2005–06 (Information Centre 2006a, 2006b; Health Statistics and Analysis Unit 1998, 2006; ISD 2006a, 2006b). The link between expectations related to aspects of health care, dissatisfaction and the propensity to complain is obscured by factors that include variable awareness of complaints mechanisms, different beliefs about the efficacy of pursuing a complaint and changes in the mechanisms for making complaints. In England in 1996, for example, a reform of complaints mechanisms was heralded as a rationalization that would benefit complainants. But seven years later – in the wake of a consultation exercise, an independent evaluation and informal discussion with NHS patients – the Department of Health itself criticized the utility of the revised complaints system (Department of Health 2003). Subsequent changes between 2004 and 2006 centred on refining local resolution procedures and passing the functions of Independent Review Panels to a national body, the Healthcare Commission (Department of Health 2004). Using complaints as an indicator of a growing consumer consciousness on the part of patients is thus not as straightforward as it first appears. And as Mulcahy (2003) notes, we should keep in mind a distinction between dissatisfaction that does not translate to action on the part of patients, 'voiced grievances', formal complaints and variation in the degree to which adverse events are attributed by patients to medical personnel or health service organizations. A focus upon recorded complaints is at best an uncertain proxy for any wider discontent.

Similarly, legal action by patients appears at first to indicate some flexing of consumerist muscle but this has to be qualified. In monetary terms, payments made to claimants by the NHS Litigation Authority in relation to clinical negligence grew from just over £70 million in 1998–9 to about £528 million in 2004–5, £560.3 million in 2005–6 and then approximately £613.3 million in 2006–7 (NHS Litigation Authority 2007a: 2). Numerically, there were 5602 recorded claims for clinical negligence and 3766 for non-clinical negligence in 2004–5 (corresponding figures in 2005–6 were 5697 and 3497 and those in 2006–7 were 5426 and 3293). Of the 40,165 clinical negligence claims dealt with by the NHS Litigation Authority (England) between 1995–6 and 2006–7, 39 per cent related to surgical procedures, just over 21 per cent to obstetrics and gynaecology and approximately 18 per cent to pharmaceuticals. Only 128 cases (less than 0.3 per cent) of claims related to general practitioners (NHS Litigation Authority 2007b: 2, 3). All these figures have, however, to be set against the fact that in England there were approximately 290 million patient consultations in general practice in 2006 and over 14.78 million finished consultant episodes in English NHS hospitals in 2006–07 (Hippisley-Cox *et al.* 2007: 2; Information Centre 2007: 7). And, as with statistics relating to complaints, the formal expression of grievances through litigation does not in itself undermine the normative and cultural basis of relations between patients and clinicians (and, by extension, between citizens and the state) that underpin a system of 'free' health care for all citizens.

Collective action

Concurrently, a concern with indicators of an individualized consumerism or an emphasis upon 'crafted' identities in strands of health policy neglects the role of mobilizations from within civil society. There is evidence of increasing activity on the part of self-help groups, patient advocacy bodies and health social movements (Brown 1997; Gabel and Peters 2004; Crossley 2006). Baggott *et al.* (2005), for example, researched 'health consumer groups' in relation to the policy and politics of five common conditions – arthritis and related complaints; heart and circulatory diseases (with a deliberate bias towards heart disease and stroke); cancer; mental health; and childbirth and maternity services. This survey revealed acceleration in the rate at which such groups have been established in recent decades. Nearly 63 per cent of the 123 organizations that were surveyed had been established since 1981 (Baggott *et al.* 2005: 81–2). This pattern is supported by Wood's (2000) research on patient associations in the United Kingdom and USA and, in terms of particular condition areas, exemplified by a study of mental health user groups in England – 75 per cent of the 318 groups studied in 2001 had been established in the preceding ten years (Sainsbury Centre for Mental Health 2003: 7).

Further analysis of the findings from the work of Baggott and his colleagues also suggests common concerns on the part of these groups despite their focus on diverse medical conditions. There tended, not surprisingly, to be a shared focus on issues pertaining to pain, loss and illness. The groups were often founded in response to a disrupted 'biographical narrative' and attempts to reconstitute major disturbances between conceptions of the self, a changed body and altered relationships with the wider world (Allsop *et al.* 2004: 741). Diverse health consumer groups thus often share an 'embodied' identity (rather than a particular political or ideological outlook) that underpins engagement with the state, science and medicine in relation to health policy and health care (Brown *et al.* 2004). Such engagement can, as in the case of some mental health 'survivor' activism, range from the confrontational to instances of collaboration (as with the co-option of AIDS/HIV treatment activists in the oversight of federal research programmes in the United States) (Crossley 2006; Milewa and Barry 2005). Gauging the impact of such mobilizations upon health care and health policy on a systematic basis is far beyond the space available in this chapter. But as Baggott *et al.* (2005) suggest, there is evidence to suggest that the 'iron triangle' (of policy makers, managers and powerful medical professional associations) that was once associated with health policy formulation is becoming more porous and fluid (Haywood and Hunter 1982).

Health care and 'the consumer'

Trends pertaining to the activities and attitudes of health service users – such as levels of reported trust, complaints, litigation and collective mobilization

– suggest an enhanced consumer consciousness on the part of these actors. But, as with the changing discourse of policy, these trends do not appear to have stimulated radical change in relationships of power and marginality between service users, the state and medical profession. Through necessity or choice the overwhelming majority of people rely upon collectively funded health care – expressions of consumerist behaviour will thus necessarily be qualified when compared to those in free market environments. Litigation, complaints and, in particular, protest arising from collective illness identities may well reflect aspects of uncertainty in relation to modern medicine and an increased willingness to contest both the medical profession's expertise and the state's competence in addressing these anxieties (Williams and Calnan 1996). But this is a long way from a fundamental and thorough-going shift towards a 'consumerist' pro-activism on the part of patients and citizens that effectively turns medical providers in the health service into businesses eager to receive the passing trade of discerning consumers.

Health care and identities in social context

The manner in which health service users have been characterized within aspects of health policy and have constituted themselves is complex and even the broadest overview is inevitably selective in terms of evidence. It is clear, however, that the British state has consciously (but perhaps not always coherently) pursued policies since the 1980s that have attempted to recast health service users in terms other than passive and marginalized actors in the health service. This can be seen in the quasi-consumerist discourse associated with the internal market within the NHS introduced in the early 1990s and, more recently, in initiatives designed to expand patient choice between providers of health care (particularly secondary care); limited training and information schemes to develop more informed and pro-active patients; a focus upon improving patient safety; enhanced surveillance of clinical practice and a concern to develop structures for systematic patient and public involvement in the planning and governance of local health services. These initiatives, particularly between 1997 and 2008, did not appear to reflect a distinct political ideology but a mixture of motives. These included the use of patient choice to encourage greater efficiency in the provision of health service, a flight from a collectivist 'one size fits all' approach to more personalized notions of care but also the inculcation of more active, occasionally quasi-communitarian, forms of citizenship practice. In parallel, potential direct indicators of an accentuated consumerism – the number of complaints and the cost of litigation instigated by NHS patients – suggest a highly qualified increase in the 'consumerist' outlook of health service users. But another indicator, the number of organized patient advocacy bodies, suggests that the rate at which such organizations have been founded accelerated considerably between the early 1980s and late 1990s.

Such statistics are, however, of limited explanatory value unless they are set against a wider appreciation of the degree to which they constitute a radical challenge to the diverse expectations surrounding relationships between health service users, providers and institutions of the state in the context of British health care (Mulcahy 2003; Allsop 2006: 624). As Parsons observed in the middle of the last century – cultural norms and practices often help to shape the means by which incomplete or ambiguous knowledge (the basis of uncertainty) is expressed and dealt with in the relationship between clinician and patient (Parsons 1951: 449). But the physiological locus of identity, the body, straddles a notional division between the public sphere of health policy and health services and the apparently private world of individual illness and well-being, particularly when access to health care is viewed as a 'right'. In this last regard, uncertainties around health care will assume an increasingly politicized hue as producers and regulators of health care are implicated in issues such as entitlement, quality and the availability of provision. Temporally and culturally specific ideas and practices – such as the right to 'free' health care, prescribed quality standards and limits placed on the individual or collective use of resources in a health system – are thus central to understanding what is meant by terms such as patient, citizen or 'consumer'.

The Expert Patient Programme, for example, was on one level a means to help patients to help themselves. Concurrently it may reflect a broader cultural and political elevation of the individual and self-responsibility that is characteristic of Western capitalism generally and, in particular, of the neo-liberal political ascendancy of the 1980s and 1990s (Castiel 2003). Similarly, the use of information and communication technologies by health service users (of their own volition or because of encouragement by doctors or the state) has been linked to identities such as the 'e-consumer' and more normatively loaded terms such as the 'responsible' or 'informed' patient (Adams and Bont 2007). Accounting for these shifting or fragmented identities thus, at one level, requires an awareness of the policies and ideas around which characterizations of the health service user can be constructed. But attention to broader contexts and contests – such as the uses to which discourses of patient safety, stakeholder involvement and personal responsibility can be put by different actors – is also necessary.

Conclusion

An understanding of the extent and significance of putative consumer identities in health care rests on two broad factors. The first, as seen, centres on the actual or aspired-to portrayal of patients and citizens in strands of health and social policy together with statistical indicators in fields such as complaints and litigation. A second, more subtle, factor encompasses the interpretations, perceptions and prescriptions on the part of health service users that underpin ideas such as trust, expectation, obligation and responsibility – ideas that help to cohere understandings of 'identity' in relation to health care and the health service. Are recorded complaints, for example, just an aggregation of individual grievances, indicative of a much wider dissatisfaction with the manner in which health care is delivered or a sign of growing societal disenchantment with the traditional power of the medical profession? Similarly, are those who become involved in the new 'spaces' of patient and public involvement motivated by personal grievances about the quality or coverage of health care or by a far more opaque sense of altruism associated with ideas of the 'active' citizen? Appreciating the relationship between aspects of health policy, choices and preferences made by health service users and wider societal expectations and interpretations is thus central to understanding the hybrid and fluid nature of consumerism in British health care.

References

Adams, S. and Bont, A. de (2007) 'Information Rx: prescribing good consumerism and responsible citizenship', *Health Care Analysis*, 15: 273–90.

Allsop, J. (2006) 'Regaining trust in medicine: professional and state strategies', *Current Sociology*, 54: 621–36.

Allsop, J., Jones, K. and Baggott, R. (2004) 'Health consumer groups in the UK: a new social movement?', *Sociology of Health & Illness*, 26: 737–56.

Appleby, J., Harrison, A. and Devlin, N. (2003) *What is the Real Cost of More Patient Choice?* London: King's Fund.

Baggott, R., Allsop, J. and Jones, K. (2005) *Speaking for Patients and Carers: health consumer groups and the policy process*, Basingstoke: Palgrave Macmillan.

Baker, R. (2004) 'Implications of Harold Shipman for general practice', *Postgraduate Medical Journal*, 80: 303–6.

Barnes, M., Newman, J. and Sullivan, H. (2007) *Power, Participation and Political Renewal: case studies in public participation*, Bristol: Policy Press.

Bate, P. and Robert, G. (2006) '"Build it and they will come" – or will they? Choice, policy paradoxes and the case of NHS treatment centres', *Policy & Politics*, 34: 651–72.

Brown, M. (1997) *RePlacing Citizenship: AIDS activism and radical democracy*, London: Guildford Press.

Brown, P., Zavestoski, S., McCormick, S., Mayer, B., Morello-Frosch, R. and Altman, R. (2004) 'Embodied health movements: new approaches to social movements in health', *Sociology of Health & Illness*, 26: 50–80.

Busfield, J. (1990) 'Sectoral divisions in consumption: the case of medical care', *Sociology*, 24: 77–96.

Calnan, M., Cant, S. and Gabe, J. (1993) *Going Private: why people pay for their health care*, Buckingham: Open University Press.

Calnan, M. and Rowe, R. (2004) *Trust in Health Care: an agenda for future research*, London: The Nuffield Trust.

Calnan, M. and Sanford, E. (2004) 'Public trust in health care: the system or the doctor?' *Quality and Safety in Health Care*, 13: 92–7.

Carr, S. (1992) 'Patient rules, OK', *Health Service Journal*, 102: 31.

Castiel, L. (2003) 'Self care and consumer health. Do we need a public health ethics?' *Journal of Epidemiology and Community Health*, 57: 5–6

Crossley, N. (2006) 'The field of psychiatric contention in the UK, 1960–2000', *Social Science and Medicine*, 62: 552–63.

Davies, C., Wetherell, M. and Barnett, E. (2006) *Citizens at the Centre: deliberative participation in healthcare decisions*, Bristol: Polity Press.

Davis, R., Jacklin, R., Sevdalis, N. and Vincent, C. (2007) 'Patient involvement in patient safety: what factors influence patient participation and engagement?' *Health Expectations*, 10: 259–67.

Department for Innovation, Universities and Skills (2008) *Drugsfutures: public consultation on the future of drug use*, London: Department for Innovation, Universities and Skills.

Department of Health (1997) *The New NHS: modern, dependable*, cm.3807, London: Department of Health.

Department of Health (2001a) *The Expert Patient: a new approach to chronic disease management for the 21st Century*, London: Department of Health.

Department of Health (2001b) *Building a Safer NHS for Patients*, London: Department of Health.

Department of Health (2003) *NHS Complaints Reform: making things right*, London: Department of Health.

Department of Health (2004) *Guidance to Support Implementation of the National Health Service (Complaints) Regulations 2004*, London: Department of Health.

Department of Health (2006) *A Stronger Local Voice*, London: Department of Health.

Department of Health (2007) *Choice Matters, 2007–08: putting patients in control*, London: Department of Health.

Department of Health (2008) *High Quality Care for All: NHS next stage review final report*, Cm. 7432, London: Department of Health.

Gabel, S. and Peters, S. (2004) 'Presage of a paradigm shift? Beyond the social model of disability toward resistance theory of disability', *Disability and Society*, 19: 585–600.

Gerrard, M. (2006) *A Stifled Voice: Community Health Councils in England, 1974–2003*, Brighton: Penn Press.

Gillett, J. (2003) 'Media activism and Internet use by people with HIV/AIDS', *Sociology of Health & Illness*, 25: 608–24.

Gubb, J. (2007) *Patient Safety: the NHS (CIVITAS online Briefing, June 2007*, London: CIVITAS. Online: www.civitas.org.uk/nhs/download/patientsafety.php (accessed 1 November 2007).

Haywood, S. and Hunter, D. (1982) 'Consultative processes in health policy in the UK: a view from the centre', *Public Administration*, 60: 143–62.

Health Statistics and Analysis Unit (1998) *Complaints to the NHS in Wales 1997–98*, Cardiff: Health Statistics and Analysis Unit.

Health Statistics and Analysis Unit (2006) *Complaints to the NHS in Wales 2005–06 (SDR 183/2006)*, Cardiff: Health Statistics and Analysis Unit.

Heller, R. (2003) *GM Nation? The findings of the public debate*, London: Department of Trade and Industry.

Hippisley-Cox, J., Fenty, J. and Heaps, M. (2007) *Trends in Consultation Rates in General Practice 1995 to 2006: analysis of the QRESEARCH database*, London: QRESEARCH and The Information Centre.

House of Commons Health Committee (2007) *Patient and Public Involvement in the NHS: third report of session 2006–07*, vol. 1, HC278-1, London: Stationery Office.

Information Centre (2006a) *Written Complaints about Hospital and Community Services in England, 1997–2005 (data-set KO41a)*, London: Information Centre.

Information Centre (2006b) *Written Complaints about Family Health Services in England, 1997–2005 (data-set KO41b)*, London: Information Centre.

Information Centre (2007) *Hospital Episodes Statistics: headline figures (December 2007)*, London: Information Centre.

ISD (2006a) *Hospital and Community Health Services Complaints Statistics*, Edinburgh: NHS National Services Scotland.

ISD (2006b) *Family Health Services Complaints*, Edinburgh: NHS National Services Scotland.

Kelleher, D. (1994) 'Self-help groups and their relationship to medicine', in J. Gabe, D. Kelleher and G. Williams (eds) *Challenging Medicine*, London: Routledge.

King, D. and Mossialos, E. (2005) 'The determinants of private medical insurance prevalence in England, 1997–2000', *Health Services Research*, 40: 195–212.

Milewa, T. (2004) 'Local participatory democracy in Britain's health service: innovation or fragmentation of a universal citizenship?' *Social Policy and Administration*, 38: 240–52.

Milewa, T. and Barry, C. (2005) 'Health policy and the politics of evidence', *Social Policy and Administration*, 39: 498–512.

Milewa, T., Valentine, J. and Calnan, M. (1998) 'Managerialism and active citizenship in Britain's reformed health service: power and community in an era of decentralisation', *Social Science and Medicine*, 47: 507–17.

MORI (2003) *Patient Choice: a presentation by Robert Worcester, 2 September 2003* (Slides), London: MORI.

Mulcahy, L. (2003) *Disputing Doctors: the socio-legal dynamics of complaints about medical care*, Maidenhead: Open University Press-McGraw-Hill Education.

National Patient Safety Agency (2007) *National Clinical Assessment Service Handbook*, fourth edition, London: National Patient Safety Agency.

NHS Litigation Authority (2007a) *Factsheet 2: financial information (August 2007)*, London: NHS Litigation Authority.

NHS Litigation Authority (2007b) *Factsheet 3: information on claims (November 2007)*, London: NHS Litigation Authority.

Office of the Prime Minister (2007) *Speech on 'Politics' to the National Council of Voluntary Organisations*, London: Office of the Prime Minister. Online: www.number10.gov.uk/output/Page13008.asp (accessed 1 June 2008).

Parkinson, J. (2004) 'Why deliberate? The encounter between deliberation and new public Managers', *Public Administration*, 82: 377–95.

Parsons, T. (1951) *The Social System*, London: Routledge and Kegan Paul.

Pickard, S., Sheaff, R. and Dowling, B. (2006) 'Exit, voice, governance and user-responsiveness: the case of English primary care trusts', *Social Science and Medicine*, 63: 373–83.

Richards, N. and Coulter, A. (2007) *Is the NHS Becoming More Patient-Centred? Trends from the national surveys of NHS patients in England 2002–07*, Oxford: Picker Institute.

Sainsbury Centre for Mental Health (2003) *The Mental Health Service User*

Movement in England, Policy Paper 2, London: Sainsbury Centre for Mental Health.

Seale, C. (2006) 'Gender accommodation in online cancer support groups', *Health* 10: 345–60.

Stationery Office (2007) *Local Government and Public Involvement in Health Act 2007*, c.28, London: Stationery Office.

Taylor, D. and Bury, M. (2007) 'Chronic illness, expert patients and care transition', *Sociology of Health and Illness*, 29: 127–45.

Timmermans, S. and Berg, M. (2003) *The Gold Standard: the challenge of evidence-based medicine and standardization in health care*, Philadelphia: Temple University Press.

Warburton, D. (2006) *Evaluation of Your Health, Your Care, Your Say: final report*, London: Department of Health.

Waring, J. (2007) 'Adaptive regulation or governmentality: patient safety and the changing regulation of medicine', *Sociology of Health and Illness*, 29: 163–79.

Williams, S. and Calnan, M. (1996) 'The "limits" of medicalization?' *Social Science and Medicine*, 42: 1609–20.

Winters, L. (2006) *Health Impact Assessment of the Patient Choice Agenda (Report)*, Liverpool: Liverpool Public Health Observatory, University of Liverpool.

Wood, B. (2000) *Patient Power? The politics of patients' associations in Britain and America*, Buckingham: Open University Press.

9 Mainstream marginality

'Non-orthodox' medicine in an 'orthodox' health service

Sarah Cant

Introduction

In the intervening period since the publication of the first edition of *The Sociology of the Health Service* (Gabe *et al.* 1991) numerous changes have occurred to the shape and practice of medical care in Britain. Arguably, one of the most significant is the proliferation and subsequent management of complementary and alternative therapies, knowledges and professions. For the purposes of this chapter these have been collectively, although not unproblematically, grouped under the heading of 'non-orthodox' care. This chapter will assess the significance of the burgeoning demand for, and ever-increasing supply of, 'non-orthodox' care for health care practice and specifically for the configuration of the health service in Britain.

There seems to be some support (McQuaide 2005; Rayner and Easthope 2001; Siahpush 1998) for the claim that 'non-orthodox' care attests to the emergence of the 'postmodern condition' (Lyotard 1979), where plural knowledge systems can co-exist and are chosen because of their practical performance in meeting the needs of clients. Drawing on the work of Giddens (1990) and Beck (1992), the attraction of 'non-orthodox' modalities might also point to the rise of a discerning and expert consumer who is increasingly sceptical of biomedical science and desires individualized care. However, having examined during the course of this chapter consumption in practice, the responses from 'orthodox' biomedicine and the state to the increased popularity of these therapies, and the demands that 'non-orthodox' care seek regulation and professionalization, it will also be suggested that such a reading is not entirely straightforward.

One difficulty in asserting that there has been major social and cultural change is that 'non-orthodox' care in Britain has been significantly shaped by 'orthodox' medicine. In particular, biomedicine has played a very strong part in determining which types of 'non-orthodox' care have gained legitimacy and has controlled their practice and modes of intervention within the NHS. Consequently, the applicability of using 'non-orthodox' care as a descriptor becomes problematic because the provision of 'non-orthodox' care within the National Health Service has been both contained by biomedical practitioners and judged by their modernist research standards.

However, analysing 'non-orthodox' care in terms of the jurisdictional battles (Abbott 1998) played out with 'orthodox medicine' is also insufficient. Whilst 'non-orthodox' medicine is often described as being built on very different ontological and epistemological premises, I will also suggest that similar structuring mechanisms and values underlie all medical practice and have shaped the development of 'non-orthodox' care. For instance, both 'orthodox' and 'non-orthodox' medical care can be seen to serve similar functions, not least in the role of surveying the population (Lowenberg and Davis 1994; Braathen 1996). Moreover, the commodification of health and the profits to be made within 'non-orthodox' care also point to the importance of the structuring mechanisms of capitalism (Navarro 1978; Han 2002) particularly as both 'orthodox' and 'non-orthodox' paradigms concentrate on the individual body/behaviour rather than social, political or economic aetiology. In this chapter, I will argue that the delivery of 'non-orthodox' medical care has been further shaped by: the rhetoric of the safe and responsible practitioner who embodies professionalism; a preferred therapeutic relationship that contrasts the client with the 'expert' and restrains the emergence of a true consumer; and the continued primacy given to 'scientific' evidence to adjudicate which practices are valid. These influences upon 'non-orthodox' care reflect a culture where uncertainty and risk is an aspect of all knowledge systems and where all practitioners, 'orthodox' or 'non-orthodox', must retain the trust of their clients (Giddens 1990). This prevailing context has maintained as much as radicalized health care provision in the United Kingdom. However, before we can engage with any of these debates, there is a need to clarify the term 'non-orthodox' care.

The problem of definition

Choosing an appropriate and collective term to describe and define this terrain is clearly difficult, not least because grouping all therapies together suggests some form of uniformity of practice and experience. In reality, the proliferation of a range of therapies, practices, professions and modalities in the last two decades defies neat packaging. This is in part because the various therapeutic modalities have distinct origins, histories and scope. For instance, homeopathy and herbalism were practised in Britain prior to, and contemporaneously, with modern biomedicine. In contrast, Ayurveda and Chinese Herbal Medicine, whilst both having long histories, have only become available in Britain as a result of migrating populations. It is estimated that there are at least 200 'non-orthodox' therapies in the UK which differ so markedly that to conceive of a single entity of 'non-orthodox' care is clearly problematic (Stone 2002). In practice, the umbrella terms 'alternative', 'complementary', 'holistic', 'traditional', 'natural', 'unconventional', 'unofficial' and 'non-orthodox' are often used interchangeably, but each carries very different connotations. In this chapter *'non-orthodox'* has been adopted, less to suggest that the practices are in some way 'out of the ordinary' or 'different', but rather to capture in the analysis the important and defining relationship with biomedicine.

Indeed, whilst a case has been made for the existence of medical pluralism in the UK (Cant and Sharma 1999), it is impossible to understand the history and co-existence of these various knowledges and practices except in relation to the dominant, state-supported, hegemonic biomedicine. It is significant that until the late 1980s 'fringe' (now defunct), 'marginal' and 'alternative' were the favoured descriptors within sociology (Inglis 1964; Wallis and Morley 1976; West 1984) and by the medical profession (BMA 1986). This was a period when the medical profession viewed the popularity of all other therapies as a cause for concern. 'Alternative' is still preferred by some (Saks 1992; Cant and Sharma 1999) because the majority of such therapies still do not receive significant support from the state or the medical establishment, despite a period of rapprochement. However, for the majority of commentators, the 1990s saw 'complementary' become the tag of choice (BMA 1993; Trevelyan and Booth 1994; Vincent and Furnham 1997), in part signifying the idea of a co-operative partnership with 'orthodox' biomedicine. Complementary and alternative (CAM) is also used as a quick shorthand and, although convenient, combines contradictory descriptions of the role and place of the therapies. More recently, 'integrated medicine' has been employed because it is felt to cement the idea of a working relationship (Rees and Weil 2001; PWFIH 2005).

However, the terms 'complementary' or 'integrative' medicine obscure the greater power differential that 'orthodox' medicine enjoys and has used to manage its interactions with other therapeutic modalities. The descriptor 'non-orthodox' care is therefore preferable but is not without its own problems. First, whilst the majority of therapists in the UK are non-medically qualified, and so there might be a case for defining them collectively as 'non-orthodox', about a fifth of practitioners are statutory registered health professionals (Mills and Budd 2000). Second, as we shall see, many 'non-orthodox' therapists have worked to professionalize their practice, to gain access to NHS settings and secure state support and so increasingly look very like 'orthodox' practitioners.

Understanding demand: consumerism and the postmodern turn?

Studying the extent of use of 'non-orthodox' care and the motivations of the users is important both to discern whether there has been a significant change in the patterning of health services, and to map cultural shifts in the expectations of health care. Certainly, the evidence of the increasing rates of diverse consumption of non-orthodox medicine is used as an indicator of societal anxiety about science (Bakx 1991), the rise of the reflexive consumer (Giddens 1990) and the ascendance of postmodern culture

(McQuaide 2005). The validity of these claims is not always easy to substantiate however, not least because of the limited and problematic evidence base.

In the first place, estimating the number of people that use 'non-orthodox' care is immensely difficult because a large[1] number of the available surveys are beset with methodological flaws (Ernst 2006) and only a minority are robust enough to be included in a valid meta-analysis (Harris and Rees 2000). Nevertheless, it is possible to conclude with some confidence that 'non-orthodox' care is increasingly popular in the UK. For example, comparison of two surveys conducted by Thomas *et al.* in 1991 and 2001 shows that there was an exponential increase in access to therapists[2] and in the amount of personal expenditure on 'non-orthodox' services and products during the 1990s. Other surveys have confirmed the continued increase in popularity of 'non-orthodox' therapies, suggesting as much as a trebling of use between 1981 and 1997 (Zollman and Vickers 1999). Recent estimates for general use within the population vary from between 6.6 per cent to 20 per cent of the population (Ong and Banks 2003). This range can be accounted for partly by the definition of 'use' employed and by the number of therapies included in the analysis. For instance, Thomas *et al.* (2001) found that 10.6 per cent of the adult population of England had visited at least one therapist providing any one of the six more established therapies[3] in the past twelve months. However, if reflexology, aromatherapy and self-care (using remedies purchased over the counter) were included the estimated proportion rose to 28.3 per cent for use in the past twelve months, and 46.6 per cent for lifetime use. The most recent study has suggested that almost half of British women (49 per cent) and just over a quarter of British men (28 per cent) have used a complementary therapy and would use it again (Mintel 2007). Despite these wide-ranging differences, it is clear that use of 'non-orthodox' care is a mainstream, not a minority, activity.

We also know that the market for 'non-orthodox' medical products is on the increase and economic explanations for the promotion of 'non-orthodox' care have become compelling. Mintel (2003) showed that £130 million was spent in the UK in 2002 (encompassing purchases from health food stores, high street retail outlets and the sales on the internet) and estimated the market would be worth £188 million by 2008. These figures were an underestimate as research in 2007 found the market to be worth £191 million and the new prediction was that this would rise to £250 million a year by 2011 (Mintel 2007). This is a substantial market, one that is largely found in the private sector as 90 per cent of users pay privately for 'non-orthodox' care rather than receiving reimbursement from private medical insurance companies or the NHS (Thomas *et al.* 2001). Consequently, there does seem to be evidence of active consumerism, albeit in part explained by increasing prosperity of the population (McQuaide 2005). To extend our understanding further we need to analyse the characteristics and motivations of users to understand why people choose 'non-orthodox' therapies and to assess whether there is evidence for broader socio-cultural shifts. It is also the case that important policy questions, not least those relating to equity, are raised through the analysis of usage patterns of 'non-orthodox' care.

All surveys confirm that the users are more likely to be women, middle aged and middle class (Thomas *et al.* 2001; Thomas and Coleman 2004; Mintel 2007), that there is substantial use amongst the elderly (Andrews 2003; Cartwright 2007) and that such usage patterns conform to those for 'orthodox' care. For McQuaide (2005), the age profile of users is instructive, constituted by the 1950s generation of 'baby-boomers' with their higher incomes and chronic disease profile. The location of 'non-orthodox' practitioners in middle-class areas and the demographic features of users (Andrews 2003; Doel and Segrott 2003; Ong and Banks 2003) also suggest important spatial differences in usage and point to some clear geographical inequalities. Inequity is also a feature of patterns of 'non-orthodox' provision in the NHS which vary according to levels of 'orthodox' medical interest and Primary Care Trust funding. Overall, then, the strong correlation between the use of 'non-orthodox' care and both gross socio-economic indicators and geographical location point to significant forms of stratification.

The evidence about cultural changes is harder to corroborate. Studies have shown that users do exhibit certain cultural value differences from non users in that they are more likely to have a holistic orientation to health, be less confident of biomedical drugs and 'orthodox' medical practices and be more committed to environmentalism and feminism (Furnham and Smith 1988; Furnham and Bragrath 1992; Sirious and Gick 2002; Hildreth and Elman 2007). It is not clear, however, whether an alternative value system preceded or resulted from use of 'non-orthodox' care. Consequently, whilst these studies give some indication of a changing orientation to health and ways in which 'orthodox' medicine may need to alter its own practice, they arguably do not give us enough insight into why people actually use 'non-orthodox' care.

Another way of assessing the value of 'non-orthodox' care is to examine what characteristics users appreciate and what that they deem to be distinctive compared with 'orthodox' medical consultations. This is again a difficult area to explore as there are many differences in motivation depending upon which therapy group is being discussed. Nevertheless, there is evidence that users appreciate the lengthy, holistic, personalized and equitable client–practitioner encounter often encouraged in 'non-orthodox' consultations (Hewer 1983; Taylor 1984) and the perceived alignment of 'non-orthodox' care with less invasive, 'natural' interventions (Power 1994). These explanations point to the importance of both the paradigm and the delivery of 'non-orthodox' care and suggest a series of changing consumer expectations of health care delivery. More than this, for McQuaide (2005), the shifts may be indicative of a postmodern cultural turn where contradictory knowledges can co-exist and where 'scientific', biomedical truth can be contested.

The importance of the consumer, as reflected in the maximization of patient choice, and the intention to provide a health service that is personalized and responsive, has of course underpinned recent policy changes within the health service (Klein 2001; DOH 2004b) (see also Milewa, Chapter 8, this volume). High levels of consumer demand for and satisfaction with 'non-orthodox' care (House of Lords 2000) might account for the greater levels of acceptance from the state and the 'orthodox' medical profession. In turn, high levels of satisfaction also point to the experiential (if not experimental) effectiveness of interventions or, more negatively, suggest that users have found some relief for conditions where 'orthodox' care has been unable to offer them any help (Ernst and White 2000). It is possible, then, that alongside the inter-personal advantages and the service orientation of the client–practitioner relationship, 'non-orthodox' care offers an important resource, providing valuable technical interventions and support, and evidence at the level of performance, where 'orthodox' medicine has less success. Specifically, 'non-orthodox' care has been perceived to offer relief for chronic conditions such as musculo-skeletal problems, stress, anxiety and depression, migraine, eczema and asthma (Sharma 1992; Mintel 2003; Ong and Banks 2003; Smallwood 2005) and to support, and sometimes alleviate, the effects of 'orthodox' cancer treatments (Bernstein and Grasso 2001). At this point, then, following Lyotard (1979), there appears to be some evidence of performative consumption in that users are making choices to consult with 'non-orthodox' practitioners on the basis of their perceived effectiveness.

However, the technical effectiveness of 'non-orthodox' care is difficult to substantiate because of the dearth of research studies, and because many interventions are deemed to be unsuitable for testing using 'scientific' biomedical methods. Nevertheless, there has been increasing pressure to validate the effectiveness of 'non-orthodox' medicine through science-based research, known as evidence-based medicine (EBM), especially through the use of randomized control trials (House of Lords 2000). Whilst an evidence base is required to justify the spending of state funds, this narrow conception of what constitutes acceptable evidence potentially serves to exclude those approaches that would claim that such testing is inappropriate. In light of the evidence that many 'orthodox' practices have not been subject to this exacting form of analysis (Jackson and Scambler 2007), it is possible to see the demands for such an evidence base as deeply political, justifying limiting integration and as countering the demands of the consumer. It has been argued that other modes of evidence might be more supportive and would highlight important elements of 'non-orthodox' care (Barry 2006).

Interestingly, the continued appeal to 'science' to legitimate 'non-orthodox' care sits alongside and contrasts with the rise of the discerning consumer who is often sceptical of scientific knowledge (Beck 1992; Giddens 1990, 1991). This scepticism might, then, underpin the motivations to use 'non-orthodox' care. Yet, the usual pattern is for users to consult and combine both 'non-orthodox' and 'orthodox' practitioners and products (Sharma 1992; Thomas and Coleman 2004), suggesting simultaneous use rather than a flight from 'orthodoxy'. Moreover, rather than reducing the use of 'orthodox' medical services, simultaneous usage patterns simply multiply consultation options. This tendency suggests that the provision of non-orthodox therapies within the NHS would be a costly option although it would facilitate communication between 'orthodox' and 'non-orthodox' practice, given that over half of users are still reluctant to tell their 'orthodox' doctor that they have used 'non-orthodox' care (Thomas and Coleman 2004). Simultaneous use does suggest, however, that consumers are content to consult both 'orthodox' and 'non-orthodox' practitioners and to mix and match medical knowledges that may be contradictory. Rather than fleeing from science, consumers are combining potentially contradictory medical systems to search for satisfactory and effective help.

The analysis of the use of 'non-orthodox' care points to some important lessons for understanding the health service. Whilst there is debate about the reality of consumerism within health care (see Milewa, Chapter 8, this volume), the turn to non-orthodox care has established that consumers are increasingly discerning and demanding and that they self-refer and appreciate health care that is individualized and personalized, where their perspective is taken seriously. There is also evidence that 'non-orthodox' care provides an important technical resource and can be used alongside 'orthodox' treatments. Yet, the option of 'non-orthodox' care is limited, at the moment, to certain sub-sections of the population, as financial constraints mean that choice is necessarily constrained whilst 'non-orthodox' care remains in the private sector.

Of course the very location of 'non-orthodox' care in the private sector might account for this individualized and personalized service, where the custom of the client must be won rather than assumed. There are resonances here with the delivery of 'orthodox' medical care prior to the development of the hospitals and state-funded health care (Jewson 1979). Overall, the changing demands of the consumer play a significant role in explaining the rise of 'non-orthodox' care as well as the changes within 'orthodox' medical practice. More than this, the changing tastes of the consumer suggest there might be some evidence of pluralism, relativism and scepticism, all associated with descriptions of the 'postmodern' condition. The 'postmodern turn' refers to more than pluralism, however, pointing in addition to changes in the way that knowledges are adjudicated. The suggestion by Lyotard (1979) was that the meta narratives of science would be replaced by judgements based on performativity. We might expect, then, that the consumers, the biomedical profession and the state would be drawn to consider the local *effectiveness* of the therapies rather than their association with science or on account of their internal discipline. By turning our attention to the experience of the therapists in Britain, we can see how the idea of a postmodern turn might be premature.

Understanding supply

The range of therapeutic modalities

It is hard to estimate the number of therapies currently available in the UK not least because the operation of common law provides a legal context where new therapies and sub-specialisms can freely emerge. Instead of trying to quantify the exact number of therapies, there have instead been attempts to classify the various therapies into common types, in itself a complex and hotly debated process. It is possible, for example, to group therapies on the basis of their type of therapeutic intervention, their underlying philosophy, their popularity, their mode of regulation, their perceived level of risk and so on (see, for example NCCAM 2004).

The House of Lords (2000) taxonomy is now the most widely used (albeit controversial, particularly within the 'non-orthodox' field) and contrasts three main groups. The first includes the so-called 'principal' therapies, those with an individual diagnostic approach and also the most commonly used (Thomas *et al.* 2001). These include osteopathy, chiropractic, homeopathy, medical herbalism and acupuncture, collectively referred to as the *'Big Five'*. Second, those therapies which are regarded as complementary to conventional medicine and which do not make claims for diagnostic skills are grouped together and include: 'aromatherapy; the Alexander technique; massage; counselling; stress therapy; hypnotherapy; reflexology and probably shiatsu; and meditation and healing' (House of Lords 2000: 2.1). The third category encompasses those disciplines which offer diagnostic information as well as treatment but are 'indifferent' to scientific principles of conventional medicine. This places together a variety of diverse practices ranging from long-established and traditional systems of health care such as Ayurvedic medicine and traditional Chinese medicine to alternative disciplines which are deemed to lack any credible evidence base such as crystal therapy and iridology.

According to the Select Committee, one of the important reasons for producing this taxonomy was to help the public make informed choices based on the *scientific* evidence base of each modality within 'non-orthodox' care, suggesting that decisions to use therapies within the third group should be harder to support in the absence of research based on the results of well designed trials (House of Lords 2000). This advice demonstrates how the requirement for scientific evidence continues to serve an important function in limiting the integration/acceptance of 'non-orthodox' care, revealing the political, if not the therapeutic, differences within the broad church of 'non-orthodox' care. From the outset, then, we can see that there is a clear division between those therapies where a working relationship can be conceived and those where collaboration is less likely, a ranking of therapies according to whether they might be conceived as valuable or as a danger. Studying the processes whereby individual therapies came to be regarded in this light is instructive. The study of the professionalization of non-orthodox care enables a description of a range of changes that have been made to the delivery and practice of 'non-orthodox' practice and reveals the criteria used to judge the various knowledge bases.

A changing product: professionalization and professionalism in 'non-orthodox' care

The history of 'non-orthodox' care in Britain teaches us that the existence of a variety of medical practices and healing modalities is nothing new. There have always been various ways of conceiving of health and illness, of the possibility of choice between a variety of health care practitioners. However, whilst many health knowledges jostled for public support in the early part of the nineteenth century, the professionalization project[4] of 'orthodox' biomedicine (Larson 1977) had a slow but significant impact on the variety of other therapeutic modalities that had previously flourished in the UK. This was because it was premised on the establishment of a monopoly over health care provision (Freidson 1970) which required the discreditation of rival health groups (Larkin 1983; Saks 1996). Legal state endorsement of biomedicine was enacted through the 1858 Medical Act (Waddington 1984), but the practical provision of a monopoly came with the passing of the NHS Act in 1946, which, through providing state funding for biomedicine, sounded the death-knell for all other therapies (with the exception of homoeopathy, if practised by biomedical doctors, which retained a minimal place in state-funded care (Nicholls 1988)).

The 'eclipse' of 'non-orthodox' medicine (Bakx 1991) was, however, short lived as a renewed popularity became apparent in the 1960s and 1970s. The renaissance came from a number of directions (Cant and Sharma 1999): those modalities that had been popular in the nineteenth and early twentieth centuries in the UK and elsewhere[5] experienced renewed interest; immigrant groups brought different health care practices to the UK; and a softening of political relations with Asia allowed the promotion of therapies such as acupuncture (Saks 1997). The study of the early configuration of these therapies (Cant 1996) has shown that until the 1980s, practices and training were localized and informal, with efforts directed at enhancing the popularity of the therapy/modality. Training was often delivered in the front rooms of charismatic and enthusiastic advocates who were passionate about simply spreading the insights of 'non-orthodox' care. Importantly, at this time, many of the practitioners believed that their approach to health was antithetical to that offered within 'orthodox' medicine, and had the potential to radicalize health care by replacing orthodox provision. Whilst the early configuration of non-orthodox care might be described as stereotypically postmodern, it was relatively short lived.

By the mid-1980s pressure from the state, the medical profession, from the consumers and from within the therapy groups themselves propagated the intense and accelerated professionalization of 'non-orthodox' care (Cant and Sharma 1999; Quah 2003; Saks 2003; Clarke *et al.* 2004; Welsh *et al.* 2004; Kelner *et al.* 2006). The ensuing changes to the training, registration and regulation of 'non-orthodox' care have been argued to be as significant as the original marginalization and exclusion of 'non-orthodox' practices in the mid-nineteenth century (Clarke *et al.* 2004). However, the consequences have varied across the 'non-orthodox' field and are found in their most developed form within the 'Big 5' therapy groups. In other words, the processes of professionalization have served to enact another axis of distinction amongst an already highly complex and differentiated 'non-orthodox' field.

During the 1980s and 1990s the majority of therapy groups, albeit with some internal dissent (see Cant and Sharma 1995), began to engage in a number of 'professionalization' strategies. First, we see radical steps to alter the delivery and codification of the various knowledge bases by the development of training schools and syllabi. In turn, the training was attached to a set of credentials; preferably ones with national recognition such as those ranging from certificates and diplomas to degree level. By 2005, 108 courses and modules in 'non-orthodox' care were running (Morgan *et al.* 2005). Some therapy groups preferred instead to employ National Occupational Standards (NOS) and to define the competences which apply to their job roles or occupations in the form of statements of performance. Nevertheless, a number of therapy groups (notably the 'Big 5') have, in a very short time frame, moved from a position where their knowledge was open to all and where boundaries between the practitioner and client where relatively fluid, to one where they are able to make claims that they possess an 'expertise'.

Second, in tandem with this strategy came attempts, with varying degrees of success, to unify the many disparate groups of practitioners that had mushroomed in the early 1980s, and to inaugurate professional bodies to administer registers, devise codes of ethics and ensure that any transgression was responded to according to established disciplinary procedures. It is estimated that there are now in excess of 170 professional associations (Mills and Budd 2000). In effect, the credentializing and registering of various groups began the process of social closure (Parkin 1974). Third, a number of the groups have included medical science in their training and, in some cases (see chiropractic and osteopathy), have used biomedical knowledge and methods as a resource to prove and account for the effectiveness of their therapy (e.g. Meade *et al.* 1990).

Fourth, there were clear attempts within some therapy groups, notably those premised on a whole diagnostic system as well as a method, to temper their knowledge claims. Within chiropractic, for example, emphasis was laid upon the musculo-skeletal aspects of their approach and the specific claim to expertise in the area of lower back pain, while wider claims for the therapy were jettisoned (Baer 1984; Willis 1992; Cant 1996). These actions, and similar tactics by other groups, constituted an active and concerted attempt to professionalize through the conscious adoption of the same strategies that were once deployed against many of them by the 'orthodox' biomedical profession.

It should be noted that not all practitioners were supportive of these changes; nor did all groups enjoy the same successes. Certainly this quick sketch has masked a great deal of local difference. For instance, there are concerns within traditional Chinese medicine that only those that have trained in China are authentic practitioners (Welsh *et al*. 2004). For some therapies, typically those that employ a limited knowledge base and do not make grand claims for their interventions, there is less evidence of the professionalization project. In aromatherapy and reflexology for instance there are still a large number of small training establishments, a variety of professional associations and training is typically short. This does not mean there have not been any concerted attempts to unify and agree on training for the purposes of voluntary self-regulation (see below), just that the steps taken have not been so far-reaching. Nevertheless, it is the case that 'non-orthodox' practice has conformed to the 'orthodox' model of organization and delivery. Far from pluralism and relativism, the field of non-orthodox care is increasingly characterized by uniformity.

The decision to copy the allopathic model of professionalization is nonetheless puzzling. This is because there have been some generic and negative, albeit unforeseen, consequences of the professionalization project that relate to the shape and form of therapeutic practice. For example, the ensuing narrowing of practice could have serious implications for the integrity of the founding principles, which comprise one of the bases for 'non-orthodox' medicine's popular support (Cant and Sharma 1996). Moreover, if the motivating factors behind these professionalization projects have been to enable the positioning of groups so that they could gain statutory self-regulation (Welsh *et al*. 2004), enhance their collaboration with the medical profession and integrate themselves into the NHS (Stone and Matthews 1996), the success of these attempts has been limited. In other words the objective of professionalization to translate knowledge and skills into economic and social rewards is hard to corroborate.

However, it is possible to make sense of these professionalizing strategies by drawing upon the new sociology of professionalism (Fournier 1999; Evetts 2006) and the appreciation of *discipline* rather than *reward*. During the period when the established profession of medicine itself may be experiencing deprofessionalization (Haug 1988) and/ or proletarianization (Oppenheimer 1973; McKinlay and Stoekle 1988), the usefulness of shifting the analysis from professionalization to professionalism (Freidson 1994) becomes apparent. The discourse of professionalism plays an important role in legitimating status (Evetts 2006), enhancing confidence in abstract systems (Giddens 1990) and trust in individual practitioners (Macdonald 1995). In this way, there are resonances with the early trait and attribute analyses of the professions which identified professionalism as a desirable occupational value, where respectability brought societal trust. However, there were problems with the teleology of the trait approach: the attributes of the professions were taken for granted and were assumed to justify the power and status of the medical profession. Within the new sociology of the professions, professionalism can be understood as serving societal functions of discipline rather than justifying the remuneration of the practitioners.

We can see, then, that during a period of diminishing trust, professionalism acts as a useful marketing device to attract and reassure customers but also as a disciplinary mechanism, a mode of self-policing of work in a largely private and free market (Fournier 1999), and as a means of controlling work practices and demarcating the competent from the incompetent. These new divisions within the field of 'non-orthodox' care serve to normalize it (Wahlberg 2007), rather than restrict or ban its practice, and re-cast it as competent and responsible. Within 'non-orthodox' care, imposing the ethic of 'professionalism' has not so much served to improve the occupations' status and rewards, but has acted to discipline a disparate number of practitioners, help maintain a client base by asserting that a trustworthy 'expert' is required and unify modes of practice. In sum, while professionalism has served to minimize pluralism and to create standardization it has not secured 'non-orthodox' care a place in the NHS or produced any special privileges, as the review of regulation and integration reveals.

Managing the market: state and voluntary regulation

The process of professionalization is not simply dependent upon what groups do to change their practice but also on the socio-political context in which the project is undertaken. History of support from the state for non-therapeutic groups through the granting of registration shows that the success of the professionalization process has been limited, as the government has maintained a laissez-faire approach to regulation (Cant and Sharma 1999; Stone and Lee-Treweek 2005).

In contrast to 'orthodox' medical care which is highly regulated in Britain, at the time of writing only two therapy groups, osteopathy and chiropractic, have gained statutory regulation (respectively in 1993 and 1994). There have been contradictory assessments of the value of state regulation, some seeing the possibility of further integration and 'orthodox' medical referrals, others worried about the scrutiny and curtailment of their practice (Cant 1996; Stone 2005). Certainly, state regulation was only possible after significant changes had been made to training and the parameters of practice and by attachment to a 'scientific' evidence base, enabling a convergence with the 'orthodox' paradigm. Within osteopathy and chiropractic, the changes made to their organization and definitions of practice were the most far-reaching and least challenging to the 'orthodox' biomedical model. The passing of the Acts to provide regulation was hailed as a great victory and it was always assumed that herbalism, acupuncture and homeopathy would quickly follow suit after resolving specific internal difficulties. Despite concerted efforts by the herbalists and acupuncturists (Stone 2005; Wahlberg 2007) and the requirement that they pursue this route because their interventions were deemed potentially harmful (House of Lords 2000; DOH 2004a), successful state registration has not yet been realized. As such, the benefits of statutory regulation have been limited, underscoring a hierarchy within 'non-orthodox' care.

Nevertheless, there has been great pressure upon all modalities to form a single, national regulatory body (House of Lords 2000) and to develop voluntary self-regulation, if not to achieve statutory conferment of a protected title. The Prince of Wales has been very vocal about the importance of integrated health care and his Foundation (The Prince's Foundation for Integrated Health (PFIH)) has organized the regulation programme, funded by the King's Fund. This programme has worked to support and encourage Regulatory Working Groups across a wide range of 'non-orthodox' practitioners, bringing disparate and often competing groups to the table. In parallel with these changes there have been consultations into the feasibility of creating a federal form of regulation (PWFIH 2006). In April 2008, the Complementary and Natural Healthcare Council was launched, providing a single regulator for 'non-orthodox' healthcare rather than a series of single-therapy regulators. However, it is still unclear who will be eligible to join and various consultation processes are ongoing. From January 2009, massage therapy and nutritional therapy were the first disciplines to enter the register with the expectation that other groups will eventually be eligible. What is clear is that as part of the requirement for some form of regulatory structure to protect the public, there is an acceptance by the state and the medical profession that registration with a single professional body confers on the practitioner the status of being 'competent, skilled and responsible' (Wahlberg 2007: 5). This marks a significant shift in the attitude towards 'non-orthodox' care, as no longer simply discredited but as heavily policed. Moreover, even in the cases of successful statutory regulation, the process does not appear to have been one that has bestowed status or, as we shall see, extended the opportunities for integrated medical care.[6]

The integration of 'non-orthodox' care within the health service

The commitment to and development of integrated health care epitomizes the most recent history of relations between 'non-orthodox' and 'orthodox' medical care and has broad support from the House of Lords (2000) and the PWFIH (2005). As a broad-brush term, integrated health care certainly encompasses the simultaneous use of 'non-orthodox' and 'orthodox' care by users. Of more significance is the extent of practical integration of 'orthodox' and 'non-orthodox' practice through the provision of 'non-orthodox' medicine by 'orthodox' practitioners, and the referral by 'orthodox' practitioners to 'non-orthodox' therapists, both within and outside the NHS (including primary and hospital settings). Whilst there is undoubtedly evidence of increasing integration of this kind, in practice it has been carefully managed, reflecting the requirement for evidence-based practice, minimal state funding and the continued dominance of 'orthodox' authority. Moreover, the question of how to enact integration in practice is conspicuous by its absence in the majority of policy documents. Instead the Department of Health has issued only very general guidance which has been subject to many local interpretations (DOH 2000, 2001).

Use by the medical and nursing professions

Research has shown an increased familiarization with and interest in 'non-orthodox' medicine from the medical profession, nurses and professions allied to medicine (Peters 2000). Whilst there are variations in survey results of doctors, the majority show considerable support and tolerance, although this is more likely for particular modalities (those that have visible regulatory and training structures and some research evidence) and is exhibited more in terms of referral patterns than personal commitment or practice (Ernst *et al.* 1995; Tovey and Broom 2007). Whilst the British Medical Association (BMA) has softened its stance towards 'non-orthodox' care (BMA 1986, 1993), it claims that there is still insufficient scientific evidence to justify compulsory training of medical students (BMA 2003). Younger general practitioners generally exhibit the most favourable attitudes to 'non-orthodox' care (Easthorpe *et al.* 2000). However, the evidence of conciliation and support may be overstated as there are also vocal, organized and high-ranking groups of 'orthodox' medical practitioners and scientists who stand in strong opposition to any use of NHS budgets for 'non-orthodox' care (*The Times* 2006). This has included lobbying health trusts, urging them to stop their funding of the Royal Homeopathic Hospitals. The BMA has also been clear that whilst it has adopted a stance of general support for 'non-orthodox' care it would resist full integration and retain the principle of referral. It believes that all 'non-orthodox' practitioners should be taught a core curriculum based on science and biomedicine (BMA 2003).

Within nursing, it has been suggested that there is a 'natural affinity' with 'non-orthodox' care (Light 1997), matching the nurses' patient-centred and more holistic approach to practice. Moreover, 'non-orthodox' care offers nurses an opportunity for career development by giving them access to a distinct medical domain that is separate from 'orthodox' medicine (Tovey and Adams 2003). Estimates suggest that nurses' use of 'non-orthodox' care is increasingly widespread, half of nurses having used some form of therapy in their practice (Rankin-Box 1997), although this is most likely in maternity and oncology wards (Mitchell *et al.* 2006). It is assumed by the Royal College of Nursing (RCN 2003) that most nurses engage in those therapies defined by the House of Lords (2000) as 'supportive techniques'. A review of the nursing journals substantiates this to some extent, although there have been no national reviews/audits of practice; for instance, there is evidence of the use of aromatherapy (Styles 1997; Hunt *et al.* 2004; Thorgrimsen *et al.* 2006), massage (McNabb *et al.* 2006), and reflexology (Quattrin *et al.* 2006). However, the literature also provides evidence that nurses additionally use approaches classed as 'complete' therapeutic systems by the House of Lords, such as acupuncture (Grabowska 2003), cranial osteopathy (Hayden and Mullinger 2006) and homeopathy (Steen and Calvert 2006).

There has been very little sociological study of nurses' use of 'non-orthodox' care but the limited research in Israel and the United Kingdom shows that such nurses do not seek to change the 'epistemological and authority boundaries' of 'orthodox' care (Shuval 2006: 1784). They also act as important gatekeepers of 'non-orthodox' practitioners, restricting their ideological claims and monitoring the patient/therapist relationship (Broom and Tovey 2007: 567). What is interesting is that when nurses practise 'non-orthodox' medicine they are deemed safe by virtue of their nurse registration alone rather than as a result of formal accreditation of training in the use of non-orthodox therapies (RCN 2003). As such, nurse provision of 'non-orthodox' care has the potential to remain unregulated, to enter the NHS via the back door and to eschew those controls that limit provision by 'non-orthodox' practitioners.

Integration of 'non-orthodox' care into primary and hospital settings

There is evidence that 'non-orthodox' medicine is available within the NHS, and it is estimated that 10 per cent of visits to the six most established[7] 'non-orthodox' therapies are funded by the NHS (Thomas *et al.* 2001). In the absence of specific policy direction, it is individual Primary Care Trusts or GP practices and individual Hospital Trusts that make local decisions about whether they will commission 'non-orthodox' care. The most recent surveys show that just over 40 per cent of Primary Care Trusts provide some access (Wilkinson *et al.* 2004). Whilst the Department of Health has published guidance on practice-based commissioning (DOH 2000), and the NHS Trusts Association[8] maintains a directory of therapists (again, those that belong to a professional association), it is not known how much money is being spent on this form of care. It is clear, however, that there are significant regional variations in provision (Smallwood 2005) and so disparities in access.

Overall, integrated care has been most successfully developed within general practice, with regional variation. Thomas *et al.* (2003) showed a steady growth in the number of general practices that provided access to therapies (an increase of 39 per cent of practices in 1995 to 50 per cent in 2000). This increase is accounted for by general practitioners' provision rather than by referral to 'non-orthodox' practitioners and suggests that provision is dependent upon both the positive attitudes and the personal interest of local 'orthodox' practitioners. At present 'non-orthodox' treatment is still most often provided by members of the primary health care team or by referrals to external 'non-orthodox' practitioners, although there is evidence of a significant number of 'non-orthodox' practitioners working within general practice (12.2 per cent) (Thomas *et al.* 2003). The provision of 'non-orthodox' care in general practice during the last twenty years marks a significant change, a reconfiguring of primary health care, but one that has occurred within the parameters of the 'orthodox' paradigm. These changes have not unsettled traditional power relations; rather, 'orthodox' medicine has contained and managed 'non-orthodox' provision.

The shift to allow 'non-orthodox' care within NHS hospital premises is also undeniably significant. However, Shuval and Mizrachi's (2002) description of the integration process in Israel as the entrance into a 'well guarded fortress' appears to be apposite for the United Kingdom. Economically, there is little support as funding for services within hospitals is more likely to come from charitable donations, or the manipulation of non-recurrent budgets or be offered free by the therapist (Heller 2005; Broom and Tovey 2007). Where there has been active encouragement of 'non-orthodox' care, notably in hospices where integration has been seen to boost the legitimacy of the service, only certain therapies have been encouraged (healing and touch therapies) and therapists are very strictly controlled in terms of what they can and cannot do (Broom and Tovey 2007). The few micro-level studies that have studied integration in practice have suggested some general trends. Again, the epistemological authority of 'orthodox' care appears intact: whilst there is evidence that 'non-orthodox' care can be used within the NHS as a response to consumer demand, even when the scientific evidence may not be forthcoming, biomedical doctors retain control over the claims made. This includes the close regulation of 'non-orthodox' practice, leaving 'non-orthodox' practitioners with lower levels of legitimacy (Broom and Tovey 2007; Mizrachi *et al.* 2005). Broom and Tovey (2007) thus describe the process as 'pseudo integration', where practices are accommodated but not encouraged. Similarly Hollenberg's (2006) study in Canada found that 'orthodox' medical practitioners continue to dominate patient charting, referrals and tests and restrict 'non-orthodox' practitioners to specific spheres of competence and appropriate 'non-orthodox' techniques. Although the integration of 'non-orthodox' care may appear to threaten biomedical authority, the practical processes of integration have ensured that the biomedical profession has retained its power and ensured the subordination, limitation and exclusion of 'non-orthodox' practices.

Overall, there appears to be significant evidence of a shift within 'orthodox' attitudes, a genuinely changing ethos. This is substantiated through the BMA's change from a position of resistance to integration, the evidence of increased training and use of non-orthodox treatments amongst doctors and nurses, and increased referrals to 'non-orthodox' practitioners. However, the movement towards integration might also be interpreted as a pragmatic response, an appeal to consumer demand that masks the control of 'non-orthodox' care in practice. Whilst the 'orthodox' medical profession has accepted 'non-orthodox' care, it has done so on its terms, deciding which therapies may be integrated, how they might practise and subjugating non-orthodox' medicine to exacting scientific scrutiny. In sum, whilst 'orthodox' medicine may no longer be able to legislate how consumers behave, it has retained a fundamental role in interpreting and shaping the field for the consumer.

Conclusion: plus ça change?

Having studied 'non-orthodox' care for the last fifteen years, I have witnessed significant changes in the health behaviour of consumers, the attitudes of the 'orthodox' medical profession and allied staff and the shape of the health service. Without doubt 'non-orthodox' care is a mainstream activity, an aspect of common experience. There is evidence of increasing integration into the health service, a product of the power of the consumer, the profitability and cost-effectiveness of the 'non-orthodox' market, and therapeutic successes in some key areas. That consumers choose amongst a variety of practices, many of which lack a scientific evidence base seems to point to medical pluralism, to the importance of experience rather than experimental research evidence. The use of 'non-orthodox' medicine suggests that consumers do desire more individualized and participative engagement. There is also evidence that the medical and nursing professions are altering their parameters of practice and that the Department of Health is open to the integration of some therapies into state-funded health care. As such the idea of a 'postmodern' turn has some credence.

Whilst the significance of these changes should not be underestimated, they do, however, mask notable continuities. Aside from continued inequalities in access, the way that 'non-orthodox' care is practised and organized has remained much the same. In the first place, there has been little change in terms of state-endorsed practice. Despite considerable governmental pressure, 'non-orthodox' care remains largely unregulated and is firmly established within the private sector. Where there is provision in NHS premises, the norm is still that this care is privately funded and is increasingly offered and managed by 'orthodox' doctors and nurses. By incorporating and restricting 'non-orthodox' medicine, potential threats have been contained and 'orthodox' medicine appears, in practice, to have sustained its jurisdictional boundaries. Further, the epistemological superiority of the biomedical model seems to have been sustained in practice, not least since 'orthodox' 'scientific' methods are used to validate or disallow 'non-orthodox' interventions. There is a dearth of sociological research in this area and further investigation of the processes whereby 'non-orthodox' therapies are integrated or excluded is necessary.

Moreover, the majority of 'non-orthodox' practitioners have, in a very short time, altered their practices, organization and knowledge transmission through processes of professionalization and social closure. Whilst this may be interpreted as a survival strategy it also points to the prevailing and pervasive importance of the idea of the 'expert' who is professionally policed, whose competence can be guaranteed and where a very specific relationship with the client can be asserted. There has also been a steady standardization of the organization and delivery of non-orthodox medicine. While this has not expanded the 'non-orthodox' share of the state-funded market to a significant degree, it has divided the 'non-orthodox' field into the *dangerous* and the *competent*.

There are, then, a number of contradictory changes within 'non-orthodox' care. Whilst there may be widespread support amongst the general public, institutional pluralism of 'non-orthodox' medicine lags behind. Specifically, 'orthodox' practitioners have integrated 'non-orthodox' care but mainly on their own terms. The 'non-orthodox' practitioners have experienced huge demand for their services but have responded to a culture of uncertainty and risk by altering their own training and practice to engender the trust of the public, state and 'orthodox' medical profession. Thus, whilst the movement of 'non-orthodox' care from the margins to the mainstream could be interpreted as a sea change, it is also possible to suggest that the great claims that 'non-orthodox' care would radicalize health care practices and policies have simply been both managed and curtailed.

Notes

1   Ernst (2006) shows that there were over 1000 surveys conducted during the last decade.
2   Mills and Budd (2000) estimated that in 2000 there were 70,000 practitioners.
3   Acupuncture, chiropractic, homoeopathy, hypnotherapy, medical herbalism, osteopathy.
4   The 'professionalization project' draws from Marxist and Weberian sociology and describes and accounts for the ways in which occupations alter their education, organization and jurisdiction (market share) in return for status and autonomy.
5   For example, homoeopathy, herbalism, osteopathy, chiropractic, naturopathy.
6   The House of Lords (2000) report recommended that only those therapies that have statutory regulation or a powerful mechanism of voluntary self-regulation should be considered for integration.
7   The same therapies as in note 3.
8   See www.nhsdirectory.org/default.aspx?page=public.

References

Abbott, A. (1998) *The System of Professions*, Chicago: University of Chicago Press.

Andrews, G. (2003) 'Placing the consumption of private complementary medicine. Everyday geographies of older people's use', *Health and Place*, 9: 337–49.

Baer, H. (1984) 'The drive for professionalisation in British Osteopathy', *Social Science and Medicine*, 19: 717–25.

Bakx, K. (1991) 'The eclipse of folk medicine in western society', *Sociology of Health and Illness*, 13: 20–38.

Barry, C. (2006) 'The role of evidence in alternative medicine: contrasting biomedical and anthropological approaches', *Social Science and Medicine*, 62: 2646–57.

Beck, U. (1992) *Risk Society*, London: Sage.

Bernstein, B. and Grasso, T. (2001) 'Prevalence of complementary and alternative medicine in cancer patients', *Oncology*, 15: 1272–83.

Braathen, E. (1996) 'Communicating the individual body and the body politic: the discourse on disease prevention and health promotion in alternative therapies', in S. Cant and U. Sharma (eds) *Complementary and Alternative Medicines. Knowledge in practice*, London: Free Association Books.

British Medical Association (1986) *Alternative Therapy*, London: BMA.

British Medical Association (1993) *Complementary Therapy. New approaches to good practice*, Oxford: Oxford University Press.

British Medical Association (2003) 'Complementary and alternative medicine – submission to public petitions committee'. Online: www.bma.org.uk/ap.nsf/Content/publicpetitioncam (accessed 9 October 2007).

Broom, A. and Tovey, P. (2007) 'Therapeutic pluralism? Evidence, power and legitimacy in UK cancer services', *Sociology of Health and Illness*, 29: 551–69.

Cant, S. (1996) 'From charismatic teaching to professional training: the legitimation of knowledge and the creation of trust in Homoeopathy and Chiropractic', in S. Cant and U. Sharma (eds) *Complementary and Alternative Medicines. Knowledge in practice*, London: Free Association Books.

Cant, S. and Sharma, U. (1995) 'The reluctant profession. Homoeopathy and the search for legitimacy', *Work, Employment and Society*, 9: 743–62.

Cant, S. and Sharma, U. (1996) 'Demarcation and transformation within homoeopathic knowledge. A strategy of professionalisation', *Social Science and Medicine*, 42: 579–88.

Cant, S. and Sharma, U. (1999) *A New Medical Pluralism? Alternative medicine, doctors, patients and the state*, London: UCL Press.

Cartwright, T. (2007) 'Getting on with life: the experiences of older people using complementary medicine', *Social Science and Medicine*, 64: 1692–703.

Clarke, D.B., Doel, M.A. and Segrott, J. (2004) 'No alternative? The regulation and professionalisation of complementary and alternative medicine in the United Kingdom', *Health and Place*, 10: 320–38.

Department of Health (2000) *Complementary Medicine: information pack for primary care groups*, London: Department of Health.

Department of Health (2001) *Government Response to the House of Lords Select Committee on Science and Technology's Report on Complementary and Alternative Medicine*, London: Department of Health.

Department of Health (2004a) *Regulation of Herbal Medicine and Acupuncture*, London: Department of Health.

Department of Health (2004b) *NHS Improvement Plan 2004: Putting people at the heart of public services*, London: Department of Health.

Doel, M.A. and Segrott, J. (2003) 'Beyond belief? Consumer culture, complementary medicine and the diseases of everyday life', *Society and Space*, 21: 739–59.

Easthorpe, G., Tranter, B. and Gill, G. (2000) 'General practitioners' attitudes toward complementary medicine', *Social Science and Medicine*, 51: 1555–61.

Ernst, E. (2006) 'Prevalence surveys. To be taken with a pinch of salt', *Complementary Therapies in Clinical Practice*, 12: 272–75.

Ernst, E. and White, A. (2000) 'The BBC survey of complementary medicine use in the UK', *Complementary Therapies in Medicine*, 8: 32–6.

Ernst, E., Resch, K.L. and White, A.R. (1995) 'Complementary medicine. What physicians think of it: a meta-analysis', *Archives of Internal Medicine*, 155: 2405–8.

Evetts, J. (2006) 'Short note: the sociology of professional groups', *Current Sociology*, 54: 133–43.

Freidson, E. (1970) *Professional Dominance*, Chicago: Atherton.

Friedson, E. (1994) *Professionalism Reborn. Theory, practice and policy*, Cambridge: Polity Press.

Fournier, V. (1999) 'The appeal to professionalism as a disciplinary mechanism', *The Sociological Review*, 47: 280–307.

Furnham, A. and Bragrath, R. (1992) 'A comparison of health beliefs and behaviours of clients of orthodox and complementary medicine', *British Journal of Clinical Psychology*, 50: 237–46.

Furnham, A. and Smith, C. (1988) 'Choosing alternative medicine: a comparison of the patients visiting a GP and a homoeopath', *Social Science and Medicine*, 26: 685–7.

Gabe, J., Calnan, M. and Bury, M. (eds) (1991) *The Sociology of the Health Service*, London: Routledge.

Giddens, A. (1990) *The Consequences of Modernity*, Cambridge: Polity Press.

Giddens, A. (1991) *Modernity and Self identity. Self and society in the late modern age*, Cambridge: Polity Press.

Grabowska, C.S. (2003) 'Provision of acupuncture in a university health centre: a clinical audit', *Complementary Therapies in Nursing and Midwifery*, 9: 14–19.

Han, G. (2002) 'The myth of medical pluralism. A critical realist perspective', *Sociological Research Online* 6(4). Online: www.socresonline.org.uk/6/4/han. html (accessed 24 July 2007).

Harris, P. and Rees, R. (2000) 'The prevalence of complementary and alternative medicine use amongst the general population: a systematic review of the literature', *Complementary Therapies in Medicine*, 8: 88–96.

Haug, M. (1988) 'A re-examination of the hypothesis of deprofessionalisation', *Milbank Quarterly*, 2: 48–56.

Hayden, C. and Mullinger, B. (2006) 'A preliminary assessment of the impact of cranial osteopathy for the relief of infantile colic', *Complementary Therapies in Clinical Practice*, 12: 83–90.

Heller, T. (2005) 'Integration of CAM with mainstream services', in T. Heller, G. Lee-Treweek, K. Katz, J. Stone, and S. Spurr (eds) *Perspectives on Complementary and Alternative Medicine*, Abingdon: Routledge.

Hewer, W. (1983) 'The relationship between the alternative practitioner and his patient: a review', *Psychotherapy and Psychosomatics*, 40: 172–80.

Hildreth, K.D. and Elman, C. (2007) 'Alternative worldviews and the utilization of conventional and complementary medicine', *Sociological Inquiry*, 77: 76–103.

Hollenberg, D. (2006) 'Uncharted ground: patterns of professional interaction among complementary and biomedical practitioners in integrative health setting, *Social Science and Medicine*, 62: 731–44.

House of Lords Select Committee on Science and Technology (2000) *Complementary and Alternative Medicine: Sixth Report*, London: The Stationery Office. Online: www.publications.parliament.uk/pa/ld199900/ldselect/ldsctech/123/12301.htm (accessed 16 September 2008).

Hunt, V., Randle, J. and Freshwater, D. (2004) 'Paediatric nurses' attitudes to massage and aromatherapy massage', *Complementary Therapies in Nursing and Midwifery*, 10: 194–201.

Inglis, B. (1964) *Fringe Medicine*, London: Faber and Faber.

Jackson, S. and Scambler, G. (2007) 'Perceptions of evidence based medicine: traditional acupuncturists in the UK and resistance to biomedical modes of evaluation', *Sociology of Health and Illness*, 29: 412–29.

Jewson, N. (1979) 'The disappearance of the sick man from medical cosmology 1770–1870', *Sociology*, 10: 225–44.

Kelner, M., Wellman, H., Welsh, S. and Boon, H. (2006) 'How far can complementary medicine go? The case of chiropractic and homeopathy', *Social Science and Medicine*, 63: 2617–27.

Klein, R. (2001) *The New Politics of the NHS*, fourth edition, London: Prentice Hall.

Larkin, G. (1983) *Occupational Monopoly and Modern Medicine*, London: Tavistock.

Larson, M.S. (1977) *The Rise of Professionalism: A sociological analysis*, Berkeley: University of California Press.

Light, K. (1997) 'Florence Nightingale and the holistic philosophy', *Journal of Holistic Nursing*, 15: 24–40.

Lowenberg, J.S. and Davis, F. (1994) 'Beyond medicalisation-demedicalisation: the case of holistic health', *Sociology of Health and Illness*, 16: 579–99.

Lyotard, J.F. (1979) *The Postmodern Condition: A report on knowledge*, Manchester: Manchester University Press.

Macdonald, K.M. (1995) *The Sociology of the Professions*, London: Sage.

McKinlay, J. and Stoekle, J. (1988) 'Corporatization and the social transformation of doctoring', *International Journal of Health Services*, 18: 191–205.

McNabb, M., Kimber, L. and Haines, A. (2006) 'Does regular massage from late pregnancy to birth decrease maternal pain perception during labour and birth? A feasibility study to investigate a programme of massage. Controlled breathing and visualisation, from 36 weeks of pregnancy until birth', *Complementary Therapies in Clinical Practice*, 12: 222–31.

McQuaide, M.M, (2005) 'The rise of alternative health care: a sociological account', *Social Theory and Health*, 3: 286–301.

Meade, T.W., Dyer, S., Browne, W., Townsend, J. and Frank, A.O. (1990) 'Low back pain of mechanical origin: randomised comparison of Chiropractic and hospital out-patient treatment', *British Medical Journal*, 300: 1431–7.

Mills, S, and Budd, S. (2000) *Professional Organisation of Complementary and*

Alternative Medicine in the United Kingdom 2000: A second report to the DOH, Exeter: Centre for Complementary Health Studies.

Mintel (2003) *Complementary and Alternative Medicine in the UK*, London: Mintel.

Mintel (2007) *Complementary Medicines in the UK*, London: Mintel.

Mitchell, M., Williams, J. and Hobbs, E. (2006) 'The use of complementary therapies in maternity services: A survey', *British Journal of Midwifery*, 14: 576–82.

Mizrachi, N., Shuval, J.T. and Gross, S. (2005) 'Boundary at work: alternative medicine in biomedical settings', *Sociology of Health and Illness*, 27: 20–43.

Morgan D., Glanville, H., Maris, S. and Nathanson, V. (2005) 'Education and training in complementary and alternative medicine: a postal survey of UK universities, medical schools and faculties of nurse education', *Complementary Therapies in Medicine*, 6: 64–70.

National Centre for Complementary and Alternative Medicine (NCCAM) (2004) 'What is complementary and alternative medicine?' Online: www.nccam.nih.gov/health/whatiscam (accessed 11 October 2007).

Navarro, V. (1978) *Class Struggle, the State and Medicine*, London: Martin Robertson.

Nicholls, P. (1988) *Homeopathy and the Medical Profession*, London: Croom Helm.

Ong, K. and Banks. B. (2003) *Complementary and Alternative Medicine: The consumer perspective*, London: The Prince's Foundation for Integrated Health.

Oppenheimer, M. (1973) 'The proletarianization of the professional', *Sociological Review Monograph*, 20: 213–37.

Parkin, F. (1974) 'Strategies of social closure in class formation', in F. Parkin (ed.) *The Social Analyses of Class Structure*, London: Tavistock.

Peters, D. (2000) 'From holism to integration: is there a future for complementary therapies in the NHS?' *Complementary Therapies in Nursing and Midwifery*, 6: 59–60.

PWFIH (2005) *A Healthy Partnership: Integrating complementary health care into primary care*, London: The Prince's Foundation for Integrated Health.

PWFIH (2006) *Exploring a Federal Approach to Voluntary Self Regulation of Complementary Health Care*, London: The Prince's Foundation for Integrated Health.

Power, R. (1994) 'Only nature heals', in S. Budd and U. Sharma (eds) *The Healing Bond*, London: Routledge.

Quah, S.R. (2003) 'Traditional healing systems and the ethos of science', *Social Science and Medicine*, 57: 1997–2012.

Quattrin, R., Zanini, A. and Buchini, S. (2006) 'Use of reflexology foot massage to reduce anxiety in hospitalised cancer patients in chemotherapy treatment: methodology and outcomes', *Journal Nursing Management*, 14: 96–105.

Rankin-Box, D. (1997) 'Therapies in practice: a survey assessing nurses' use of complementary therapies', *Complementary Therapies in Nursing and Midwifery*, 3: 2–99.

Raynor, L. and Easthope, G. (2001) 'Postmodern consumption and alternative medications', *Journal of Sociology*, 37: 157–76.

Rees, L. and Weil, A. (2001) 'Integrated medicine', *British Medical Journal*, 322: 119–20.

RCN (2003) *Complementary Therapies in Nursing, Midwifery and Health Visiting Practice*, London: RCN.

Saks, M. (1992) 'Introduction', in M. Saks (ed.) *Alternative Medicine in Britain*, Oxford: Clarendon Press.

Saks, M. (1996) 'From quackery to complementary medicine: the shifting boundaries between orthodox and unorthodox medical knowledge', in S. Cant and U. Sharma (eds) *Complementary and Alternative Medicines. Knowledge in practice*, London: Free Association Books.

Saks, M. (1997) 'East meets West: the emergence of a holistic tradition', in R. Porter (ed.) *Medicine: A history of healing*, London: The Ivy Press.

Saks, M. (2003) *Orthodox and Alternative Medicine: Politics, professionalisation and health care*, London: Sage.

Sharma, U. (1992) *Complementary Medicine Today*, London: Routledge.

Shuval, J. (2006) 'Nurses in alternative health care: integrating medical paradigms', *Social Science and Medicine*, 63: 1784–95.

Shuval, J. and Mizrachi, N. (2002) 'Entering the well guarded fortress: alternative practitioners in hospital settings', *Social Science and Medicine*, 55: 1745–55.

Siahpush, M (1998) 'Postmodern values, dissatisfaction with conventional medicine and popularity of alternative therapies', *Journal of Sociology*, 31: 58–70.

Sirious, F.M. and Gick, M.L. (2002) 'An investigation of the health beliefs and motivations of complementary medicine clients', *Social Science and Medicine*, 55: 1025–37.

Smallwood, C. (2005) *The Role of Alternative and Complementary Medicine in the NHS*, London: PWFIH.

Steen, M. and Calvert, J. (2006) 'Homeopathy for childbirth: remedies and research', *RCM Midwives Journal*, 9: 438–40.

Stone, J. (2002) *An Ethical Framework for Complementary and Alternative Therapists*, London: Routledge.

Stone, J. (2005) 'Regulation of CAM practitioners: reflecting on the last 10 years', *Complementary Therapies in Clinical Practice*, 11: 5–10.

Stone, J. and Matthews, J. (1996) *Complementary Medicine and the Law*, Oxford: Oxford University Press.

Stone, J. and Lee-Treweek, G. (2005) 'Regulation and control', in G. Lee-Treweek, T. Heller, H. MacQueen, J. Stone, and S. Spurr (eds) *Complementary and Alternative Medicine: Structures and safeguards*, Abingdon: Routledge.

Styles, J.L. (1997) 'The use of aromatherapy in hospitalized children with HIV disease', *Complementary Therapies in Nursing and Midwifery*, 3: 16–20.

Taylor, C.R. (1984) 'Alternative medicine and the medical encounter in Britain and the United States', in W.J. Salmon (ed.) *Alternative Medicines. Popular and policy perspectives*, London: Tavistock.

The Times (2006) Letter. Online: www.timesonline.co.uk/tol/news/uk/health/article 723787.ece (accessed 9 November 2007).

Thomas K.J. and Coleman, P. (2004) 'Use of complementary or alternative medicine in a general population in Great Britain. Results from the National Omnibus Survey', *Journal of Public Health* 26: 152–7.

Thomas, K.J., Coleman, P. and Nicholl, J.P. (2003) 'Trends in access to complementary or alternative medicines via primary care in England: 1995–2001. Results from a follow up national survey', *Family Practice*, 20: 575–7.

Thomas K.J., Nicholl J.P. and Coleman P. (2001) 'Use and expenditure on complementary medicine in England: a population based survey', *Complementary Therapies in Medicine*, 9: 2–11.

Thomas, K.J., Carr, J., Westlake, L. and Williams, B. (1991) 'Use of non-orthodox and conventional health care in Great Britain', *British Medical Journal*, 302: 207–10.

Thorgrimsen, L., Spector, A. and Orrell, M. (2006) 'The use of aromatherapy in dementia care: a review', *Journal of Dementia Care*, 14: 33–6.

Trevelyan, J. and Booth, B. (1994) *Complementary Medicine for Nurses, Midwives and Health Visitors*, London: Macmillan.

Tovey, P. and Adams, J. (2003) 'Nostalgic and nostophobic referencing and the authentication of nurses' use of complementary therapies', *Social Science and Medicine*, 56: 1469–80.

Tovey, P. and Broom, A. (2007) 'Oncologists and specialist cancer nurses' approaches to complementary and alternative medicine and their impact on patient action', *Social Science and Medicine*, 64: 2550–64.

Vincent, C. and Furnham, A. (1997) *Complementary Medicine. A Research Perspective*, Chichester: Wiley.

Waddington, I. (1984) *The Medical Profession in the Industrial Revolution*, London: Gill and Macmillan.

Wahlberg, A. (2007) 'A quackery with a difference – new medical pluralism and the problem of dangerous practitioners in the UK', *Social Science and Medicine*, 65: 2307–16.

Wallis, R, and Morley, P. (1976) *Marginal Medicine*, London: Owen.

Welsh, S., Kelner, M., Wellman, B. and Boon, H. (2004) 'Moving forward? Complementary and alternative practitioners seeking self regulation', *Sociology of Health and Illness*, 26: 216–41.

West, R. (1984) 'Alternative medicine: prospects and speculations', in N. Black, D. Boswell, A. Gray, S. Murphey and J. Popay (eds) *Health and Disease. A Reader*, London: Open University Press.

Wilkinson, J., Peters, D. and Donaldson, J. (2004) *Clinical Governance for Complementary and Alternative Medicine in Primary Care*, London: University of Westminster.

Willis, E. (1992) *Medical Dominance*, Sydney: Allen and Unwin.

Zollman, C. and Vickers, A. (1999) 'Complementary medicine and the doctor', *British Medical Journal*, 319: 1558–61.

10 Social care
Relationships, markets and ethics

Caroline Glendinning

Introduction

This chapter discusses the provision of care to people who, because of illness, impairment or ageing, require help with personal tasks, help with practical everyday living tasks and/or supervision, guidance and emotional support. It is therefore concerned with help that is given *over and above* that normally given within close family relationships to non-disabled partners, children or other relatives. The chapter takes forward the Hilary Land's analysis of community care policies in the first edition of this text.

The aims of the chapter are three-fold. First, it provides an overview of theory and debate about the nature of 'care'. It describes the development of major bodies of feminist and philosophical theory on care, and the growing salience of care as a key dimension of welfare state policy and analysis. The chapter then offers insights into the provision of social care in England, first of all by close relatives and friends providing 'informal' care to disabled, ill or frail elderly people; and second, by formally organized social care services. Third, the chapter focuses on the troubled history of relationships between social care and the National Health Service (NHS); the raft of initiatives introduced since the late 1990s aimed at improving those relationships are described. The chapter concludes by noting the potential divergence between NHS and social care policies aimed at increasing, respectively, patient and user choice. The chapter argues that this divergence risks threatening some of the improvements in inter-sectoral and inter-agency collaboration that have been achieved since the late 1990s; introducing new instabilities in the governance of social care and the nature of citizenship; and marginalizing the interests of by far the largest group of providers of social care – close relatives and friends.

What is 'social care'?

One starting point for defining 'social care' is to see it as a primarily organizational construct whose roots lie in the institutional structures of the English post-war welfare state. These structures assigned responsibility for 'treatment' and 'cure' to the newly established NHS, with local government providing longer-term personal and practical services to older and disabled people. Thus while the NHS provided for the 'ill' and 'sick', the 1948 National Assistance Act made local authorities responsible for providing residential and other services for people in need of 'care and attention' (Means and Smith 1998). This division of responsibilities was underpinned by different funding and accountability mechanisms, which have remained fundamentally unchanged since the late 1940s. NHS services, funded from general taxation, remain largely free at the point of delivery and directly accountable to central government. In contrast, local authority services are funded through a mixture of central and locally raised taxation, plus significant contributions of means-tested co-payments from service users. While the accountability of local authority social care services to central government has increased over the past fifty years through an extensive range of financial controls and performance management mechanisms, these services nevertheless also retain a degree of accountability to locally elected politicians. (The implications of these structural differences are discussed later in this chapter.)

Unlike NHS services, about half of all expenditure on social care services comes from private sources: the means- and assets-tested co-payments required by local authorities from users of residential and domiciliary services; or the payments made by people who purchase their care services privately. This private expenditure was estimated to be £5.9 billion in 2005–6 (CSCI 2008). Yet even this significant contribution of private resources to overall expenditure on social care is minuscule by comparison with the massive volume of unpaid social care contributed 'in kind' by close kin and friends, as the next section of this chapter will explain.

Although the concept of social care can be traced back to the origins of the welfare state, simply defining it as the product of social care services is both tautologous and unhelpful. It is also imprecise, because the boundaries between the responsibilities of the NHS and local authority social care services have shifted considerably over time – and with them the definition of social care (Lewis 2001; Glendinning and Means 2004). Since the late 1940s the NHS has withdrawn from providing non-medical care for a wide range of people with long-term support needs. In some cases, for example people with severe learning disabilities, the redefinition of their support as 'social care' is widely acknowledged to have been entirely appropriate, particularly when the shifting boundary was accompanied by some transfer of resources. In other instances it has proved more controversial. For example, during the 1970s a series of central government circulars defined older people with ever higher levels of frailty and ill-health as 'appropriate' for local authority residential care, so that those considered to need social 'care and attention' came to include people with severe cognitive impairments, who were bed-bound, or who were in the final stages of terminal illness (Means and Smith 1998). Similarly, since the mid-1990s, a series of legal challenges and government directives have attempted to restrict long-term NHS services only to people whose health care needs are intensive and/or highly unpredictable (Glendinning and Lloyd 1998; Glasby and Littlechild 2004).

Institutional or service-based definitions of social care may therefore vary considerably over time (and indeed, between different welfare states). However, there is an extensive body of research and theory on the social and philosophical meanings of social care, and the implications of these meanings for the respective responsibilities of individuals, families and the state. Much of this work was originally prompted by research into the 'social' (i.e. largely non-treatment-based) care provided on a predominantly unpaid basis by close relatives to adults, children and older people who are disabled, chronically ill or elderly – what is commonly termed 'informal' care.

The nature of care

Care is a complex phenomenon. It can include caring *for* – the work involved in tending and sustaining another person – and caring *about* – love, concern and other affective dimensions (Graham 1983). It may include emotional labour – working on and through the feelings of others, with the aim of affecting their emotional state (Hochschild 1983). It is unusual for boundaries to be imposed on the range or duration of activities or responsibilities which constitute a care-giving relationship. Care, whether provided by close kin or paid care workers, is also generally a very private activity, often taking place within the confines of the home and involving intimate 'transgressive' bodily contact (Twigg 2000).

Theorizing about the nature of care has its origins – and continuing roots – in traditions of feminist scholarship. Initially feminists aimed to make visible the unpaid work performed by women within the private sphere of the family. As early as 1978, Hilary Land argued that family policies failed to address the unequal contributions of women and men to the well-being of families; this failure had significant consequences for women's financial independence and risks of poverty (Land 1978). Subsequently, feminist critiques were extended to contemporary policies of community care and the implicit assumption that care within 'the community' in effect meant care within the family – again to be provided predominantly by women (Finch and Groves 1980, 1983; Graham 1983; Dalley 1988; Lewis and Meredith 1988). Feminists also pointed to the close alignment between the nature of 'care' and assumptions about femininity and women's 'natural' roles: 'In general, caring relationships are those involving women; it is the presence of a woman . . . which marks out a relationship as . . . a caring one' (Graham 1983: 15).

Early feminist writers on care aimed to render explicit and visible the work involved in care. Much of this research therefore emphasized the material, physical and emotional demands associated with caring; the consequent personal, material and opportunity costs; and the disproportionate impact of these costs on women (Fine and Glendinning 2005). From this starting point, research on care has developed a number of different strands.

One major strand of research has explored how care is 'inherently defined by the relations within which it [is] carried out, relations that tended to be characterized by personal ties of obligation, commitment, trust and loyalty' (Daly and Lewis 2000: 283). The relational nature of care is also emphasized by ethical theorists such as Gilligan (1982) and Tronto (1993), who have highlighted the interconnectedness and interdependency that characterizes the close relationships, often between close family members or characterized by quasi-kinship features, within which care is typically given and received. They point out that these relationships, which are universally experienced in different ways throughout the life course, are fundamental both to individual identity and to the production and reproduction of society.

The relationships within which care is given and received are framed by strong normative and moral dimensions. Confirmation of the distinctive nature of the kin relationships which frequently form the context for care is given by Finch and Mason's research, which shows how kinship responsibilities and commitments develop over time, through iterative processes of interaction and negotiation. Moreover, 'through negotiations about giving and receiving assistance, people are being constructed and reconstructed as moral beings' (Finch and Mason 1993: 70). Consideration of the normative dimensions of care have led to arguments that the allegedly 'feminine' qualities from which the concept and practice of 'care' have been constructed (Graham 1983) should be positively valued and universalized. Care – and the values on which it is based – is argued to be threatened by the male, scientific, bureaucratic and market-based rationalities that typically shape public policy (Wærness 2006). In contrast, it is argued that the 'important values attributed to women but traditionally confined to the domestic sphere can provide a broad moral compass for public life' (Fine 2007: 37). This body of theory, termed an 'ethics of care', has built upon the positive valuation of women's role in caring that was provided by earlier feminist writing and has argued for the extension into the public sphere of the virtues and activities involved in care. Tronto (1993), for example, argued that the values associated with care need to be recognized as providing a set of principles about responsibility for the well-being of others that should shape both public and private life. Furthermore, if public policies fail to recognize and support these responsibilities, those involved in providing care to people who are in some way dependent risk serious threats to their social citizenship (Kittay 1999).

These important strands of feminist-inspired theory and research into the nature of care have not gone unchallenged. The association between gender and care has been questioned: Arber and Gilbert (1989) and Arber and Ginn

(1999) have drawn attention to the prevalence of care provided by men, particularly for their partners and parents. Another powerful critique has come from disabled people themselves, who have argued for a social model of disability that focuses on the social and environmental barriers that impede equality and citizenship (Swain *et al.* 1993); from this perspective the very language of care is problematic, connoting as it does dependency and a lack of agency and autonomy. From this perspective too, feminist researchers who have emphasized the 'burdens' of care are criticized for contributing to the objectification and disempowerment of disabled people, and for failing to acknowledge the agency and care-giving activities of many disabled people themselves (Morris 1991, 1993). Other writers, from both disability and feminist perspectives, have also drawn attention to the reciprocity and interdependency that exists within care-giving relationships, and to the difficulties surrounding the use of 'care' as a key analytic concept (Fine and Glendinning 2005). Thus Shakespeare (2000a, 2000b) argues that the concept of care is negatively loaded and should be replaced by that of 'help'; help opens up the possibility of a wide range of alternative sources of social support and informal community networks, underpinned by moral values of altruism and friendship. This is also the basis of feminist political theorist Selma Sevenhuijsen's (2000) argument that care is an essentially relational activity; consequently, the recognition and support of human interdependency needs to replace the ideals of independence and autonomy as the basis of social and public policies:

> A democratic ethic of care starts from the idea that everybody needs care and is (in principle at least) capable of care giving, and that a democratic society should enable its members to give both these activities a meaningful place in their lives if they so want.
>
> (Sevenhuijsen 2000: 15)

Similarly, Kittay (1999) proposes public policies based on the concept of 'doulia' – an obligation on the wider social order to support the relationships involved in protecting and nurturing dependent and vulnerable people.

Care as an analytic tool

Critiques of social and public policies through the 'lens' of social care, underpinned by the gender-based and feminist perspectives outlined above, constitute a growing strand of political, economic and sociological analysis, both in England and elsewhere. Moreover, the extent to which public policies recognize and support care is increasingly far more than just a moral and philosophical issue. Population ageing affects dependency ratios (fewer working age people to support growing proportions of economically inactive people), at the same time as generating growing pressures for the provision of care and support for frail older people. Global economic pressures generate additional demands for high levels of economic activity on the part of working age populations. A growing challenge for social policies, therefore, is to find ways of encouraging labour market participation at the same time as supporting care-giving. (This particular issue is discussed further in the next section.)

Thus Daly and Lewis (2000) use care as an analytic tool to explore a complex set of activities and relations that lie at the intersections of the state, market and family. Daly and Lewis argue that the concept of care makes explicit the gender dimensions of social policies; helps to overcome fragmentation in conventional policy analysis between the provision of cash support and services; and identifies new trajectories of change (see also Daly 2002). Policies in Britain and the USA have been analysed to see how far they support both those giving *and* those receiving care, in order to avoid risks to the well-being, opportunities and citizenship rights of both (see for example Kittay 1999; West 2002; Glendinning and Kemp 2006; Beckett, 2007). In contrast, Nordic analyses of social care have extended to paid as well as unpaid care, drawing attention to the incompatibility between the managerialist imperatives that currently shape the organization of paid care work and the action, reason and feelings that are key elements in the provision of good quality care (Wærness 2006). Economists writing from an 'ethic of care' perspective have also generated critiques of mainstream economic theory for failing to recognize the distributional conflicts that can occur if the 'costs' of care are not properly recognized (Folbre 2004). These negative distributional effects increasingly include a 'care drain' as workers (usually women) move from poorer South to richer North countries to fill low-paid care posts – a trend which helps to perpetuate the low economic value placed on paid care work (Wærness 2006; Da Roit *et al.* 2007).

In summary, care is a complex, multi-dimensional concept which cuts across conventional dichotomies and divisions between rationality and emotion, public and private domains, paid and unpaid work, and which is characterized by strong normative frameworks of obligation and responsibility. Since the 1970s, it has been the focus of research and theorizing by feminists, disability writers, political theorists, ethicists, sociologists and policy analysts. Consequently, care is no longer viewed as 'just' a 'women's issue', but one that raises fundamental questions about the moral and ethical basis of social relationships; about the conditions under which societies produce and reproduce themselves; and about the role of the state in creating appropriate conditions to support these relationships. These questions are becoming increasingly acute as demographic and globalizing pressures converge to place multiple demands on the adult population to combine paid work and care. The next section of this chapter shows how these issues are currently addressed in the organization of informal and formal social care.

Social care – the private and the public

Informal care

Given the foregoing analysis, it is not surprising that most social care for ill, disabled and elderly people is provided on a largely unpaid basis by close kin – partners, children and parents. According to the 2001 Census, there were almost 6 million carers (one in ten of the population) in the UK. Of these, 3,952,572 provided up to 20 hours a week care to sick, disabled or older people (care of non-disabled children was not included); 659,069 provided 20–49 hours care a week; and 1,247,291 provided 50 or more hours a week care. It is estimated that the value of this care across the UK in 2007 amounted to just over £87 billion – slightly more than the total annual UK NHS budget and more than four times the level of annual local authority spending on social services (Carers UK 2007).

Although people aged 45–59 are most likely to be carers, as the population ages so the numbers of older carers are also increasing. Across the UK, there are 1.5 million carers aged 60-plus; of these almost 350,000 are 75 and over and more than 8,000 are aged 90-plus. Also with population ageing, the numbers of male carers and the amount of care they provide are both increasing; above age 85, over half of male carers and almost half of female carers provide at least 50 hours of care each week.

A majority of working age carers (72 per cent of men carers and 62 per cent of women carers) now combine care-giving with paid work. Working carers face high risks of wage discrimination and consequent opportunity costs; recent research demonstrates that these risks have increased over time (Heitmueller and Inglis 2007). Carers who exercise their rights to request flexible working arrangements under the 2002 Employment Act receive no financial compensation for any time taken off work. Moreover, without adequate support, the dual pressures of paid work and care-giving can lead to serious health problems (Buckner and Yeandle 2006). Yet withdrawing from paid employment risks even more serious financial disadvantage, in both the shorter and the longer terms. Carers Allowance, the main social security benefit for carers, is one of the lowest benefits in the UK and is wholly inadequate for replacing lost earnings. Carers' incomes in their own old age are also affected, as their contributions to state, occupational or private pensions are reduced by interrupted labour market participation and/or depressed earnings (see Arksey *et al.* 2005, for a summary of evidence on carers' employment, earnings, income and pensions). Again, state pension arrangements only partially compensate for these losses.

While local authorities have had powers since 1995 to conduct assessments of carers' needs and some central government funding has been allocated (and ring-fenced) specifically for the development of carers' services, services for carers remain fragmented, locally variable[1] and often dependent on the voluntary sector. Services for carers are most likely to consist of respite care facilities to give carers a break, or cash payments on a regular or one-off basis to help carers purchase whatever additional help they need. Additional funding was announced in 2006 for local authorities to develop services for carers experiencing a sudden crisis or emergency. The creation of a national telephone information and advice service for carers and an 'Expert Carer' programme to provide training for carers in managing their own health and that of the person they care for are also in progress.

Carers are a highly diverse population, varying by age, gender, employment status and relationship to the person they care for, among other key variables. For some, caring is short and intensive – for example, when looking after a terminally ill partner. For others, such as for parents of severely disabled children, it is a very long-term experience. Carers commonly report difficulties in obtaining help, support and information. Moreover the services that are available, such as respite care, are not necessarily acceptable to either carers or the people they care for. At the same time, policies aimed at increasing choice and personalization of services for older and disabled people themselves may inadvertently have adverse consequences for carers (Arksey and Glendinning 2007a); this risk will be discussed further in the final section of this chapter. Major challenges remain to develop policies that can effectively support the very diverse population of carers, particularly in the context of an increasingly tight labour market where demands for their skills remain high (see Arksey and Glendinning (2007b), for further discussion of policies for carers in Britain).

Social care – public funding and organization

As noted above, responsibility for funding and commissioning formal social care services for adults lies with local authorities.[2]

From its origins in the discretionary Poor Law welfare responsibilities of local government, adult social care remains seriously under-funded, despite growing demographic pressures from an ageing population: 'the legacy of the Poor Law can still be seen in the way long-term care is provided today' (Robinson 2001: 3). This under-funding is particularly apparent in relation to social care services for older people, which are governed by high eligibility thresholds and lower cost ceilings than for younger adults. Changes in levels of spending also vary between different groups of adults, with social care spending on older people and adults with mental illness growing at only 4.1 or 4.2 per cent in real terms between 2003–4 and 2004–5, compared with growth rates of 7.2 per cent in social care spending on adults with learning disabilities and 6.3 per cent for adults with physical or sensory disabilities (CSCI 2006a).

One consequence of this underfunding has been the gradual withdrawal since the early 1990s by adult social care services from the provision of practical help such as cleaning and from low-level preventive interventions for people whose support needs are not yet substantial (see for example Clarke *et al*. 1998). This represents another 'redrawing' of the definitional boundaries of local authority social care services which, so far as older people are concerned, now largely consist of help with, or supervision of, personal care tasks only; other elements of social care provision fall to informal carers or private purchase.

Like the NHS, a split between the purchasing and provision of social care services was introduced in the early 1990s. However, unlike the NHS, the introduction of quasi-markets within social care was from the start characterized by a 'mixed economy' of provision. This reflected a strong suspicion on the part of the (then) Conservative government about the role of local authorities as direct providers of welfare services (Means *et al*. 2002). Thus voluntary, for profit and non-profit organizations were involved from the start of the quasi-market in providing social care services and their role has grown exponentially in the subsequent fifteen years, particularly in England. The majority of both residential and home care services, whether funded by local authority adult social care departments or through private purchase, are now provided by voluntary or for-profit organizations.

Since the early 1990s, there has been a consistent decline in permanent admissions to residential care (nursing and care homes), as, indeed, would be expected from policies encouraging 'community'-based care. However, temporary or short-stay admissions have increased, either for 'intermediate care' (to support older people following early discharge from hospital) or as 'respite care' for people with high support needs, to give family carers a break. During the same period, there has been a marked decline in local authorities' own provision of residential care. By March 2006, almost three-quarters of residential care homes were owned by private sector providers and a further 19 per cent by voluntary sector organizations (all figures from CSCI 2006a). Private and voluntary sector operators therefore receive a very large proportion of the estimated £3 billion spent by local authorities in England on residential provision (Hirsch 2005), in addition to the resources spent by private purchasers of residential care. The residential care market has been subject to significant changes since the early 1990s as large, sometimes multi-national organizations have bought out smaller, family operators and as the former have themselves been subject to further buy-outs and take-overs. 'Residential care is now a commodity and . . . is there to be traded and exploited for its surplus value like any other commodity' (Scourfield 2007a: 162). The concentration of provision in the hands of a few large providers means that around 20 per cent of all older people in residential homes live in homes owned by the top ten biggest providers such as BUPA, Southern Cross, Four Seasons and Westminster Health Care – a trend exacerbated by the very large size of many nursing homes (although the speed of merger and take-over activity within the residential care market means that the precise identity of dominant provider groups undergoes frequent change).

These developments have had a number of consequences. They strengthen providers' power vis-à-vis local authority commissioners and government regulators; for example, in resisting compliance with potentially costly improvements in standards. They also compromise the rights and choices of users, who have dramatically reduced options to 'exit' from an unsatisfactory service (Marquand 2004); and they blur lines of accountability between service users and shareholders (Drakeford 2006).

The provision of home care services has similarly seen a major shift from in-house to private sector organizations; however, this shift is both more recent and more dramatic. In 1992 only two per cent of home care hours were delivered by independent sector providers; by 2005 this had mushroomed to more than 73 per cent (CSCI 2006b). Also in contrast to the residential care sector, most domiciliary care providers are relatively small: 'most of the industry still has the characteristics of a "cottage industry" dominated by small providers' (CSCI 2006b: 27). There is considerable turnover within this particular sector, with between one-fifth and a tenth of home care agencies being registered or deregistered each year.

Although the process of divesting local authorities of their roles as direct providers of social care was begun by pre-1997 Conservative administrations, it has continued unabated by successive Labour governments in an on-going ideological belief in the role of markets and competition in improving service quality and efficiency. Moreover, regulation and inspection – the new mode of 'state intervention in order to promote and protect the public interest' (Drakeford 2006: 940) has failed to live up to this promise – at the very least its application to the residential care market has been flawed.

As noted above, growing pressures on social care budgets have led to a marked concentration of publicly funded social care services on people with high levels of personal care needs; these pressures are clearly apparent in the changing patterns of home care. Between 1992 and 2005 the total number of households receiving local authority-funded home care services fell from over 500,000 to 354,500 – despite demographic trends and changes in the boundaries of NHS responsibilities, both of which were likely to increase overall demand. However, the average weekly hours of home care received by these households tripled during the same period, from 3.2 to 10.1 hours (CSCI 2006b). There is relatively little information on the use of home care services by people who purchase these services privately, but some reports suggest that private demand is increasing, a trend which would be consistent with both demographic trends and the tightening of eligibility criteria for local authority-funded home care (Wanless 2006; CSCI 2008).

Social care services are very labour intensive and staff costs represent a significant proportion of total costs. Yet, consistent with the continuing association of care with 'women's work', social care remains a low paid and low status employment sector, with considerable problems of recruitment, retention and career progression. Not surprisingly, given the structure of social care services outlined above, significant proportions of the total workforce are employed in the private and voluntary sectors, about which information is particularly scarce (Wanless 2006). Vacancy rates in the sector are high, both among social care professionals such as social workers and occupational therapists and among semi-skilled home carers and care assistants; together vacancy rates in social care are about twice as high as those in private and public sector businesses as a whole. With an increasingly tight labour market, the social care workforce may be increasingly sourced from immigrant labour (Wanless 2006).

Since 1998, local authorities have been able to offer cash payments ('direct payments') instead of services in kind to disabled and older adults (see Leece and Bornat 2006). Direct payments were introduced in response to demands by younger disabled people for greater choice and control over their support arrangements (Morris 2006). They are typically used to employ someone (not a close co-resident relative) as a personal assistant, who can provide flexible help at the time and in the manner preferred by the disabled/older employer. However, take-up of direct payments has been low, and highly variable between different groups of social care service users and individual local authorities (Fernández *et al.* 2007).

Despite this apparent lack of demand, and evidence of considerable organizational and cultural barriers within local authorities (Ellis 2007), social care has been a particular focus for new policy discourses of consumerism and personalization (Glendinning 2008). Further opportunities for social care users to exercise greater choice and control over their own support arrangements through the new concept of 'individual budgets' were announced in a report from the Cabinet Office Strategy Unit (2005) and a Green Paper on adult social care (DH 2005). Individual budgets were piloted in thirteen English local authorities between 2005 and 2007, with the expectation that this approach will be adopted by other local authorities as the means of enabling people to fashion their own, highly individual, social care support arrangements. Individual budgets aim to bring together, for any individual, resources from a number of different funding streams to which s/he is entitled. In addition to resources from adult social care services, other resources include equipment, home adaptations and support for employment. The aim of the pilots is that these resources are pooled and spent flexibly on whatever personal support (including payments to friends and relatives for help given), equipment and services will contribute to meeting individual needs and priorities (Glendinning *et al.* 2008).

To the extent that individual budgets are expected eventually to transform the landscape of social care, they suggest some significant new risks for older and disabled people. While user movements have played a major role in shaping new patterns of social care, particularly direct payments (Morris 2006), it is not clear that this involvement can successfully be extended to enjoining users as active participants in the construction, production and management of their own social care. Yet individual service users will increasingly be expected to take responsibility for managing their own services and achieving agreed outcomes, possibly supported by their families – the 'transformation of citizens into both managers and entrepreneurs' (Scourfield 2007b: 112). Such roles require easily accessible information, on-going support and a range of decision-making skills, none of which may be available to at least the more disadvantaged users of social care services. Other risks that may be transferred from local authorities to users include responsibility for managing finite public resources; responsibility for maximizing efficiency and effectiveness in the use of those resources; and risks arising from shortfalls in the supply of desired social care commodities, with the consequent danger 'that individuals will end up in competition with each other over limited resources, an obvious example being personal assistants, who are in scarce supply' (Scourfield 2007b: 120).

Social care and health services – a long and troubled relationship

This section of the chapter outlines the history of relationships between social care and NHS services, focusing particularly on recent measures to improve collaboration and partnership between the two sectors.

As noted above, a salient feature of the construction of the post-war welfare state was the division between NHS and local government responsibilities for 'health' and 'social' care respectively. However, both sectors soon experienced rapid increases in demand for services and this quickly led to arguments, particularly over their respective responsibilities for older people. Thus hospitals alleged that local authorities, unable to provide sufficient residential care places, were refusing to accommodate older people 'in need of care and attention', while local authorities complained of being pressurized to look after people with long-term health needs, but without a corresponding transfer of resources. The response of central government during the 1950s was to confirm that the responsibilities of social care services extended to a much wider group of older people than had been intended by the 1948 National Assistance Act (Means and Smith 1998; Lewis 2001).

Both health and welfare services underwent major reorganizations during the early 1970s, within the context of a relationship that was already troubled. Following the Seebohm Report (1968), local authorities' fragmented mental health, children's and older people's welfare services were brought together in 1971 into integrated social services departments. Three years later another major reorganization transferred a large number of community health services – including health visiting, school health, vaccination and immunization, family planning, chiropody, home midwifery, health education and ambulance services – to the NHS. Although this latter reorganization was intended to improve the integration of local health services, it also deepened the division between health and social care services – and between health services and other local authority services that contribute to health and well-being. For example, opportunities for social workers to work closely with community nursing and other health professionals were reduced, while the public health responsibilities of local authorities were reduced by the transfer of the role of medical officer of health to the NHS (Glendinning *et al.* 2005).

As policies of deinstitutionalization ('community care') developed during the 1980s, difficulties over the respective responsibilities of each sector continued, culminating in a highly critical Audit Commission (1986) report and the subsequent recommendation by Sir Roy Griffiths (1988) of a clear lead role for local authority social services in the planning and delivery of social care. This recommendation was enacted in the 1990 NHS and Community Care Act and eventually implemented in 1993 – a move that is argued to have provided the NHS with yet another opportunity to withdraw from the provision of long-term care (Glendinning *et al.* 2005).

The history of relationships between health and social care services up to the late 1970s can therefore be summarized as a series of attempts to delineate the boundaries between, and respective responsibilities of, each sector. However, these attempts were repeatedly thwarted by demographic changes (particularly the growing numbers of people needing complex, long-term health and social care support) and, especially from 1976 onwards, by severe budgetary constraints that increased pressures to shift demand and costs to the other sector.

On top of these difficulties, from the early 1980s onwards strong quasi-market features were introduced into the organization of, first social and then health care (see Le Grand and Bartlett 1993). Quasi-markets created additional problems. It might be assumed that collaboration is a prerequisite for the effective joint planning and delivery of services between health and social care sectors. In contrast, effective quasi-markets involve a number of mechanisms that are profoundly inimical to collaboration (Wistow and Hardy 1996). They rely on incentives for purchasers to maximize their market shares and cost-shunt responsibilities; and on competition between providers for the business of purchasers. Moreover, the use of contracts as the dominant co-ordinating mechanism within quasi-markets involves clear specifications of service responsibilities and remits, thus further sharpening organizational and service boundaries and creating and legitimizing concepts of the 'core businesses' of health and social care. Market-based welfare also requires more explicit regulation and performance management mechanisms (Clarke *et al.* 2000). Thus inspection, accounting, regulation and performance management regimes were strengthened within each sector, but working to different agendas and priorities (Newman 2001).

This was the challenge facing the Labour government in 1997. Early ministerial references to dismantling the 'Berlin Wall' and ending the 'border patrols' between health and social care were quickly followed with a commitment to partnerships as the means of overcoming these barriers.

A plethora of measures to promote, incentivize and facilitate closer collaboration was introduced; 'partnership, co-operation and collaboration were emphasized and mandated at every turn' (Paton 1999: 69). Measures included statutory obligations on NHS organizations and local authorities to work in partnership; 'ring-fenced' central government funding from 1998 to 2001 to enable local authority social services departments to develop services in collaboration with NHS partners; joint planning objectives; national service frameworks that set benchmarks across the two sectors; and partnership 'flexibilities' – the relaxation of legal barriers to closer organizational collaboration (see Glendinning *et al.* 2005, for further details of these various measures).

The vigour with which collaboration between NHS and social care services was promoted, particularly during Labour's first two terms of office, was unprecedented. Rather than collaboration being a marginal activity, Labour established a clear strategic framework for the delivery of services that encouraged (and from time to time required) collaboration between health and social care services (Sullivan and Skelcher 2002). Moreover, these measures contained the potential for deepening partnerships along a continuum (Hudson *et al.* 1999) from isolation, through encounter, communication and collaboration to full organizational integration in the form of Care Trusts (Glasby and Peck 2004).

The encouragement, exhortations and resources that have been directed since 1997 to reducing problems at the interface between NHS and social care services have been significant. There have undoubtedly been many new developments resulting from these collaborative imperatives, particularly in relation to services for older people and people with severe mental health problems and in relation to the high profile policy area of admissions to and discharges from acute hospital care. For example, intermediate care services to support early hospital discharge have been established in most English localities, often jointly commissioned and funded by NHS and local authority partners and employing a range of therapist and care staff (University of Leeds 2005). Moreover, collaboration and partnership are now mainstream rather than marginal activities, particularly for senior managers in both sectors. However, two rather more cautious conclusions also need to be drawn. First, the promotion of health and social care partnerships since 1997 has utilized mainly structural, organizational and funding levers. Far less policy attention has been paid to the professional socialization and operational routines that both shape and constrain the behaviours of front-line professionals and practitioners. Different professional groups have different ideologies, culture, values and views about the interests of service users. Moreover, these differences are legitimated by external professional bodies and internal management practices alike. For example, Miller and Freeman (2003) examined the impact of central government policy priorities, translated into management practices, on the operation of multi-professional teams working in health and social care. They concluded that: 'Interpersonal relationships were undermined by power structures and differences in beliefs about team working and were challenged further where professionals' roles needed to be reconstructed in the light of new policy' (Miller and Freeman 2003: 123–4).

Yet it is changes in the activities of front-line practitioners that are likely to impact most on the experiences of health and social care service users. An overview of a series of studies on the 'modernization' of adult social care found repeated emphasis on the need for training and development; communication and leadership; champions to lead change management processes; and the development of networks to support cross-boundary working (Newman *et al.* 2008). The focus on organizational solutions to problems at the health–social care interface and the failure to address their human resource dimensions have been termed the 'Achilles heel' of partnerships (Hudson 2002).

Second, despite a plethora of advice on how to make partnerships work (Ling 2000), evidence of their 'success' is mixed (El Ansari *et al.* 2001). One review of evidence on partnerships between health and social care in England since 1997 distinguished between the processes of partnership working and their outcomes – the benefits in terms of improved services or better experiences for users (Dowling *et al.* 2004). Many studies have demonstrated 'success' in relation to partnership processes, including the creation of trust, reciprocity and respect; agreement about purpose and aims; and satisfactory audit, accountability and leadership arrangements. However, there is far less evidence on the impact of partnerships – improvements in the accessibility, equity and efficiency of services; in user and carer experiences; or in health status and quality of life. Even where research has attempted to assess the outcomes of partnership, the causal relationships involved are often far from conclusive; it is therefore not clear whether or in what ways 'successful' partnership processes might contribute to 'successful' partnership outcomes at the levels of service users, although other valuable but less instrumental outcomes may often be generated (Boydell *et al.* 2008).

Conclusions

This chapter has tried to capture the complexity of social care. Institutionally based definitions are far from adequate, not least because of the complexity of the concept of 'care' and its embeddedness within private, familial and often intimate relationships. Indeed, Scandinavian sociologists have argued that the 'rationality of caring' is entirely incompatible with the economic and managerialist logics underpinning the modernization of formal social care services (Wærness 2006). Moreover, the boundaries of publicly funded and formally organized social care services have moved significantly over the past half century. Thus social care services now include a substantial number of activities that were formerly the responsibility of the NHS, including long-term support for older people, people with mental health problems and people with learning disabilities, all of whom were likely to have been accommodated in long-stay hospitals some fifty years ago. Social care services also no longer include many of the activities, and cover fewer of the people, than they previously did. Domestic help, help with other practical activities and support to engage with activities outside the home are now rarely provided through publicly funded social care services, particularly for older people. Moreover, the volume of social care provided by close family members, on a largely unpaid basis, overwhelms that provided by local authority social care services, while further major amounts of social care services are purchased privately by older and disabled people or their families.

Given the extensive spread of social care across private and public domains, between families and formal services, and involving public, private and voluntary providers, the specific interface between social care and health is a relatively small part of the overall picture. However, it is a part that has been extensively researched and subject to repeated policy interventions, with only limited evidence of success in improving the accessibility, equity, responsiveness or efficiency of services or the outcomes for service users.

Policies for both health and social care have increasingly taken a consumerist approach (Clarke *et al.* 2007; Needham 2007; Newman *et al.* 2008), emphasizing the importance of individual choice as the key organizing concept in public service reform. Within social care, this has taken the form of arguments for self-directed services:

> which allocate people budgets so that they can shape, with the advice of professionals, the support and services they need. This participative approach delivers highly personalized, lasting solutions to people's needs for social care . . . at lower cost than traditional, inflexible and top-down approaches.
>
> (Leadbeater *et al.* 2008: 9)

Underpinning this rhetoric lies a continuing belief in the role of competition within social care markets to generate increases in efficiency and quality (Glendinning 2008). However, so far the introduction of greater choice has taken different forms in social care and health services. In the former, direct payments and individual budgets devolve resources and purchasing power to individual service users; in the latter, command over resources remains largely in the hands of professionals, particularly general practitioners. There is already evidence of problems at the boundaries, with people receiving direct payments experiencing restrictions on their use to purchase health-related services, despite the fact that both 'health' and 'social' tasks are embraced within users' overarching conceptualizations of personal care (Glendinning *et al.* 2000). Even though there are suggestions that direct payments could be extended to health care (Le Grand 2007), it is not unreasonable to assume that professional assessments and advice over the use of those payments may continue to play a major role. It is therefore far from clear that, once commodified, users will wish, or be able to, play similar roles in relation to the purchase of their health and their social care services.

One of the arguments for greater consumer choice is that this places pressure on providers to increase their responsiveness. However, there is so far little evidence of this effect. Since the early 1990s the 'mixed economy' market of social care has been shaped by the activities of local authority purchasers, who have been able to exert considerable leverage over prices and quality through their 'bulk' purchasing role. Individual purchasers, with far less purchasing power, are unlikely to be able to exercise the same leverage and secure appropriate and desired responses from providers (Glendinning 2008). It will be important to examine the impact of extended individualized purchasing in social care before similar measures are introduced into the NHS. It will also be vitally important to examine the implications and impact of consumer choice on the close kin and friends who currently – and will continue to – provide the greatest proportion of social care.

Notes

1 Since devolution, the governments of England, Scotland, Northern Ireland and Wales have been responsible for policies for disabled and older people and carers. Additional variations exist between local authorities within each country.
2 Social care for children is the responsibility of integrated children's departments at local level and the Department for Children, Schools and Families at government level.

References

Arber, S. and Gilbert, N. (1989) 'Men: the forgotten carers', *Sociology*, 23: 111–18.
Arber, S. and Ginn, J. (1999) 'Gender differences in informal caring', in G. Allen (ed.) *The Sociology of the Family: a reader*, Oxford: Blackwell.
Arksey, H. and Glendinning, C. (2007a) 'Choice in the context of informal care-giving', *Health and Social Care in the Community*, 16: 165–75.
Arksey, H. and Glendinning, C. (2007b) ' Informal welfare', in M. Powell (ed.), *Understanding the Mixed Economy of Welfare*, Bristol: Policy Press.
Arksey, H., Kemp, P., Glendinning, C., Kotchetkova, I. and Tozer, R. (2005) *'Carers' Aspirations and Decisions around Work and Retirement'*, Research Report 290, London: Department for Work and Pensions.
Audit Commission (1986) *Making a Reality of Community Care*, London: Audit Commission.
Beckett, C. (2007) 'Women, disability and care; good neighbours or uneasy bedfellows?' *Critical Social Policy*, 27: 360–80.
Boydell, L., Hoggett, P., Rugösa, J. and Cummins, A.M. (2008) 'Intersectoral partnerships, the knowledge economy and intangible assets', *Policy and Politics*, 36: 209–24.
Buckner, L. and Yeandle, S. (2006) *Who Cares Wins*, London: Carers UK.

Cabinet Office (2005) *Improving the Life Chances of Disabled People*, London: Cabinet Office Strategy Unit.

Carers UK (2007) 'Carers save UK £87 billion per year', September. Online: www.carersuk.org/Newsandcampaigns/News/1190237139 (accessed 5 February 2008).

Clark, H., Dyer, S. and Horwood, J. (1998) *'That Bit of Help'. The High Value of Low Level Preventive Services for Older People*, Bristol: The Policy Press.

Clarke, J., Gewirtz, S., Hughes, G. and Humphrey, J. (2000) 'Guarding the public interest? The rise of audit and inspection', in J. Clarke, S. Gewirtz and E. McLaughlin (eds), *New Managerialism, New Welfare?* London: Sage.

Clarke, J., Newman, J., Smith, N., Vidler, E. and Westmarland, L. (2007) *Creating Citizen-Consumers. Changing publics and changing public services*, London: Sage Publications.

CSCI (2006a) *The State of Social Care in England, 2005–06*, London: Commission for Social Care Inspection.

CSCI (2006b) *Time to Care?* London: Commission for Social Care Inspection.

CSCI (2008) *The State of Social Care in England, 2006–07*, London: Commission for Social Care Inspection.

Daly, M. (2002) 'Care as a good for social policy', *Journal of Social Policy*, 31: 251–70.

Daly, M. and Lewis, J. (2000) 'The concept of social care and the analysis of contemporary welfare states', *British Journal of Sociology*, 51: 281–89.

Dalley, G. (1988) *Ideologies of Caring. Rethinking community and collectivism*, London: Macmillan.

Da Roit, B., Le Bihan, B. and Österle, A. (2007) 'Long-term care policies in Italy, Austria and France', *Social Policy and Administration*, 41: 653–71.

DH (2005) *Independence, Well-being and Choice. Our vision for the future of adult social care in England*, London: Department of Health.

Dowling, B., Powell, M. and Glendinning, C. (2004) 'Conceptualising successful partnerships', *Health and Social Care in the Community*, 12: 309–17.

Drakeford, M. (2006) 'Ownership, regulation and the public interest: the case of residential care for older people', *Critical Social Policy*, 26: 932–44.

El Ansari, W., Phillips, C. and Hammick, M. (2001) 'Collaboration and partnerships: developing the evidence base', *Health and Social Care in the Community*, 9: 215–27.

Ellis, K. (2007) 'Direct payments and social work practice; the significance of "street-level bureaucracy" in determining eligibility', *British Journal of Social Work*, 37: 405–22.

Fernández, J-L., Kendall, J., Davey, V. and Knapp, M. (2007) 'Direct payments in England: factors linked to variations in local provision', *Journal of Social Policy*, 36: 97–121.

Finch, J. and Groves, D. (1980) 'Community care and the family: a case for equal opportunities?' *Journal of Social Policy*, 9: 487–514.

Finch, J. and Groves, D. (eds) (1983) *A Labour of Love. Women, work and caring*, London: Routledge.

Finch, J. and Mason, J. (1993) *Negotiating Family Responsibilities*, London: Routledge.

Fine, M.D. (2007) *A Caring Society? Care and the dilemmas of human service in the 21st Century*, Basingstoke: Palgrave Macmillan.

Fine, M. and Glendinning, C. (2005) 'Dependence, independence or inter-dependence? Revisiting the concepts of 'care' and 'dependency', *Ageing and Society*, 25: 602–21.

Folbre, N. (2004) 'Questioning care economics', in K. Wærness (ed.) *Dialogue on Care*, volume 16, Bergen: Centre for Women's and Gender Research, pp. 11–14.

Gilligan, C. (1982) *In a Different Voice*, Cambridge, MA: Harvard University Press.

Glasby, J. and Littlechild, R. (2004) *The Health and Social Care Divide: The experiences of older people;* revised second edition, Bristol: The Policy Press.

Glasby, J. and Peck, E. (eds) (2004) *Care Trusts: Partnership working in action*, Oxford: Radcliffe Medical Press.

Glendinning, C. (2008) 'Increasing choice and control for older and disabled people: a critical review of new developments in England', *Social Policy and Administration*, 42: 451–69.

Glendinning, C., Halliwell, S., Jacobs, S., Rummery, K. and Tyrer J. (2000) *Buying Independence. Using direct payments to integrate health and social services*, Bristol: The Policy Press.

Glendinning, C., Hudson, B. and Means, R. (2005) 'Under strain? Exploring the troubled relationship between health and social care', *Public Money and Management*, 25: 245–52.

Glendinning, C. and Kemp, P.A. (eds) (2006) *Cash and Care: policy challenges in the welfare state*, Bristol: The Policy Press.

Glendinning, C. and Lloyd, B. (1998) 'The implications of the continuing care guidelines for primary and community health services', *Health and Social Care in the Community*, 6: 181–6.

Glendinning, C. and Means, R. (2004) 'Rearranging the deckchairs on the Titanic of long-term care – is organizational integration the answer?' *Critical Social Policy*, 24: 435–57.

Glendinning, C., Challis, D., Fernández, J.L., Jacobs, S., Jones, K., Knapp, M., Manthorpe, J., Moran, N., Netten, A., Stevens, M. and Wilberforce, M. (2008) *Evaluation of the Individual and Budget Pilot Programme: Final Report*, York: University of York, Social Policy Research Unit.

Graham, H. (1983) 'Caring: a labour of love', in J. Finch and D. Groves (eds) *A Labour of Love. Women, work and caring*, London: Routledge.

Griffiths, R. (1988) *Community Care: an agenda for action*, London: HMSO.

Heitmueller, A. and Inglis, K. (2007) 'The earnings of informal carers: wage differentials and opportunity costs', *Journal of Health Economics*, 26: 821–41.

Hirsch, D. (2005) *Facing the Cost of Long-Term Care*, York: Joseph Rowntree Foundation.

Hochschild, A. (1983) *The Managed Heart: commercialisation of human feeling*, Berkley: University of California Press.

Hudson, B. (2002) 'Interprofessionality in health and social care: the Achilles' heel of partnership?', *Journal of Interprofessional Care*, 16: 7–17.

Hudson, B., Hardy, B., Henwood, M. and Wistow, G. (1999) 'In pursuit of inter-agency collaboration in the public sector', *Public Management*, 1: 235–60.

Kittay, E.F. (1999) *Love's Labour: Essays on women, equality and dependency*, New York: Routledge.

Land, H. (1978) 'Who cares for the family?' *Journal of Social Policy*, 7: 357–84.

Leadbeater, C., Bartlett, J. and Gallagher, N. (2008) *Making it Personal*, London: Demos.

Leece, J. and Bornat, J. (2006) *Developments in Direct Payments*, Bristol: The Policy Press

Le Grand, J. (2007) *The Other Invisible Hand. Delivering public services through choice and competition*, New Jersey: Princeton University Press.

Le Grand, J. and Bartlett, W. (eds) (1993) *Quasi-Markets and Social Policy*, Basingstoke: Macmillan.

Lewis, J. (2001) 'Social services departments and the health/social care boundary; half a century of hidden policy conflict', *Social Policy and Administration*, 35: 343–59.

Lewis, J. and Meredith, B. (1988) *Daughters who Care*, London: Routledge.

Ling, T. (2000) 'Unpacking partnership: the case of healthcare', in J. Clarke, S. Gewirtz and E. McLaughlin (eds) *New Managerialism, New Welfare?* London: Sage.

Marquand, D. (2004) *Decline of the Public*, Cambridge: Policy Press.

Means, R. and Smith, R. (1998) *From Poor Law to Community Care: The development of welfare services for elderly people*, Bristol: The Policy Press.

Means, R., Morbey, H. and Smith, R. (2002) *From Community Care to Market Care?* Bristol: Policy Press.

Miller, C. and Freeman, M. (2003) 'Clinical teamwork: the impact of policy on collaborative practice', in A. Leathard (ed.) *Interprofessional Collaboration; from policy to practice in health and social care*, Hove: Brunner-Routledge.

Morris, J. (1991) *Pride against Prejudice*, London: Women's Press.

Morris, J. (1993) *Independent Lives: community care and disabled people*, Basingstoke: Macmillan.

Morris, J. (2006) 'Independent living: the role of the disability movement in the development of government policy', in C. Glendinning and P.A. Kemp (eds) *Cash and Care: Policy challenges in the welfare state*, Bristol: The Policy Press.

Needham, C. (2007) *The Reform of Public Services under New Labour. Narratives of consumerism*, Basingstoke: Palgrave Macmillan.

Newman, J. (2001) *Modernizing Governance: New Labour, policy and society*, London: Sage.

Newman, J., Glendinning, C. and Hughes, M. (2008) 'Beyond modernisation? Social care and the transformation of welfare governance', *Journal of Social Policy*, 37: 531–58.

Paton, C. (1999) 'New Labour's health policy: the new healthcare state', in M. Powell, (ed.) *New Labour, New Welfare State? The third way in British social policy*, Bristol: The Policy Press.

Robinson, J. (2001) 'Long-term care in the twenty-first century', in J. Robinson (ed.), *Towards A New Social Compact for Care in Old Age*, London: Kings Fund.

Scourfield, P. (2007a) 'Are there reasons to be worried about the "cartelization" of residential care?' *Critical Social Policy*, 27: 155–80.

Scourfield, P. (2007b) 'Social care and the modern citizen: client, consumer, service users, manager and entrepreneur', *British Journal of Social Work*, 37: 107–22.

Seebohm Report (1968) *Report of the Committee on Local Authority and Allied Personal Social Services*, Cmnd 3703, London: HMSO.

Sevenhuijsen, S. (2000) 'Caring in the Third Way: the relation between obligation, responsibility and care in Third Way discourse', *Critical Social Policy*, 20: 5–37.

Shakespeare, T. (2000a) 'The social relations of care', in G. Lewis, S. Gewirtz and J. Clarke (eds) *Rehinking Social Policy*, London: Sage.

Shakespeare, T. (2000b) *Help*, Birmingham: Venture Press.

Swain, J., Finkelstein, V., French, S. and Oliver, M. (1993) *Disabling Barriers, Enabling Environments*, London: Sage.

Sullivan, H. and Skelcher, C. (2002) *Working across Boundaries*, Basingstoke: Palgrave.

Tronto, J. (1993) *Moral Boundaries. A political argument for an ethic of care*, London: Routledge.

Twigg, J. (2000) *Bathing. The body and community care*, London: Routledge.

University of Leeds (2005) *An Evaluation of Intermediate Care for Older People: Final Report*: Institute of Health Sciences and Public Health Research, University of Leeds.

Wanless, D. (2006) *Securing Good Care for Older People: Taking the long-term view*, London: Kings Fund.

Wærness, K. (2006) 'Research on care: what impact on policy and planning?' in C. Glendinning and P.A. Kemp (eds) *Cash and Care: Policy challenges in the welfare state*, Bristol: Policy Press.

West, R. (2002) 'The right to care', in E.F. Kittay and E.K. Feder (eds) *The Subject of Care: Feminist perspectives on dependency*, Lanham, MD: Rowman and Littlefield Publishers Inc.

Wistow, G. and Hardy, B. (1996) 'Competition, collaboration and markets', *Journal of Interprofessional Care*, 10: 5–10.

11 Equalizing the people's health
A sociological perspective

Jennie Popay and Gareth Williams

We have no doubt that greater equality of health must remain one of our foremost national objectives and that in the last two decades of the twentieth century *a new attack upon the forces of inequality has regrettably become necessary and now needs to be concerted.*
(From the introduction to the original *'Black Report'*, Department of Health and Social Security, 1980: 1; emphasis added)

Introduction

Anthony Giddens, a sociologist perhaps best known as the 'Third Way' adviser to the 'New Labour' government that came to power in the UK in 1997, has argued that *dynamism* is the defining characteristic of late modern societies (Giddens 1991). Notwithstanding the frequent portrayal of this dynamism as broadly positive in its impact, deep and widening inequalities in life circumstances persist: globally, nationally, regionally and locally. Indeed, some people argue that inequality is an inherent feature of a dynamism which serves a global 'oligarchy of the rich' (Gray 2003: 162) populated by 'greedy bastards' (Scambler 2002). In this chapter we move away from the sociology of health care and health professionals to explore the relationship between society and population health, and policy and practice related to this. With the unequivocal words of Sir Douglas Black ringing in our ears, we aim to develop a sociological perspective on the health dimensions of these inequalities, that is, a perspective that emphasizes the relationships between social structure and experiences of health inequalities in everyday life. For reasons of space, we focus particularly on class and income inequalities, and leave the very important issues of gender and ethnicity to one side. We then go on to explore the ways in which our understanding of inequalities influences public health policy and practice – the domain of public policy whose role it is to address health inequalities.

The chapter develops through three stages. First, we explore the dominant paradigmatic 'ways of knowing' and explaining health inequalities and how these have changed over time. We consider in particular social epidemiological approaches, focusing on the life-course and on psycho-social pathways to ill health and on the relationship between people and places. While social epidemiology since Black has made a major contribution to our knowledge of health inequalities, it has sometimes excluded alternative, more fully sociological ways of approaching these issues; though in recent years a more explicitly Durkheimian frame of reference has helped to enliven some social epidemiology. Second, therefore, we briefly consider two less visible paradigms for research on health inequalities: neo-Marxist analyses of the political economy of social and health inequalities which have a global scope; and interpretivist analyses providing a micro gaze on how ordinary people make sense of and deal with the impact of inequalities in their everyday lives. Taken together these two sociological approaches form a powerful critique of the myopias evident in dominant ways of knowing about health inequalities and provide the foundation for a more integrative approach to knowledge. Finally, we look at how the domains of public health policy and practice have responded to the challenge of reducing health inequalities, considering in particular the influence of the causal explanations and whether devolution has triggered new, locally situated ways of framing and acting to reduce health inequalities.

Explaining health inequalities

For more than a hundred years the experience of mortality and morbidity has been consistently worse in lower than in higher socio-economic groups: a global phenomenon found both within and between all countries (Davey Smith *et al.* 2001). The evidence for this has been thoroughly reviewed, and for that reason we do not spend time on it here (Bartley 2004; Siegrist and Marmot 2006; Graham 2007). Defining health inequalities has become a complex scientific enterprise. As Graham (2004) has shown, health inequalities are defined in three different ways in policy and academic work: as the health status of a group defined as 'poor'; as the 'health gap' between a group defined as 'poor' and another group, such as the richest 10 per cent, or the average for the population as a whole; or as the gradient in mortality or morbidity tracked across all socio-economic positions in an entire population. In the UK all three approaches can be identified in work on health inequalities spanning at least 150 years (Davey Smith *et al.* 2001). Yet, in spite of all the analysis and argument, social and spatial inequalities in health defined in terms of a gap or gradient are significant and are now greater than they have been since records have been kept; and notwithstanding high-profile policy initiatives, the evidence suggests that: 'Under the first 10 years of the New Labour government, inequalities in mortality rose relentlessly' (Dorling *et al.* 2007: 42).

In the UK Black Report on health inequalities – commissioned by a Labour government and born and buried in 1980 by the new Conservative administration – social class was still the core analytical unit of social stratification. The cross-sectional nature of the data on which the analysis was based opened it up to criticism, but what was important about the Black Report was not the robustness of the data but the attempt to 'test' four possible 'theoretical explanations' of social inequalities in health: artefact explanations, natural or social selection, materialist, and cultural-behavioural. The Black committee came down firmly in favour of materialist explanations: improvements in health overall were argued to be as a result of improved material living standards whilst inequalities in health were argued to be caused by inequalities in access to socially acceptable standards of living: to incomes that allowed people to live decent lives, to have good quality homes, to engage in social interaction, to access and use education and health care, and so on. Only materialist explanations, Black and his colleagues argued, could simultaneously account for the improvements in the general health of the population and the persistence of social class differences in health.

Both social selection and artefact explanations have been largely discredited since 1980, although there remains some debate over the relative contribution of these to the interpretation of the social class gradient in health (Carr-Hill and Chalmers-Dixon 2008). Moreover, while some have found the lure of a relatively simple behavioural approach to understanding health inequalities difficult to resist, 'risk factor' epidemiology, which crudely seeks associations between premature mortality, social position and unhealthy behaviours, has lost its force as a major explanatory framework (Steptoe 2006). For example, whilst there is clear evidence that smoking is a risk factor for early death, neither smoking nor other individual risks such as cholesterol or blood pressure adequately explain socio-economic differences in mortality (Shaw *et al.* 1999). In contrast, there has been a growing body of work supporting 'materialist' explanations since the Black Report was published (Whitehead 1987; Department of Health 1998a; Shaw *et al.* 1999; Bartley 2004). Notwithstanding the *prima facie* plausibility of cultural and behavioural factors, this work has shown that the key to explaining differences in both 'risky' behaviours and health outcomes lies with a better understanding of the influence of material and 'neo-material' factors (Bartley 2004).

While materialism remains the epistemological frame of reference for many, the meaning of 'materialism' is far from settled within health inequalities research. The Black Report's approach to materialism, shared by more recent commentators, explicitly encompassed an individual's 'socio-economic position' alongside 'other dimensions of social class': the social structure within which people live in industrial–capitalist societies, including the 'security and stability' provided in a mature social democracy with a welfare state (see Chung and Muntaner 2006, 2008; Graham 2007; and Mackenbach and Bakker, 2002 for recent commentaries on this issue). In addition, Black's materialist explanation included personal experiences associated with 'material security and advantage' such as 'self fulfilment and job satisfaction'. In other words, the Black Report contained within it a sharp macro-sociological critique of neo-liberalism and a clear micro-sociological recognition that there were important subjective dimensions to any fully rounded materialist analysis. Since Black, the word 'materialist' has often been interpreted in narrower ways, to include only physical material things (Siegrist and Marmot 2006). Although it has been argued that a softer version of this approach to explaining health inequalities can include the psychosocial (Macintyre 1997), this remains contested (Lynch *et al.* 2000). In more recent years there have been advances in three key areas of research on the causes of health inequalities.

Life-course effects

The availability of longitudinal data from birth cohorts in particular and linked analytical developments has enabled research into the complex interactions between individuals' health experiences and their environments – from the womb to the tomb (Kuh and Ben-Shlomo 2004; Power and Kuh 2006). The particular strengths of this approach are in introducing a crucial temporal element into explanations and allowing careful forensic work on causal pathways for different diseases and health problems. This allows social epidemiologists to demonstrate that different aspects of 'people's social biographies matter for their health' (Graham 2007: 145). In epidemiology, what this means is that we can view people's lives in a 'socio-economic life course': 'the journey from the socio-economic environment of the natal family (usually indexed by father's occupation) to adulthood (own occupation)' (Graham 2007: 145). As Blane vividly describes it, the life-course approach:

> sees a person's biological status as a marker of their past social position and, through the structured nature of social processes, as liable to selective accumulation of future advantage or disadvantage.
>
> (Blane 1999: 64)

There are, as Graham (2007: 145) stresses, 'formidable methodological challenges' for epidemiology in relating these journeys to specific health risks and health outcomes. However, the evidence indicates a strong correlation between sustained hardship and poor health which it would be difficult to see as anything other than the cumulative impact of social processes on health outcomes, well into adult life. At an individual level, for example, the cross-generational and cumulative effects of poverty and disadvantage have been shown in the effects of maternal malnourishment and low birth-weight over time (Power and Kuh 2006) which is in turn correlated with poor health in adult life (Kuh *et al.* 2004). This burgeoning body of work is demonstrating that in a powerful sense 'history is what you live' (Williams 2006). There is much more to be done, but what is required is not only more and better life-course epidemiology, but also an 'historical materialist' sociology which re-connects the now highly sophisticated but reductive, nominalist work of epidemiologists – research that reduces knowledge to measurable, supposedly concreted entities – to a broader interpretation of the generative mechanisms of social structures and historical processes (Williams 2003).

The importance of place

While the perspective of the life course reminds us of the importance of time and history, the clustering of advantages and disadvantages at particular points in specific localities indicates the significance of place and geography. There has been a long interest within what used to be called medical geography in the spatial patterns of disease, but more sociological work within geography has increasingly used aggregate, asset-based data, such as housing tenure and car ownership on individuals to develop area-based deprivation measures and explore the link between these measures and health outcomes (Macintyre *et al.* 2002). However, most of this work is 'compositional', looking at the relationship between health experiences and the characteristics of individuals living within certain boundaries rather than on the characteristics of the places themselves. In much of this work, location remains: 'the canvas on which events happen, but the nature of the locality and its role in structuring health status and health-related behaviour is neglected' (Jones and Moon 1993: 515).

The proposition that ' . . . the characteristics of places may be as important as the characteristics of people for an understanding of particular patterns of health' (Phillimore 1993), remains very difficult to test, notwithstanding the rapid developments in geographical data-handling technology and associated techniques of multi-level modelling (Pickett and Pearl 2001; Smyth 2008). In addition to the complexities already referred to, there is the problem of health-related migration which leaves concentrations of poor people with poor health in poor neighbourhoods (Brimblecombe *et al.* 2000; Norman *et al.* 2005).

In spite of the difficulties, there is evidence that some areas (former coal-mining and port communities, for example), have higher rates of ill-health than other areas with equally disadvantaged residents with similar ways of life (Joshi *et al.* 2001). However, more importantly from our point of view, it may be that the rather rigid epidemiological framing of place excludes precisely those place-based qualities which have an impact on health. Places need to be conceptualized in much 'thicker' and richer ways, and this approach to place has been invigorated by the extraordinary rise and expansion of the concept of 'social capital' and the rediscovery of Durkheimian ideas about the importance of 'social cohesion' to health over the last ten to fifteen years (Kawachi and Kennedy 1997; Kennedy *et al.* 1999; Fone *et al.* 2007).

It is probably true to say that the concept of social capital has increasingly been asked to bear too great a weight as an explanation for population level health and health inequalities (Muntaner *et al.* 2008). Nonetheless, the concept has helped to foreground the idea that the connections between an unequal society and unequal risks of poor health pass through more than empty space. Spaces are places that contextualize the impact of 'material' circumstances (Frohlich *et al.* 2001, 2002; Williams 2003) and class differences (Stephens 2008); context needs to include attention to the normative dimensions of place, what a 'proper place' ought to be (Popay *et al.* 2003), as well as the opportunity structures and material features of the 'landscape' (Curtis and Rees Jones 1998) and threats, hassles and hazards such as crime, vandalism and dog dirt (Gatrell *et al.* 2001; Popay *et al.* 2003; Macintyre *et al.* 2002; Sooman and Macintyre 1995). In other words, context includes not only the networks, relationships and give-and-take of Putnamesque social capital but also the unequal economics of everyday life.

This 'thickening' of notions of context opens up the possibility of incorporating into explanations for health inequalities an understanding of the impact of the socio-economic history of places alongside biographical time (Mallinson *et al.* 2003). Whilst such research is under-developed, the cumulative effects of economic disinvestments and social decline over generations, as well as the characteristics of individuals, can be expected to be important parts of a fuller sociological understanding of the dramatic area variations in mortality and morbidity that research is highlighting (Joshi *et al.* 2001; Phillimore 1993; Shaw *et al.* 1999; Williams 2006).

Psychosocial processes

The third important development takes this argument forward by exploring how relative poverty or relative social position in an affluent society or population has the impact it does on differences in mortality and life expectancy. Richard Wilkinson (1996, 2005), one of the leaders of this exploration, argues that while simple materialist approaches can explain some of the health gap between the poorest groups and the rest of the population in affluent societies, they cannot explain all of it; and they cannot explain health gradients across whole societies in which most of the population are not seriously disadvantaged (Williams, S. *et al.* 2007). From this perspective, the main effect of living standards and social circumstances on health is not 'direct' but mediated by psychological responses to relative deprivation and relative social status and manifest in people's psychological responses to these: worry, stress, insecurity, lack of control and vulnerability (Wilkinson 1996, 1999a).

Wilkinson argues that the effect of material factors on health inequalities in relatively wealthy societies is 'indirect' – that it is not to do with poverty and deprivation:

The importance of income distribution implies that we must explain the effect of low income on health through its social meanings and implications for social position rather than through the direct physical effects which material circumstances might have independently of their social connotations in any particular society.

(Wilkinson 1996: 176)

Wilkinson argues that societies with more equitable distributions of income and wealth are more socially cohesive. This in turn means less stress and fewer negative emotions leading to better population health and narrowing health inequalities. In short, 'part of the association between low social status and poor health springs from the experience of low social status or subordination itself' (Wilkinson 2000: 999).

Other forms of understanding

These developments in research on health inequalities have opened up the possibility of new theoretically informed analyses of the relationships between individual lives and social structures, including 'materially informed' ways of thinking about the contribution of 'individual lifestyle' factors to health inequalities (Bartley 2004). Although primarily emanating from social epidemiology, the dominant research paradigm in the health inequalities field is increasingly characterized, as Wilkinson (2005) himself has recently argued, by more integrative approaches to explanation, bringing together insights from biology, psychology, geography, anthropology and sociology and taking account of time, space and history. However, much of the research described above is restricted by its focus on individual-level measures of socio-economic position.

The Black Report itself pointed to a number of ways in which the social sciences in general and sociology in particular, in contrast to social medicine or social epidemiology, might contribute to our understanding of health inequalities. 'Sociology', the Black Report argues:

> is concerned with the social production of understanding, meanings, knowledge; with social structure and process; and with the behaviour of people.
>
> (Townsend *et al.* 1988: 36–7)

With few exceptions, this sociological strand from the Black Report has remained unclaimed. Most social epidemiology has failed to develop an adequate (sociological and/or political) analysis of 'class' and its relationship to other social and material forces (Veenstra 2006). As a result, few social epidemiological studies have moved beyond 'the rather tame and tedious hunt for statistical associations' (Scambler 2002: 88) to postulate explanatory and interpretive theories through which a sociologically convincing 'causal narrative' can be developed (Prandy 1999). Concern over how to research and represent structure as something more than an aggregation of individuals, and agency as something more than individual behaviours, and then to make sense of the relationship between them is central to sociology in general and, increasingly, to medical sociology (Cockerham 2007). Such a sociology of population health would require much greater attention to political economy perspectives, exploring the generative determinants of socio-economic inequalities operating at a global level. It would also need to draw more deeply on the resources of sociology to theorize more adequately the relationship between social structures and individual agency. In this context, one of most significant problems with the dominant body of health inequalities research is that there is no attempt to consider the point of view of those who experience what Bourdieu *et al.* (1999) have referred to as 'the weight of the world'. Importantly, as we describe below, there are bodies of work that can help in the construction of a more adequate causal narrative but these are relatively invisible in debates about the evidence for health inequalities.

Materialism re-considered

Wilkinson's relationship to materialism remains ambiguous. As we have seen, in his early work, and particularly his first book, Wilkinson (1996) ties his growing interest in psychosocial processes to material circumstances, broadly defined to include both poverty or income deprivation and the pressures of hierarchy, whether in workplaces or in society as a whole. More recently he has appeared to distance himself from anything approaching a materialist analysis; and, when provoked (Muntaner and Lynch 1999), he appears to dismiss any notion that social class is a direct cause of health inequalities, accusing his critics of 'clinging to a misconceived materialism' (Wilkinson 1999b). This de-centring of materialist notions of social class as the key unit of social stratification linking public issues to personal troubles is part of a wider postmodern 'turn' in sociology which has seen two leading academics asking rhetorically: 'Is there any writer now more dated, more of a "dinosaur" than Marx?' (Lash and Urry 1994: 1). New materialists such as Muntaner and Lynch acknowledge the sociological approach of Wilkinson which leads away from oversimplified notions of individual behaviour and focuses on income inequality as something which frames relations between individuals. However, in laying to one side a fuller class analysis, it remains the case that mid-stream concepts such as social cohesion and social hierarchy can still lead to community-level victim blaming, and fall back on under-theorized 'culture of poverty' narratives.

Wilkinson is not alone in this reluctance to become engaged in Marxist dialectics. There is now a considerable programme of work on the relationship between socio-economic status and health (Bartley 2004; Graham 2007). However, the means of production, 'the means by which income, education and occupational prestige are accumulated in society have received relatively short shrift in the health literature' (Veenstra 2006: 111), and anything approaching '("hard") class theory, as opposed to ("soft") class analysis has all but disappeared from medical sociology' (Scambler 2002: 98). After all, who wants to be seen dancing with a dinosaur? The failure of the health inequalities literature to engage with more robust forms of Marxist theory is partly political: a vague sense that we are living through 'the end of history' (Fukyama 1992), and that anything beyond minor 'Third Way' modifications of neo-liberalism is impossible; and partly methodological: a positivist anxiety about contemplating 'the deeper relations of class that are "real", even if they are not directly observable, empirically speaking' (Williams, S. *et al.* 2007: 57).

However, Simon Williams *et al.* (2007: 57) argue that the work of Scambler and others represents 'a distinctly post-positivist position within the inequalities in health debate centred on a reinvigorated class agenda'. These explanatory approaches locate the causes of health inequalities in neo-liberal economic policies, the associated global adherence to free markets, unrestricted capital and labour movements and a restricted role for the state in welfare provision. Coburn (2000) argues that these changes have led to both greater inequalities in income and wealth and reduced social cohesion in many countries. For him, differences in population health and health inequalities between countries reflect the degree to which national governments have been willing and/or able to resist the imposition of these neo-liberal changes. These writers also alert us to the crucial influence of the oligarchy of the rich or the 'capitalist–executive class' as a key driver of inequalities (Scambler 2002). From this perspective explanations that place in the foreground psycho-social pathways are focusing downstream on the impact of these upstream global drivers of inequality.

The importance of a materialist approach, therefore, is twofold. It keeps the global influence of capital in the frame while also preventing the transformation of an analysis based on inequality into an analysis of the culture of poverty. It does this by focusing on the material qualities of neighbourhood or community, placing in the foreground issues such as levels of economic investment in local infrastructures, policy decisions about land-use patterns in post-industrial communities and housing need, and levels of citizen participation in the policy-making process (Duranceau and McCall 2007). Although this is sometimes presented as an analysis based on Marx, a properly articulated Durkheimian analysis of social inequality would be equally critical of the reduction of society to aggregations of individual feelings and behaviours. Social capital, in this sense, is not just a feeling of belonging, but a field of social struggle over the connections to economy, society, political power and cultural influence (Bourdieu 1993; Turner 2003; Stephens 2008).

Meaning and agency

The absence of class analysis from much epidemiological literature on health inequalities is matched by the failure of research in this area to engage with qualitative explorations of the everyday lives of the subjects of these inequalities. While much of the work we have described above is important because it reminds us of the 'indebtedness of agency to structure' (Scambler 2002: 95), it is also important to acknowledge the indebtedness of structure to agency: 'the social production of understanding, meanings and knowledge' (Townsend *et al.* 1988: 36).

We have explored the relationship between structure and agency through the concept of 'lay knowledge' elsewhere (Popay *et al.* 1998; Williams and Popay 2001). Our basic proposition is simple:

> Attention to the meanings people attach to their experience of places and how this shapes social action could provide a missing link in our understanding of the causes of inequalities in health. In particular, the articulation of these meanings – which we refer to as 'lay knowledge' – in narrative form could provide invaluable insights into the dynamic relationships between human agency and wider social structures that underpin inequalities in health.
>
> (Popay *et al.* 1998: 636)

The importance of understanding the world of the 'knowing subject' who develops understanding through 'knowledgeable narratives' (Williams 2000) about self, place and wider structures is clearly important if we are to understand the way in which inequalities 'work' in everyday life. Without this we reduce the people whose health is being unequally affected to unthinking bearers of various assets, deficits and risks.

All the explanatory approaches described above exclude the insights into causality and effective action for change that are provided by experiential or lay knowledge about health and inequalities. While Wilkinson's work moves towards 'social meanings', he makes no attempt to step outside the methodological frame of social epidemiology to think about how this might be done. While the social epidemiological approach to health inequalities will remain central, it is clearly the case that opportunities for developing our understanding require very different, additional (though not necessarily complementary) approaches: ones which explore people's own understandings of their situation. The emotional experiences described by Wilkinson as psychosocial processes linking structural inequality, societal breakdown and health inequalities – experiences of humiliation, rejection and disrespect, or what Sennett and Cobb (1973) referred to as the 'hidden injuries of class'– are experiences about which people themselves have points of view; and these points of view constitute bodies of knowledge which will inform the impact of these things upon them, and what action, if any, they feel able to take.

The work of Popay *et al.* (2003) demonstrated the complex ways in which people construct an understanding of health inequalities that acknowledges the differential impact of social and economic circumstances, but resists the moral judgements implied by ideas about failure to cope and unhealthy behaviours. As Simon Williams *et al.* (2007: 53) argue, lay knowledge provides 'a lived as well as a theoretical bridge between structure and agency, people and places, composition and context', opening a unique window on the 'duality of structure': the idea that social structures make social action possible and social action creates those very structures.

Lay knowledge, and the narrative forms in which it is expressed, provide a distinctive mode of what, in the context of Ancient Greek society, Aristotle referred to as 'practical wisdom' – the complex responsiveness to the concrete situations in which people find themselves. Discussing Aristotle's notion of practical wisdom the philosopher Martha Nussbaum argues that:

> Even more in our own time than in his, the power of 'scientific' pictures of practical rationality affects almost every area of human social life, through the influence of the social sciences and the more science-based parts of ethical theory on the formation of public policy. We should not accept this situation without assessing the merits of such views against those of the most profound alternatives.
>
> (Nussbaum 1990: 55)

The practical wisdom embedded in experiential or lay knowledge is a 'profound alternative' to the dominant scientific–technical rationality of epidemiological approaches to understanding health inequalities. One important aspect of this alternative way of 'knowing' is the emotion which lay knowledge may embody. Conventionally, emotion is seen as antithetical to rationality, whereas the Aristotelian view articulated by Nussbaum is that emotions and the imagination fed by them are central to a fuller and more grounded understanding of how knowledge of human predicaments is articulated. As Nussbaum puts it elsewhere, 'cognitive appraisals' are often emotional, but it is precisely the emotionality of lay responses to concrete situations of deprivation and exclusion that gives them 'a high degree of focussed attention to the world . . . there is no contradiction at all between analysing emotions as cognitive appraisals and insisting that they embody a sense of importance and urgency' (Nussbaum 2001: 108). Rather than bracketing these as residuals in the analysis of health inequalities, it would be more fully rational to include them as components in a 'passionate epistemology' for a 'critical' public health (Krieger 2000).

From this perspective the emotionality embedded in lay knowledge about the causes and consequences of experiences of health inequalities points to the significance of the experience to the people involved; but the articulation of these experiences can also highlight causal pathways within which different kinds of intervention or action might be developed.

Action to reduce inequalities: public health policy and practice

Although we have described an evolution in our understanding of health inequalities to more complex epistemological forms, the most enduring characteristic of public health policy and practice in the UK has been the emphasis on individual behaviour as a primary target for action (Spencer and Dowler 2007). In the UK, the Conservative government of Margaret Thatcher in the 1980s is often seen as the starting point for a new philosophy of individual responsibility in all areas of social life. The notion of 'lifestyle'-dominated public health policy and practice: a concept connecting smoothly to a stripped-down idea which it is easy to read off certain assumptions about people's *freedom to choose* the lives they lead and to take responsibility for the style in which they do it (see Beattie 1991, for a critical discussion of this). Far from being a new development, however, the 1980s lifestyle discourse embodies a variation on the theme of 'possessive individualism' (Macpherson 1964) that had been part of political thinking generally about health and other aspects of social life long before Thatcher's government.

Prior to the election of the first New Labour government, Margaret Whitehead (1995) had undertaken a comprehensive review of policy initiatives to tackle health inequalities within the UK and beyond. Developing the thinking that informed the justifiably celebrated 'rainbow' model of the social determinants of health (Dahlgren and Whitehead 1991), she identified four policy levels at which responses, initiatives or programmes could take effect, from empowering individuals (level one) to revolutionizing global social and economic structures (or at least regulating the 'greedy bastards' more rigorously) in level four. Not surprisingly, but always disappointingly, her review suggested that nearly all the attention was focused at level one, and within those:

> Some efforts also require a health warning: although they purport to empower individuals or communities, they risk being patronising and victim-blaming if not undertaken with skill and sensitivity.
>
> (Whitehead 1995: 51)

The election of the New Labour government in 1997 marked a key moment for many in the public health community. For the first time in eighteen years a government made an explicit commitment to reducing health inequalities (Berridge and Blume 2003). There was a sense of hope that public health policy would move from a primary emphasis on personal responsibility and life-styles to address the wider social determinants of health inequalities through what an earlier, pre-New Labour report had referred to as 'the organised efforts of society' (Acheson 1988: 1). These hopes were reinforced by some early, pragmatic left-of-centre rhetoric about patient and public participation (Forster and Gabe 2008), the appointment of a public health minister who argued, in her first public speech, for primary attention to the social/material determinants of unhealthy behaviour (Jowell 1997) and the publication of a challenging Green Paper that included a focus on the material causes of health inequalities (Department of Health 1998b). The findings of the Labour-commissioned Acheson Report (Department of Health 1998a) reinforced the Black Report's broadly materialist perspective on health inequalities, while building on some of the new findings from research on the life-course and psychosocial processes which we discussed in the previous section.

There were also formal changes in the ways in which the processes of policy were conceived. In particular, a focus on 'wicked problems' (Hunter 2003) or cross-cutting and interlinked policy issues became characteristic themes of policy development, with a growing emphasis on how 'delivery' could be assured (Newman 2001). As Cropper and Goodwin note:

> New Labour's programme identified a set of interlinked social issues, each complex, each deeply rooted and enduring, and for each, the question is how best to catalyse and coordinate action that has demonstrable impact.
>
> (Cropper and Goodwin 2007: 30)

What policy analysis might refer to as the 'problem structure' of health inequalities is complex with both 'clarity about goals' (Graham 2004: 127) and appropriate means of monitoring and evaluating strategies being necessary (Petticrew *et al.* 2003). Additional complexity was added by the multiple departments of government that would be implicated and the proliferation of various partnerships and community involvement initiatives designed to address these. The consequence of this was that there was uncertainty within government about both goals or ends and the means necessary to achieve them (Cropper and Goodwin 2007).

Whether the complexity was just too complex, or other agendas and moral panics dominated, the early interest of the incoming New Labour government in socio-economic determinants has regressed to an emphasis on behaviour change that is no less focused on personal responsibility than the policies of the Thatcher years (for example, Department of Health 2004). Behaviour change and downstream interventions, leavened with area-based initiatives with time-limited funding, and the intensification of a target culture, form the hallmarks of the approach to health inequalities at the UK government level (Porter *et al.* 2007). Indeed, looked at alongside other policy initiatives on crime and work, the policies of New Labour can be argued to be the climax of Thatcherism, with a relentless focus on changing individual beliefs and behaviours.

However, this general picture has been rendered more complex by devolution which, as a 'process not an event' (Davies 1999), has only gradually revealed its impact on development and implementation in specific policy fields. A manifesto commitment to devolution had been a key aspect of the policy portfolio of New Labour, and was established by the Government of Wales Act and the Scotland Act in 1998. Despite the limited nature of political devolution (especially in Wales), it was welcomed by many as opening up 'the potential for the development of radically different social policies' (Mooney *et al*. 2006: 483; Mooney and Williams 2006: 610). With a limited history of self-government in modern times, it takes time and new capacity to create and re-direct institutional and political structures and cultures. Against this background, some of the expectations regarding the emergence of three separate 'policy laboratories' have probably been overblown, and the impact of devolution remains the subject of much debate (Mooney and Scott 2005; Silburn 2004; Stewart 2004).

There is consensus that policy makers in the devolved governments have responded to 'their particular [health] problems and debates in ways that vary territorially and produce territorial policy divergence that matters' (Greer 2005: 501). This thesis is widely cited (Chaney and Drakeford 2004; Keating 2005; Mooney and Scott 2005) and has led to claims that we are now experiencing a natural policy experiment in the health arena (Smith and Babbington 2006). However, these analyses focus almost entirely on *health care* policies. This is particularly surprising given that public health has become a key concern of all three mainland British countries and Ireland. Health inequalities are particularly interesting to explore from the perspective of devolution because, as we have suggested, they constitute a 'wicked issue' with no obvious solution: one might therefore expect different policy-making contexts to approach the problem in contrasting and experimental ways (Blackman *et al*. 2006; Smith *et al*. 2009).

In the event, and particularly after 2003, the 'policy problem' of health inequalities has been framed in a relatively consistent manner across the territories: as a 'health gap' between deprived areas or communities and the rest of the population. As Graham and Kelly (2004) emphasize, framing the problem in this way invites responses which focus on trying to improve the health of the poorest people (or people in the poorest areas and groups), rather than broader, societal responses. There is some evidence that, rhetorically at least, the early public health 'White Paper' in Wales – *Better Health, Better Wales* (Welsh Office 1998) was more radical in emphasizing wider social determinants of health inequalities than equivalent policy documents in England or Scotland (Greer 2003; Chaney and Drakeford 2004). But none of these early policy documents contained a strong materialist or structuralist agenda.

Around 2003 there was a marked rhetorical move towards clinical interventions and health promotion: a move that is paradoxically more overt in Wales. In England the most recent English White Paper, *Choosing Health* (Department of Health 2004) promulgates the introduction of lay trainers, aimed at informing and advising other local people about health and health care. This provides a vivid illustration of a regressive poverty of policy ideas with regard to the implementation of an analysis that emphasizes socio-economic determinants. While the Welsh Assembly Government has been vocal in declaring its commitment to addressing the social determinants of health, much of its action has been directed at changing individual or family behaviour. Indeed, the online strategy *Health Challenge Wales* (Welsh Assembly Government 2004) fails to mention inequalities in health at all, focusing instead on creating a climate of healthy behaviours in relation to food and drink, sex, alcohol and drugs (Porter *et al.* 2007).

Alongside all this there were some initiatives that attempted to implement forms of social action rather different from individual behaviour change. In England the most important example of this was the Health Action Zones (HAZs), 'established in 1998 to serve as trailblazers for a concerted attempt to modernise the NHS and to tackle health' (Bauld and Judge 2008: 93). Each of the zones had geographical boundaries and time-limited funding, a broad remit that included traditional health concerns as well as community cohesion and capacity building, and operated through partnership building and the setting of targets (Benzeval and Meth 2002): partnership has been a guiding concept across Wales, Scotland and England. HAZs were just one example of a clutch of initiatives developed by New Labour, and by no means the only one to include the determinants of health as part of its remit – Sure Start, local programmes focusing on the health and social development of children in deprived areas in England were another and the major urban renewal initiative – New Deal for Communities – also included a health theme. Evaluation was also built to a greater or lesser extent into these developments, often proving no less complex and contentious than the initiatives themselves (Barnes *et al.* 2005; Belsky *et al.* 2007; Bauld and Judge 2008).

In Wales, the Communities First programme was set up in 2001 to bring resources into 132 of the most deprived communities in Wales (based on the Welsh Index of Multiple Deprivation). Although this was not a health intervention, it was expected to have an impact on the determinants of health within local settings. It was also based on a 'partnership approach', but was mired from the beginning in contested definitions of this, and concerns over the leadership role of local authorities (Welsh Assembly Government 2006a). Possibly the most innovative development, first highlighted in the *Better Health – Better Wales* strategy (Welsh Office, 1998), was the Sustainable Health Action Research Programme (SHARP) 'designed to show the most effective ways of breaking the cycle of poor health in Wales [and] to establish a programme of action research to support and strengthen evidence on the effectiveness of interventions in health determinants' (Porter *et al.* 2007: 59). In contrast to the other initiatives mentioned, therefore, SHARP was unusual in being research-driven – indeed, higher education institutions were central to each of the seven initiatives funded by the Welsh Assembly Government under that scheme (Cropper *et al.* 2007).

For those attempting to develop a more socio-economic approach to health inequalities, these initiatives were a welcome break from unrelenting instructions to eat five a day and do impossible amounts of aerobic exercise. However, they had their difficulties, partly because of structural constraints which are difficult for national governments to control. They neither addressed the big issues of de-industrialization and widening economic inequalities, nor did they for the most part provide the quick behavioural improvements craved by politicians. Moreover, as examples of complex, community-based interventions designed 'to tackle configurations of long-standing social problems' (Bauld and Judge 2008: 101), they are not easily tested by randomized controlled trials or other forms of social experiment: the inputs are composite, the contexts are complex and the outcomes are often multiple. Nonetheless, if we develop the lines of argument of this chapter, they do represent attempts to look at structural and material factors at their point of impact; and treat seriously the need to understand social lives not just as a series of behaviours to be manipulated, but as complex situations of values, knowledge and action within which scientific and political experts have to work (Williams *et al.* 2007).

Conclusion

The dominant approaches to explaining population health and health inequalities are not necessarily mutually exclusive. As we have seen, for example, whilst behaviours are implicated in the genesis of ill-health, they are themselves embedded in material contexts. So the key to effective action to change behaviours is to develop a more adequate contextual understanding of the well-springs of human agency. Similarly, it appears that increasing polarization of societies is important in understanding increasing health polarization, but the key for action is to understand the drivers of social polarization – the changing nature of global markets, their effects on inequalities in income and wealth and the rise of an oligarchy of the rich, not to focus exclusively down-stream on the psychosocial consequences. Life-course perspectives – interweaving biological, biographical, and historical time – add other layers of complexity to the explanatory framework needed to inform policy and action to address health inequalities. Multi-level modelling of the relationship between people and place also adds important insights into causal pathways. What has been missing until recently has been any attempt to connect these powerful changes in economic and social conditions to what Raymond Williams long ago referred to as 'structures of feeling' through which people can articulate the meaning of the impact of these powerful changes in their lives (Williams 1965; Smith 2008).

It is, of course, national governments and international agencies which will have most impact on processes of de-industrialization, economic insecurity and rising social inequality. However, there is a vital need for informed public debate about the role and scope of public welfare as a mechanism to reduce health inequalities. The post-war welfare consensus that has characterized Western industrialized countries was built upon some redistribution of income and wealth with a view to creating fairer, more equal societies which would be more socially cohesive; alongside universal provision to meet basic needs for health care, housing and socially adequate incomes. The authoritarian individualism implicit in some of these services is problematic but the new 'conditional' welfare – with services and benefits provided only on condition that people adopt professionally defined 'appropriate' behaviours – is a poor substitute for the universalist action that has contributed much to population health improvement over time (Townsend 2007).

There is also a continuing and vital role for local action in neighbourhoods and in communities of place and interest as well as for global social movements (such as the labour and anti-poverty movements). The potential for local social action is something that the Welsh Assembly Government addressed in its first plan for health services in Wales, articulating the need to develop strategies in which 'the values of *citizenship* and collective action can grow . . . replacing élite policy making by *participative* policy development' (2001: 5 – emphasis in the original). The young government in Wales put at least some of its money where its mouth is, through a number of initiatives that were designed to encourage policy that was evidence based, while putting in place initiatives to ensure the involvement of local communities and their lay knowledge (Cropper *et al.* 2007; O'Neill and Williams 2008). Similarly, the early years of New Labour in England saw bold 'experiments' in public involvement in policy development and their implementation in Health Action Zones, for example, and Healthy Living Centres (Bauld and Judge 2008). However, these and other policy initiatives aimed at greater community engagement have joined the other burnt out policy tanks that litter the road from Whitehall. In Wales, notwithstanding more general political arguments for 'citizen-centred services' (Welsh Assembly Government 2006b), the radical health agenda of the early years of devolution seems to have evolved into more easily measurable and manageable behavioural approaches to health improvement (Welsh Assembly Government 2004).

The history of policy responses to health inequalities in the UK is not marked by success. Notwithstanding the build-up of evidence providing broad support for the original findings of the Black Report, governments seem to be more reluctant than ever to engage in an 'attack upon the forces of inequality' in public health policy and practice. A fuller understanding of inequalities in life chances and health chances – why they persist and what is to be done about them – requires a far more extensive application of the sociological imagination than is currently evident in research on health inequalities. Only by linking personal experiences of inequality to public issues of social structure, and by seeing national social structure in a global context, will adequate understanding for action on health inequalities be achieved.

References

Acheson, D. (1988) *Public Health in England: the report of the committee of inquiry into the future development of the public health function*, Cm 289, London: HMSO.

Barnes, M., Bauld, L., Benzeval, M., Judge, K., McKenzie, M. and Sullivan, H. (2005) *Health Action Zones: partnerships for health equity*, London: Routledge.

Bartley, M. (2004) *Health Inequality: an introduction to concepts, theory and methods*, Cambridge: Polity Press.

Bauld, L. and Judge, K. (2008) 'Strong theory, flexible methods: evaluating complex, community-based initiatives', in J. Green and R. Labonté (eds) *Critical Perspectives in Public Health*, London: Routledge.

Beattie, A. (1991) 'Knowledge and control in health promotion', in J. Gabe, M. Calnan and M. Bury (eds) *The Sociology of the Health Service*, London: Routledge.

Belsky, J., Barnes, J. and Melhuish, E. (2007) *The National Evaluation of Sure Start: does area-based early intervention work?* Bristol: Policy Press.

Benzeval, M. and Meth, F. (2002) 'Innovation', in L. Bauld and K. Judge (eds) *Learning from Health Action Zones*, Chichester: Aeneas Press.

Berridge, V. and Blume, S. (eds) (2003) *Poor Health: social inequality before and after the Black Report*, London: Frank Cass.

Blackman, T., Elliott, E., Greene, A., Harrington, B., Hunter, D.J., Marks, L., McKee, L. and Williams, G. (2006) 'Performance assessment and wicked problems: the case of health inequalities', *Public Policy and Administration*, 21: 66–80.

Blane, D. (1999) 'The life course, the social gradient and health', in M. Marmot and R.G. Wilkinson (eds) *Social Determinants of Health*, Oxford: Oxford University Press.

Bourdieu, P. (1993) *Sociology in Question*, London: Sage.

Bourdieu, P. (ed.) *et al.* (1999) *The Weight of the World: social suffering in contemporary society*, Cambridge: Polity.

Brimblecombe, N., Dorling, D. and Shaw, M. (2000) 'Migration and geographical analysis of inequalities in health in Britain', *Social Science and Medicine*, 50: 861–78.

Carr-Hill, R. and Chalmers-Dixon, P. (2008) *The Public Health Observatory Handbook of Health Inequalities Measurement*, Oxford: South-East Public Health Observatory. Online: www.sepho.org.uk/extras/rch_handbook.aspx# chapters.

Chaney, P. and Drakeford, M. (2004) 'The primacy of ideology: social policy and the first term of the National Assembly for Wales', in N. Ellison, L. Bauld and M. Powell (eds), *Social Policy Review, 16: Analysis and Debate in Social Policy, 2004*, Bristol: The Policy Press.

Chung, H. and Muntaner, C. (2006) 'Political and welfare state determinants of infant and child health indicators: an analysis of wealthy countries', *Social Science and Medicine*, 63: 829–42.

Chung, H. and Muntaner, C. (2008) 'Welfare regime types and global health: an emerging challenge', *Journal of Epidemiology and Community Health*, 62: 282–3.

Coburn, D. (2000) 'Income inequality, social cohesion and the health status of populations: the role of neoliberalism', *Social Science and Medicine*, 51: 135–46.

Cockerham, W.C. (2007) *Social Causes of Health and Disease*, Cambridge: Polity.

Cropper, S. and Goodwin, M. (2007) 'Policy experiments: policy making, implementation and learning', in S. Cropper, A. Porter, G.H. Williams *et al.* (eds) *Community Health and Wellbeing: action research on health inequalities*, Bristol: Policy Press.

Cropper, S., Porter, A., Williams, G., Carlisle, S., Moore, R., O'Neill, M., Roberts, C. and Snooks, H. (eds) (2007) *Community Health and Wellbeing: action research on health inequalities*, Bristol: Policy Press.

Curtis, S. and Rees Jones, I. (1998) 'Is there a place for geography in the analysis of health inequality?' in M. Bartley, D. Blane and G. Davey Smith (eds) *The Sociology of Health Inequalities*, Oxford: Blackwell.

Dahlgren, G. and Whitehead, M. (1991) *Policies and Strategies to Promote Social Equity in Health*, Stockholm: Institute of Futures Studies.

Davey Smith, G., Dorling, D. and Shaw, M. (eds) (2001) *Poverty, Inequality and Health in Britain, 1800–2000: a reader*, Bristol: Policy Press.

Davies, R. (1999) *Devolution: a process not an event*, Cardiff: Institute for Welsh Affairs.

Department of Health (1998a) *Independent Inquiry into Inequalities in Health – Report* (Acheson Report), London: HMSO.

Department of Health (1998b) *Our Healthier Nation: a contract for health* (Green Paper), London: HMSO.

Department of Health (2004) *Choosing Health: making healthier choices easier*, Cm 6374, London: The Stationery Office.

Department of Health and Social Security (1980) *Inequalities in Health: report of a research working group*, London: DHSS.

Dorling, D., Shaw, M. and Davey Smith, G. (2007) 'Inequalities in mortality rates under New Labour', in E. Dowler and N. Spencer (eds) *Challenging Health Inequalities*, Bristol: The Policy Press.

Duranceau, R. and McCall, D. (2007) 'Setting the stage: the influence of place on health', *Health Policy Research Bulletin*, 14: 1–5.

Fone, D., Dunstan, F., Lloyd, K., Williams G., Watkins, J. and Palmer, S. (2007) 'Does social cohesion modify the association between area income deprivation and mental health?' *International Journal of Epidemiology*, 36: 338–45.

Forster, R. and Gabe, J. (2008) 'Voice or choice? Patient and public involvement in the National Health Service in England under New Labour', *International Journal of the Health Services*, 38: 333–56.

Frohlich, K.L., Corin, E. and Potvin, L. (2001) 'A theoretical proposal for the relationship between context and disease', *Sociology of Health and Illness*, 23: 776–97.

Frohlich, K.L., Potvin, L., Chabot, P. and Corin, E. (2002) 'A theoretical and empirical analysis of context: neighbourhoods, smoking and youth', *Social Science and Medicine*, 54: 1401–17.

Fukyama, F. (1992) *The End of History and the Last Man*, New York: Free Press.

Gatrell, A., Thomas, C., Bennett, S., Bostock, L., Popay, J., Williams, G. and Shahtahmasebi, S. (2001) Understanding health inequalities: locating people in geographical and social spaces, in H. Graham (ed.) *Understanding Health Inequalities*, Buckingham: Open University Press.

Giddens, A. (1991) *Modernity and Self Identity: self and society in the late modern age*, Cambridge: Polity Press.

Graham, H. (2004) 'Tackling inequalities in health in England: remedying health disadvantages, narrowing health gaps or reducing health gradients', *Journal of Social Policy*, 33: 115–31.

Graham, H. (2007) *Unequal Lives: health and socioeconomic inequalities*, Maidenhead: McGraw-Hill/Open University Press.

Graham, H. and Kelly, M.P. (2004). *Health inequalities: concepts, frameworks and policy* (Briefing Paper), London: HDA.

Gray, J. (2003) *Straw Dogs: thought on humans and other animals*, London: Granta.

Greer, S. (2003) 'Health: how far can Wales diverge from England?' in J. Osmond (ed.) *Second Term Challenge: can the Welsh Assembly hold its course?* Cardiff: Institute for Welsh Affairs.

Greer, S. (2005) 'The territorial bases of health policy making in the UK after devolution', *Regional and Federal Studies*, 15: 501–18.

Hunter, D.J. (2003) *Public Health Policy*, Cambridge: Polity.

Jones, K. and Moon, G. (1993) 'Medical geography: taking space seriously', *Progress in Human Geography*, 17: 515–24.

Joshi, H., Wiggins, R.D., Bartley, M., Mitchell, R., Gleave, S. and Lynch, K. (2001) 'Putting health inequalities in the map: does where you live matter and why'? in H. Graham (ed.) *Understanding Health Inequalities*, Buckingham: Open University Press.

Jowell, T. (1997) Speech at the Conference of the Faculty of Public Health Medicine, Liverpool, 26 June.

Kawachi, I. and Kennedy, B. (1997) 'Health and social cohesion: why care about income inequality'? *British Medical Journal*, 314: 1037–9.

Keating, M. (2005) 'Policy convergence and divergence in Scotland under devolution', *Regional Studies*, 39: 453–63.

Kennedy, B., Kawachi, I. and Brainerd, E. (1999) 'The role of social capital in the Russian mortality crisis', *World Development*, 26: 2029–43.

Krieger, N. (2000) 'Passionate epistemology, critical advocacy and public health: doing our profession proud', *Critical Public Health*, 10: 287–94.

Kuh, D. and Ben-Shlomo, Y. (eds) (2004) *A Life Course Approach to Chronic Disease Epidemiology*, second edition, Oxford: Oxford University Press.

Kuh, D., Power, C., Blane, D. and Bartley, M. (2004) 'Socio-economic pathways between childhood and adult health', in D. Kuh, and Y. Ben-Shlomo (eds) *A Life Course Approach to Chronic Disease Epidemiology*, second edition, Oxford: Oxford University Press.

Lash, S. and Urry, J. (1994) *Economies of Signs and Space*, London: Sage.

Lynch, J.W., Davey Smith, G. and Kaplan, G. (2000) 'Income inequality and mortality: importance to health of individual income, psychosocial environment, or material conditions', *British Medical Journal*, 320: 1200–4.

Macintyre, S. (1997) 'The Black Report and beyond: what are the issues?' *Social Science and Medicine*, 44: 723–45.

Macintyre, S., Ellaway, A. and Cummins, S. (2002) 'Place effects on health: how can we conceptualise, operationalise and measure them?' *Social Science and Medicine*, 55: 125–39.

Mackenbach, J. and Bakker, M. (eds) (2002) *Reducing Inequalities in Health: a European perspective*, London: Routledge.

Macpherson, C.B. (1964) *The Political Theory of Possessive Individualism: from Hobbes to Locke*, Oxford University Press.

Mallinson, S., Popay, J., Elliott, E., Bennett, S., Bostock, L., Gatrell, A., Thomas, C. and Williams G.H. (2003) 'Historical data for health inequalities research: a research note', *Sociology*, 37: 771–80.

Mooney, G. and Scott, G. (eds) (2005) *Exploring Social Policy in the 'New' Scotland*, Bristol: Policy Press.

Mooney, G. and Williams, C. (2006) 'Forging new "ways of life"? Social policy and nation building in devolved Scotland and Wales', *Critical Social Policy*, 26: 608–29.

Mooney, G., Scott, G. and Williams, C. (2006) 'Introduction: rethinking social policy through devolution', *Critical Social Policy*, 26: 483–97.

Muntaner, C. and Lynch, J. (1999) 'Income inequality, social cohesion and class relations: a critique of Wilkinson's neo-Durkheimian research programme', *International Journal of Health Services*, 29: 59–81.

Muntaner, C., Lynch, J. and Davey Smith, G. (2008) 'Social capital and the third way in public health', in J. Green and R. Labonté (eds) *Critical Perspectives in Public Health*, London: Routledge.

Newman, J. (2001) *Modernising Governance: New Labour, policy and society*, London: Sage.

Norman, P., Boyle, P. and Rees, P. (2005) 'Selective migration and deprivation: a longitudinal analysis', *Social Science and Medicine*, 60: 2755–71.

Nussbaum, M. (1990) *Love's Knowledge: essays on philosophy and literature*, Oxford: Oxford University Press.

Nussbaum, M. (2001) *Upheavals of Thought: the Intelligence of Emotions*, Cambridge: Cambridge University Press.

O'Neill, M. and Williams, G. (2008) 'Developing community and agency engagement in an action research study in south Wales', in J. Green and R. Labonté (eds) *Critical Perspectives in Public Health*, London: Routledge.

Petticrew, M., Whitehead, M., Macintyre, S., Graham, H. and Egan, M. (2003) 'Evidence for public health policy on inequalities, 1: the reality according to policy makers', *Journal of Epidemiology and Public Health*, 58: 811–16.

Phillimore, P. (1993) 'How do places shape health? Rethinking locality and lifestyle', in S. Platt, H. Thomas, S. Scott, and G.H. Williams (eds) *Locating Health: sociological and historical explorations*, Aldershot: Avebury.

Pickett, K.E. and Pearl, M. (2001) 'Multilevel analyses of socioeconomic context and health outcomes: a critical review', *Journal of Epidemiology and Community Health*, 55: 111–22.

Popay, J., Williams, G., Thomas, C. and Gatrell, A.C. (1998) 'Theorising inequalities in health: the place of lay knowledge', in M. Bartley, D. Blane and G. Davey Smith (eds) *The Sociology of Health Inequalities*, Oxford: Blackwell.

Popay, J., Thomas, C., Williams, G., Bennett, S., Gatrell, A. and Bostock, L. (2003) 'A proper place to live: health inequalities, agency and the normative dimensions of space', *Social Science and Medicine*, 57: 55–69.

Porter, A., Roberts, C. and Clements, A. (2007) 'Policy innovation to tackle health inequalities', in S. Cropper, A. Porter, G. Williams *et al.* (eds) *Community Health and Wellbeing: action research on health inequalities*, Bristol: Policy Press.

Power, C. and Kuh, D. (2006) 'Life course development of unequal health', in J. Siegrist and M. Marmot (eds) *Social Inequalities in Health: new evidence and policy implications*, Oxford: Oxford University Press.

Prandy, K. (1999) 'Class, stratification and inequalities in health: a comparison of the Registrar General's social classes and the Cambridge Scale', *Sociology of Health and Illness*, 21: 466–84.

Scambler, G. (2002) *Health and Social Change: a critical theory*, Buckingham: Open University Press.

Sennett, R. and Cobb, J. (1973) *The Hidden Injuries of Class*, New York: Vintage.

Shaw, M., Dorling, D., Gordon, D. and Davey Smith, G. (1999) *The Widening Gap: health inequalities and policy in Britain*, Bristol: The Policy Press.

Siegrist, J. and Marmot, M. (eds) (2006) *Social Inequalities in Health: new evidence and policy implications*, Oxford: Oxford University Press.

Silburn, R. (2004) 'An introduction to devolution: how much difference has it made?' *Benefits*, 12: 163–8.

Smith, D. (2008) *Raymond Williams: a warrior's tale*, Cardigan, Wales: Parthian.

Smith, K., Hunter, D.J., Blackman, T., Williams, G.H., McKee, L., Harrington, B.E., Elliott, E., Marks, L. and Greene, A. (2009), 'Divergence or convergence? The post-devolution health policies of England, Scotland and Wales', *Critical Social Policy*, 29.

Smith, T. and Babbington, E. (2006) 'Devolution: a map of divergence in the NHS', *Health Policy Review*, 1: 9–40.

Smyth, F. (2008) 'Medical geography: understanding health inequalities', *Progress in Human Geography*, 32: 119–27.

Sooman, A. and Macintyre, S. (1995) 'Health and perceptions of the local environment in socially contrasting neighbourhoods in Glasgow', *Health and Place*, 1: 15–26.

Spencer, N. and Dowler, E. (2007) 'Introduction', in E. Dowler and N. Spencer (eds) *Challenging Health Inequalities*, Bristol: The Policy Press.

Stephens, C. (2008) 'Social capital in its place: using social theory to understand social capital and inequalities in health', *Social Science and Medicine*, 66: 1174–84.

Steptoe, A. (2006) 'Psychobiological processes linking socioeconomic position with health', in J. Siegrist and M. Marmot (eds), *Social Inequalities in Health: new evidence and policy implications*, Oxford: Oxford University Press.

Stewart, J. (2004) 'Scottish solutions to Scottish problems? Social welfare in Scotland since devolution', in N. Ellison, L. Bauld, M. Powell (eds) *Social Policy Review, 16: analysis and debate in social policy, 2004*, Bristol: The Policy Press.

Townsend, P. (2007) *The Right to Social Security and National Development: lessons from OECD experience for low income countries* (Issues in Social Protection, Discussion Paper 18), London: International Labour Office.

Townsend, P., Davidson, N. and Whitehead, M. (eds) (1988) *Inequalities in Health: the Black Report and the Health Divide*, Harmondsworth: Penguin.

Turner, B. (2003) 'Social capital, inequality and health: the Durkheimian revival', *Social Theory and Health*, 1: 4–20.

Veenstra, G. (2006) 'Neo-Marxist class position and socio-economic status: distinct or complementary determinants of health', *Critical Public Health*, 16: 111–29.

Welsh Assembly Government (2001) *Improving Health in Wales: a plan for the NHS and its partners*, Cardiff: Welsh Assembly Government.

Welsh Assembly Government (2004) *Health Challenge Wales*. Online: http://new.wales.gov.uk/hcwsubsite/healthchallenge/?lang=en.

Welsh Assembly Government (2006a) *Interim Evaluation of Communities First: final report*, Cardiff: Welsh Assembly Government.

Welsh Assembly Government (2006b) *Beyond Boundaries: citizen-centred services for Wales. Review of local service delivery: report to the Welsh Assembly government* (Chair: Sir Jeremy Beecham), Cardiff: Welsh Assembly Government.

Welsh Office (1998) *Better Health – Better Wales*, Cm 3922, Cardiff: The Stationery Office.

Whitehead, M. (1987) *The Health Divide*, London: Health Education Council.

Whitehead, M. (1995) 'Tackling health inequalities: a review of policy initiatives', in M. Benzeval, K. Judge and M. Whitehead (eds) *Tackling Inequalities in Health: an agenda for action*, London: King's Fund.

Wilkinson, R.G. (1996) *Unhealthy Societies: the afflictions of inequality*, London: Routledge.

Wilkinson, R.G. (1999a) 'Putting the picture together: prosperity, redistribution, health and welfare', in M. Marmot and R. Wilkinson (eds) *The Social Determinants of Health*, Oxford: Oxford University Press.

Wilkinson, R.G. (1999b) 'Income inequality, social cohesion and health: clarifying the theory – a reply to Muntaner and Lynch', *International Journal of Health Services*, 29: 525–43.

Wilkinson, R.G. (2000) 'Deeper than "neo-liberalism": a reply to David Coburn', *Social Science and Medicine*, 51: 997–1000.

Wilkinson, R.G. (2005) *The Impact of Inequality: how to make sick societies healthier*, London: Routledge.

Williams, G. (2000) 'Knowledgeable narratives', *Anthropology and Medicine*, 7: 135–40.

Williams, G. (2003) 'The determinants of health: structure, context and agency', *Sociology of Health and Illness*, 25: 131–54.

Williams G. (2006) 'History is what you live: understanding health inequalities in Wales', in P. Michael and C. Webster (eds) *Health and Society in Twentieth-Century Wales*, Cardiff: University of Wales Press.

Williams, G. and Popay, J. (2001) 'Lay health knowledge and the concept of the life world', in G. Scambler (ed.) *Habermas, Critical Theory and Health*, London: Routledge.

Williams, G., Cropper, S., Porter, A. and Snooks, H. (2007), 'Beyond the experimenting society', in S. Cropper, A. Porter, G. Williams *et al.* (eds) *Community Health and Wellbeing: action research on health inequalities*, Bristol: Policy Press.

Williams, R. (1965) *The Long Revolution*, Harmondsworth: Penguin.

Williams, S., Calnan, M. and Dolan A. (2007) 'Explaining inequalities in health: theoretical, conceptual and methodological agendas', in E. Dowler and N. Spencer (eds) *Challenging Health Inequalities: from Acheson to 'Choosing Health'*, Bristol: Policy Press.

Index